Forensic Ballistics in Court

Forensic Ballistics in Court

Interpretation and Presentation of Firearms Evidence

Brian J. Heard

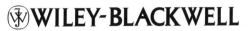

A John Wiley & Sons, Ltd., Publication

This edition first published 2013 © 2013 by John Wiley & Sons, Ltd

Wiley-Blackwell is an imprint of John Wiley & Sons, formed by the merger of Wiley's global Scientific, Technical and Medical business with Blackwell Publishing.

Registered office: John Wiley & Sons, Ltd, The Atrium, Southern Gate, Chichester, West Sussex, PO19 8SQ, UK

Editorial offices: 9600 Garsington Road, Oxford, OX4 2DQ, UK

The Atrium, Southern Gate, Chichester, West Sussex, PO19 8SQ, UK

350 Main Street, Malden, MA 02148-5020, USA

For details of our global editorial offices, for customer services and for information about how to apply for permission to reuse the copyright material in this book please see our website at www.wiley.com/wiley-blackwell.

Library of Congress Cataloging-in-Publication Data

Heard, Brian J.
  Forensic ballistics in court : interpretation and presentation of firearms evidence / Brian J. Heard.
    pages cm
  Includes index.
  ISBN 978-1-119-96267-0 (cloth) – ISBN 978-1-119-96268-7 (pbk.) 1.   Forensic ballistics. 2.   Firearms–Identification.
  3.   Bullets–Identification. 4.   Criminal investigation. I. Title.
  HV8077.H4293 2013
  363.25'62–dc23

                                                                                2012042783

A catalogue record for this book is available from the British Library.

Cover image: Images supplied by iStock
Cover design by Dan Jubb

Wiley also publishes its books in a variety of electronic formats. Some content that appears in print may not be available in electronic books.

Set in 10/12pt Times-Roman by Thomson Digital, Noida, India
Printed and bound in Singapore by Markono Print Media Pte Ltd

1   2013

Contents

About the Author

Brian Heard started his career as a forensic firearms examiner in the New Scotland Yard Forensic Science Laboratory in 1966. He rose to become Deputy Head of the firearms section before joining the Ballistics and Firearms Identification Bureau in the Royal Hong Police Force. In 1996, he was promoted to Director of what was then called the Forensic Firearms Examination Bureau of the Hong Kong Police Force.

He was awarded the Distinguished Service Medal and the Police Meritorious Service Medal for his work in forensic science.

He retired in 2001 and now works as a consultant and lecturer in Forensic Firearms Examinations.

Introduction

An expert may be used in, basically, two different capacities: for consultation or for testimony.

These are derived from five general categories of expertise:

1. **Lay people:** common sense and life long experience.

2. **Technician/examiner:** limited area experience and concentrated training, applies known techniques, works in a system and taught with the system (e.g. investigator and supervisors (observers and viewers)). The technician is generally taught to use complex instruments (gas chromatograph, infrared spectrophotometer, mass spectrophotometer) or even 'simple' breath alcohol testing equipment as 'bench operators', who have only a superficial understanding of what the instrument really does and how the readout is generated. Bench operators, who qualify as expert witnesses, are not competent to explain the instrumentation used unless it is established that they received the training and education necessary to impart a thorough understanding of the underlying theories.

3. **Practitioner:** material and information analysis and interpretation.

4. **Specialist:** devoted to one kind of study or work with individual characteristics.

5. **Scientist:** conducts original empirical research, then experiments to verify the validity of the theory; designs and creates instrumentation and applied techniques; is published in own field with peers; and advances his/her field of knowledge.

In court, the proffered witness must be assessed as to his/her:

- **Expertise.** Courts rely heavily on forensic evidence to convict the guilty and to protect the innocent. The presentation of flawed forensic evidence has obvious implications for individual cases, but raises questions about the integrity of the entire criminal justice system. Innocent people may be wrongly convicted and people may lose trust in the justice system. This is not unknown,, as a number of recent high profile cases have proved.

- **Training.** What sets an expert apart from a novice? How does forensic expertise develop over time? Does the speed of expert decision-making influence performance? How does memory for forensic information relate to matching accuracy? Can training time be reduced without compromising performance? What is the best way to provide feedback to examiners about their performance? Do examiners know when to ask for help? How much should examiners rely on instructions from a textbook, compared to practical experience?

- **Testimony.** What can examiners reasonably claim when testifying in court? What is the most effective way to present forensic evidence to juries? On what basis should judges admit forensic testimony? Should examiners report opinions or statistics?

Judges also have to consider the following factors in determining the manner in which expert testimony should be presented to a jury and in instructing the jury in its evaluation of expert scientific testimony in criminal proceedings:

1. Whether experts can identify and explain the theoretical and factual basis for any opinion given in their testimony and the reasoning upon which the opinion is based.

2. Whether experts use clear and consistent terminology in presenting their opinions.

3. Whether experts present their testimony in a manner that conveys, accurately and fairly, the significance of their conclusions, including any relevant limitations of the methodology used.

4. Whether experts explain the reliability of evidence and address problems fairly with evidence, including relevant evidence of laboratory error, contamination or sample mishandling.

5. Whether expert testimony of individuality or uniqueness is based on valid scientific research.

6. Whether the court should prohibit the parties from tendering witnesses as experts and should refrain from declaring witnesses to be experts in the presence of the jury.

7. Whether to include in jury instructions additional specific factors that might be especially important to a jury's ability to assess fairly the reliability of, and weight to be given to, testimony on particular issues in the case.

Many of the reported problems with forensic science evidence have resulted from the failures of trial legal representatives to investigate thoroughly forensic science evidence, the misunderstandings concerning the nature of that evidence, and mis-statements concerning the weight to be attributed to that evidence. Until an elevation in the knowledge base of trial legal representatives is achieved, the adversarial system will continue to falter with respect to the proper presentation of forensic science evidence.

In investigating, assessing and presenting forensic science evidence, the legal representatives should consider the following:

- The extent to which a particular forensic science discipline is founded on reliable scientific methodology that gives it the capacity to analyse accurately the evidence and to report findings.

- The extent to which examiners in a particular forensic science discipline rely on human interpretation.

- The extent to which the examiner using the particular forensic science technique in the case has followed established procedures and standards in examining the evidence.

By keeping these considerations in mind during the investigation and presentation of forensic science evidence, legal representatives will better inform the jury of the relevant contested forensic science issues in the case. The evidence presented that is relevant to these considerations will also provide the underlying basis for instructions to the jury concerning the consideration of the forensic scientist.

Experts frequently testify that they have made a match 'to the exclusion of all other firearms.'[1] This is simply another way of claiming uniqueness. In United States v. Green,[2] the court questioned such testimony: *'O'Shea* [the expert] *declared that this match could be made "to the exclusion of every other firearm in the world". .... That conclusion, needless to say, is extraordinary, particularly given O'Shea's data and methods.'*[3]

Further, in 2008, a year before the National Academy of Science (NAS) report on forensic science was issued, a different NAS report, one on computerised ballistic imaging, addressed this issue. The report cautioned: *'Conclusions drawn in firearms*

---

[1] *See* Giannelli, P.C. & Imwinkelried, E.J. (2007). *Scientific Evidence* (4th ed., citing *FBI Handbook of Forensic Sciences* 57 (rev. ed. 1994)), § 14.01, at 706 n.1. Albany, NY: Lexis Publishing Co.

[2] United States v. Green, 405 F. Supp. 2d 104 (D. Mass. 2005).

[3] *Ibid.* at 107 (citations omitted).

identification should not be made to imply the presence of a firm statistical basis when none has been demonstrated.[4] In particular, that report was concerned about testimony cast 'in bold absolutes', such as that a match can be made to the exclusion of all other firearms in the world: '*Such comments cloak an inherently subjective assessment of a match with an extreme probability statement that has no firm grounding and unrealistically implies an error rate of zero.*' Some courts are in accord.[5]

The court should consider whether additional factors such as those set forth below might be especially important to a jury's ability to fairly assess the reliability of and the weight to be given testimony on particular issues in the case.[6]

1. The extent to which the particular forensic science technique or theory used in the analysis is founded on a reliable scientific methodology that gives it the capacity to accurately analyse evidence and report findings.

2. The extent to which the forensic science examiner followed, or did not follow, the prescribed scientific methodology during the examination.

3. The extent to which the particular forensic science technique or theory relies on human interpretation that could be tainted by error.

4. The extent to which the forensic science examination in this case may have been influenced by the possibility of bias.

5. The extent to which the forensic science examination in this case uses operational procedures and conforms to performance standards established by reputable and knowledgeable scientific organisations.

6. The extent to which the forensic science examiner in this case followed the prescribed operational procedures and conformed to the prescribed performance standards in conducting the forensic science examination of the evidence.

7. The qualifications of the person(s) conducting the forensic science examination.

8. Whether the handling and processing of the evidence that was tested was sufficient to protect against contamination or alteration of the evidence.

9. The extent to which the particular forensic science technique or theory is generally accepted within the relevant scientific community.

10. The reasons given by the forensic science examiner for the opinion.

11. Whether the forensic science examiner has been certified in the relevant field by a recognised body that evaluates competency by testing.

12. Whether the facility is accredited by a recognised body, if accreditation is appropriate for that facility.

13. The extent to which the forensic science examiner has complied with applicable ethical obligations.

14. Whether the physical observations made by the forensic science examiner are observable by others.

15. Other evidence of the accuracy of the forensic science examiner's conclusions.

16. The extent to which the forensic science technique or theory has undergone validation.

---

[4] National Research Council, National Academy of Sciences, *Ballistic Imaging* **82** (2008).

[5] *See* United States v. Alls, slip opinion, No. CR2-08-223(1) (S.D. Ohio Dec. 7, 2009) ('Although Ms. McClellan may testify as to her methodology, case work, and observations in regards to the casing comparison she performed for this case, she may not testify as to her opinion on whether the casings are attributable to a single firearm to the exclusion of all other firearms.'); *Diaz*, 2007 WL 485967, at *1.

[6] The court should instruct the jurors only on the factors relevant to the specific forensic science evidence in the case as presented by the parties. Not all factors will be relevant in every case. Parties should consider limiting the instruction to the most probative contested factors to avoid overwhelming the jury with a 'laundry list' of factors that may diminish the jury's consideration of the most probative evidence.

17. The known nature of error associated with the forensic science technique or theory.

18. The fact that the nature and degree of error associated with the forensic science technique or theory (why, and how often, incorrect results are obtained) cannot be, or has not been, determined.

19. The estimation of uncertainty (the range of values encompassing the correct value at a defined confidence interval) associated with the forensic science technique or theory.

As a consequence of advances in analytical technology and limitations on the way in which suspect interrogation is carried out, there has been an increasing necessity for courts of law to rely on expert testimony. Scientific proof has therefore become a necessity in reconstructing the sequence of events at a crime scene. Such 'scientific proof' covers a large range of disciplines, varying in value from the indisputable to that of very dubious value.

Data obtained in a forensic laboratory has no meaning or worth until presented to a court of law.

It is the expert witness who must serve as the vehicle to present this scientific data effectively to the court in a manner understandable to the layman.

Unfortunately, it is often the interface between the lawyer and the expert that breaks down, leaving the court with a somewhat myopic view of the evidence available. This lack of intelligible dialogue with the expert will often result in both the defence and prosecution failing to utilise the testimony of the expert fully and to their best advantage.

At times, it is the lawyer's lack of scientific knowledge which is at fault, while at others it is the expert's inability to present his testimony in a clear and precise manner.

It must be stated that it is not the role of the defence – or, for that matter, the prosecution – to verbally batter the expert into submission. This could easily destroy a perfectly well-qualified expert's career and alienate the court towards the lawyer concerned. What is required is for the lawyer to qualify the expert, seek out the relevance of his or her experience and qualifications to the matter in question, and then delve into the probative value of the evidence tendered.

About the companion website

This book is accompanied by a companion website:

www.wiley.com/go/heard/forensicballistics

The website includes:
- Powerpoints of all figures from the book for downloading
- PDFs of tables from the book

1.0

Firearms History

1.0.1 Introduction

It may seem that a history of firearms is an illogical way to begin this book, but any competent forensic firearms examiner needs to have a good working knowledge of this subject matter. As such, it should form part of the court qualification process at the beginning of any trial. Having said that, though, it would be unreasonable to expect a firearms examiner with many years' experience to be able to give, for example, a precise date for the introduction of the Anson and Deeley push button fore-end. Such an esoteric piece of firearms history may have formed part of the examiner's training many years ago, but unless s/he had a particular interest in shotgun history it would be unlikely that s/he would remember little other than an approximate date or period.

Knowledge of the subject matter will also add gravitas to the presentation and examination of witnesses by the legal team. It may not help the case, but it will show that the solicitor or barrister is familiar with the history and workings of the presented firearm and can pose knowledgeable questions without the fear of being bamboozled by an expert witness.

It should also be appreciated that there is a very large market in replica 'antique' firearms. Some of these are only approximate reproductions of the original weapon, while others are made to the exact measurements of the original. A working knowledge of what these particular weapons look like and how their mechanisms work is therefore a perquisite.

While a history of firearms should start with the earliest of hand cannons, progressing through the wheel lock, miquelet and so on. For this book, however, it will start at the flintlock, as it is unlikely that anything earlier would be encountered in everyday case work. A much more comprehensive history of firearms is offered in Appendix 4.

1.0.2 The flintlock (Figure 1.0.1)

The flintlock ignition system really signalled the advent of an easy-to-use firearm with a simple mechanism for the discharge of a missile via a powdered propellant. In this type of weapon, the propellant was ignited via a spark produced by striking a piece of flint against a steel plate. The piece of flint was held in the jaws of a small vice on a pivoted arm, called the *cock*. This is where the term 'to cock the hammer' originated.

The steel, which was called the *frizzen*, was placed on another pivoting arm opposite the cock, and the pan containing the priming compound was placed directly below the frizzen. When the trigger was pulled, a strong spring swung the cock in an arc so that the flint struck the steel a glancing blow. This glancing blow produced a shower of sparks which dropped into the priming pan, igniting the priming powder. The flash produced by the ignited priming powder travelled through the touch hole, situated at the breech end of the barrel, igniting the main charge in the barrel and thus discharging the weapon.

Forensic Ballistics in Court: Interpretation and Presentation of Firearms Evidence, First Edition. Brian J. Heard.
© 2013 John Wiley & Sons, Ltd. Published 2013 by John Wiley & Sons, Ltd.

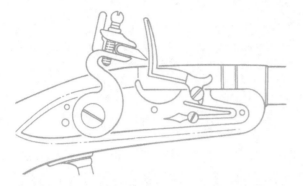

Figure 1.0.1   The flintlock.

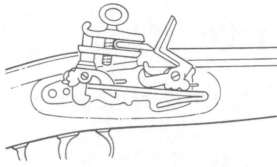

Figure 1.0.3   The miquelet.

The flintlock represented a great advance in weapon design. It was cheap, reliable and was not overly susceptible to damp or rainy conditions. Unlike the complicated and expensive wheel lock, this was a weapon that could be issued in large numbers to foot soldiers and cavalry alike.

As in the case with most weapon systems, it is very difficult to pinpoint an exact date for the introduction of the flintlock system. There are indications of it being used in the middle of the 16th century, although its first widespread use cannot be established with acceptable proof until the beginning of the seventeenth century.

Three basic types of flintlock were made:

Snaphaunce (Figure 1.0.2)

A weapon with the mainspring inside the lock plate and a priming pan cover which had to be manually pushed back before firing.

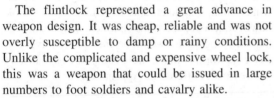

The snaphaunce was used from about 1570 until modern times (in North African guns), but by about 1680 it was out of fashion everywhere except Northern Italy, where it persisted until the 1750s.

Miquelet (Figure 1.0.3)

A weapon with the mainspring outside of the lock plate, but with a frizzen and priming pan cover all in one piece. In this type of lock mechanism, the pan cover was automatically pushed out of the way as the flint struck the frizzen. The great advantage of this type of lock is that the gunpowder in the priming pan is covered up until the point of ignition by a spring loaded plate, thus allowing the weapon to be used in adverse weather conditions.

It is generally thought that the miquelet was introduced after the disastrous campaign of Algiers (1541), where 'wind and rain' prevented firing, firstly by blowing away the gunpowder and/or secondly by wetting the gunpowder. In less than three decades, a lock did appear that is known today as the miquelet lock.

True flintlock (Figure 1.0.4)

A weapon with a mainspring on the inside of the lock plate and with the frizzen and priming pan cover in one piece. This also had a half cock safety position, enabling the weapon to be safely carried with the barrel loaded and the priming pan primed with powder. This system was probably invented by

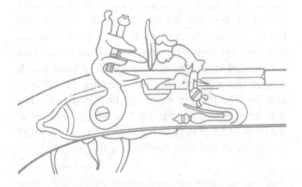

Figure 1.0.2   The snaphaunce.

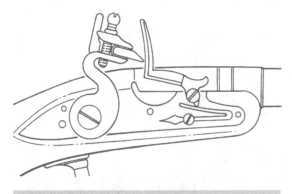

Mann Le Bourgeoys, a gun maker for Louis XIII of France, in about 1615.

1.0.3   The percussion system (Figure 1.0.5)

The flintlock continued to be used for almost 200 years. It was not until 1807 that a Scottish minister, Alexander John Forsyth, revolutionised the ignition of gunpowder by using a highly sensitive compound which exploded on being struck. When struck by a hammer, the compound, *mercury fulminate*, produced a flash which was strong enough to ignite the main charge of powder in the barrel. A separate sparking system and priming powder was now no longer required. With this invention, the basis for the self-contained cartridge was laid down and a whole new field of possibilities opened up.

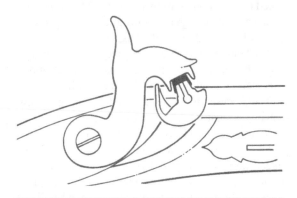

Figure 1.0.5   The percussion lock.

Once this type of ignition, known as *percussion priming*, had been invented, it was still some time before ways for it to be applied practically were perfected.

From 1807 to 1814, a wide range of systems were invented for the application of the percussion priming system, including the Forsyth scent bottle, pill locks, tube locks and the Pauly primer cap.

The final form of the percussion cap was claimed by a large number of inventors. It is, however, probably attributable to Joshua Shaw, an Anglo-American living in Philadelphia in 1814. Shaw employed a small iron cup, into which was placed a small quantity of mercury fulminate. This was placed over a small tube, called a *nipple*, projecting from the breech end of the barrel. When the hammer struck the cap, this detonated the mercury fulminate, causing a strong flame to travel down the nipple and thus igniting the main charge in the breech end of the barrel.

1.0.4   The pinfire system (Figure 1.0.6)

Introduced in the United Kingdom at the Great Exhibition in London in 1851 by Lefaucheux, the pinfire was one of the earliest true breech-loading weapons, using a self-contained cartridge in which the propellant, primer and missile were all held together in a brass case.

In this system, the percussion cup was inside the cartridge case, while a pin, which rested on the open end of the percussion cup, protruded through the side of the cartridge case. Striking the pin with the weapon's hammer drove the pin into the priming cup, causing the mercury fulminate to detonate and so ignite the main charge of propellant powder. The pin, which protruded through a slot in the side of the weapons chamber, not only served to locate the round in the correct position, but also aided the extraction of the fired cartridge case.

The pinfire was at its most popular between 1890 and 1910 and was still readily available in Europe until 1940. It had, however, fallen out of favour in England by 1914 and was virtually unobtainable by 1935. Boxes of old ammunition can, however, still be purchased in shooting quantities, from specialised ammunition dealers. This could place into question

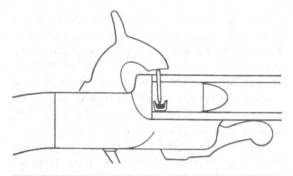

Figure 1.0.6   The pinfire.

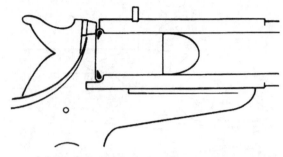

Figure 1.0.7   The rimfire system.

the placing of this type of weapon into the category of 'Antique' rather than that of a firearm requiring certification.

Calibres available for pinfire revolvers were 5, 7, 9, 12 and 15 mm, while shotgun and rifle ammunition in 9 mm and 12 bore and other various calibres were also available.

The really great advance of the pinfire system was, however, not just the concept of it being a self contained cartridge, but *obturation,* the ability of the cartridge case under pressure of firing to swell and so seal the chamber preventing the rearward escape of gases.

1.0.5   The rimfire system (Figure 1.0.7)

Although the pinfire system was a great step forward, it did have a number of drawbacks, not least of which was the tendency for the cartridge to discharge if dropped onto its pin. The problem was all but eliminated by the rimfire system which, like the pinfire, was exhibited at the Great Exhibition in 1851.

The rimfire system consists of a thin walled cartridge with a hollow flanged rim. Into this rim is spun a small quantity of a priming compound. Crushing the rim with a firing pin causes the priming compound to explode, thus igniting the propellant inside the case.

The initial development was made by a Paris gunsmith, Flobert, who had working examples of it as early as 1847. It was some time before it gained acceptance, however, and it was not until 1855 that

Smith and Wesson manufactured the first revolver to fire rim fire cartridges. This was a .22" calibre weapon in which the barrel tipped up by means of a hinge on the top of the frame. This enabled the cylinder to be removed for loading and unloading the weapon.

Although the rimfire was a great step forward, the rimfire cartridge was only suitable for high pressure weapons in small calibres. With any calibre above .22", the soft rim necessary for the ignition system resulted in cartridge case failures.

1.0.6   The Dreyse needle fire system (Figure 1.0.8)

The Dreyse needle gun was a military breech-loading rifle famous as the main infantry weapon of the Prussian army, who adopted it for service in 1848 as the Dreyse Prussian Model 1848. Its name, the 'needle gun', comes from its needle-like firing pin, which passed through the cartridge case to impact on a percussion cup glued to the base of the bullet.

The Dreyse rifle was the first breech-loading rifle to use a bolt action to open and close the chamber, executed by turning and pulling the bolt handle.

The Dreyse rifle was invented by the gunsmith Johann Nikolaus von Dreyse (1787–1867) and it was first produced as a fully working rifle in 1836. From 1848 onwards, the new weapon was gradually introduced into the Prussian service, then later into the military forces of many German states. The employment of the needle gun radically changed military tactics in the 19th century.

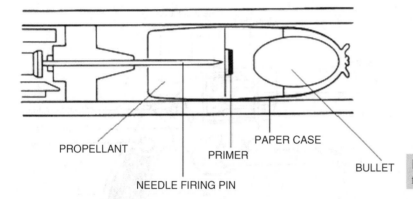

PROPELLANT
PAPER CASE
PRIMER
BULLET
NEEDLE FIRING PIN

Figure 1.0.8 The Dreyse needle fire.

The cartridge used with this rifle was a self-contained paper case containing the bullet, priming cup and black powder charge. The bullet, which was glued into the paper case, had the priming cup glued to its base. The upper end of the case was rolled up and tied together. Before the needle could strike the primer, its point had to pass through the paper case, then through the powder charge, before striking the primer cup on the base of the bullet. The theory behind the placement of the primer was that it would give a more complete ignition and, thus, combustion of the charge of propellant. Unfortunately, this led to severe corrosion of the needle, which then either stuck in the bolt or broke off, rendering the rifle useless. It was, however, a major step forward in the production of a modern rifle firing a self-contained cartridge.

1.0.7 The centre fire system (Figure 1.0.9)

This was the great milestone in weapon and ammunition development. In centre fire ammunition, only the primer cup needed to be soft enough to be crushed by the firing pin. The cartridge case could thus be made of a more substantial material, which would act as a gas seal (obturation) for much higher pressures than could be obtained with rimfire ammunition.

Once again, the exact date for the invention of the first centre fire weapon is difficult to ascertain, although a patent was issued in 1861 for a Daws centre fire system.

Probably no invention connected with firearms has had such an impact on the principles of firearms development as the obturating centre fire cartridge case. Although invented around 1860, the principles are still the same and they are utilised in every type of weapon, from the smallest handgun up to some of the largest artillery pieces.

Rocket-propelled bullets (the Gyrojet), caseless ammunition, hot air ignition and many other esoterica have come and gone. However, for simplicity, reliability and ease of manufacture, the centre fire ignition system in an obturating cartridge case has not been excelled.

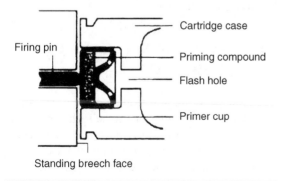

Firing pin
Cartridge case
Priming compound
Flash hole
Primer cup
Standing breech face

Figure 1.0.9 The centre fire system.

1.0.8 The revolver (Figure 1.0.10)

A revolver is a weapon that has a revolving cylinder containing a number of firing chambers (basically a revolving magazine) which may be successively lined up and discharged through a single barrel.

In the long history of revolvers, no name stands out more strongly than that of Samuel Colt. However, despite his claims to the contrary, Colt did not invent the revolver.

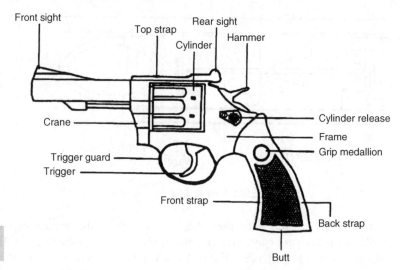

Figure 1.0.10 Major parts of a typical solid frame revolver.

The earliest forms of the revolver include a snaphaunce revolver made in the days of King Charles I, said to have been made before 1650, and an even earlier weapon made during the reign of Henry VIII, some time before 1547.

Those early revolvers were, surprisingly enough, practically identical to the actions covered in Colt's early patents. The actions for those early patents are still in use today in the Colt Single Action Army or Frontier model.

Colt's original patent, dated 1835, dealt with revolving of the cylinder via a ratchet and pawl arrangement. The original patents belonging to Colt were so tightly worded that no other manufacturer had any real impression on the market until these patents ran out in 1850. After this, the market opened up, with Dean-Adams in 1851, Beaumont in 1855, and Starr and Savage in 1865 all bringing out innovative designs. These were, however, still all muzzle-loading percussion systems.

It was not until the advent of the rimfire in 1851 that breech-loading revolvers really started to appear. Even then, it was not until 1857 that Smith and Wesson introduced the first hinged frame .22″ rim fire revolver. The patent for bored-through chambers and the use of metallic cartridges gave Smith and Wesson the market until 1869.

With the passing of the Smith and Wesson patents, there was a flood of breech-loading arms in calibres from .22″ to 50″. However, except for .22″ target shooting, the days of the rimfire were

numbered, thanks to the introduction of the centre fire system.

The first centre fire Colt revolver to be patented was the Colt Single Action Army Model 1873. In 1880, Enfield produced a .476″ hinged frame revolver, but it was a design monstrosity and was soon superseded by the now familiar Webley top latching hinged frame design in 1887. In 1894, this was modified slightly and it became the standard Webley Mk.1 British Army service revolver. In 1889, the US Government officially adopted a Colt .38″ revolver, using the now familiar swing-out cylinder system.

A multitude of variations on the Smith and Wesson and Colt designs followed, but little has really changed in the basic design of the revolver mechanism since then. It would seem that little can be done to improve on the efficiency of the basic Smith and Wesson and Colt designs.

1.0.9 The self-loading pistol (Figure 1.0.11)

The principle of the self-loading pistol was grasped long ago. It is reported in Birche's History of the Royal Society for 1664 that a mechanic had made a claim of being able to make a pistol which could 'shoot as fast as presented and stopped at will'. However, without the necessary combination of a self-contained cartridge, smokeless propellant and

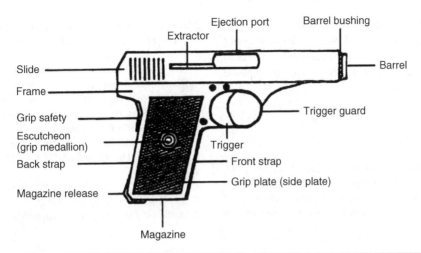

Ejection port Barrel bushing

Extractor

Slide

Frame

Grip safety

Escutcheon
(grip medallion)

Back strap

Magazine release

Barrel

Trigger guard

Trigger

Front strap

Grip plate (side plate)

Magazine

Figure 1.0.11   Major parts of a typical self-loading pistol.

metallurgical advances, it was not possible to utilise these principles in a practical way.

While patent records from 1863 show numerous attempts to develop a self-loading pistol, it was not until 1892 that the first successful weapon appeared. This was a weapon patented by the Austrian Schönberger, and made by the company Steyr. It was a blowback design and made for the 8 mm Schönberger, a very powerful cartridge.

The first commercially successful design was by an American, Hugo Borchardt. Unable to finance his design, he took it to Germany to have it manufactured there. Although clumsy, this weapon was of radical design, containing the first magazine to be held in the grip and the 'knee-joint' toggle locking system. It was this design which was slightly modified by Luger to become Germany's first military self-loading pistol, the Walther P08.

In 1893, Bergman produced a whole range of pistols, one of which, the 1897 8 mm 'Simplex', is of particular interest as the cartridge became the .32″ Colt Automatic Pistol (ACP) cartridge.

In 1896, the story of the truly successful self-loading pistol really began with the introduction of the 7.63 mm calibre Mauser 'broom handle' pistol (Mauser Model C96 pistol). This was the pistol made famous by Winston Churchill, who purchased one for use during the Sudan campaign of 1898. Churchill credited the weapon with saving his life when he shot his way out of a native trap, 'killing several

fuzzy-wuzzies'! I have lost count of the number of Mauser C96 pistols I have examined which have had 'Winston Churchill' engraved on the side. So far not one has proved to be genuine!

In 1898, the German factory of DWM brought out the first model of the famous Luger pistol in 7.65 mm Parabellum calibre. In 1904, the weapon was made available in 9 mm Parabellum, which was the calibre adopted for the German service pistols.

In 1897, John Browning, the greatest of all American small arms designers, produced his first patent. This was finally introduced as the Model 1900 Colt .38″ automatic.

Webley made a few unsuccessful forays into the self-loading pistol market, with their .455″ calibre 1904 model, the .45″ 1905 model, the 1910 .38″ calibre and the .455″ Navy model in 1913. The Webley design was not, however, very successful and never became popular.

Probably the most successful pistol ever to be introduced was the Colt Model 1911. This was designed by Browning and was placed into military service as the Colt Government Model in .45″ calibre. With minor modifications, as the Model 1911A1, the weapon was the standard issue military weapon for the USA until the late 1980s.

Since then, the main innovations have been in the use of lightweight aluminium and plastics for the weapons frame, the move towards smaller calibres and higher velocity bullets, the development of magnum handgun ammunition and the use of gas-operated locking systems. These are, however, only variations on a theme and, as with revolvers, it would seem that there is little that can be done to improve on the basic design.

Further reading

1 Chase, K. (2003), *Firearms: A Global History to 1700*, Cambridge University Press, ISBN 0-521-82274-2.
2 Myatt, F. *An Illustrated History of the Development of the World's Military Firearms During the 19th Century.*
3 Fowler, W., North, A. & Stronge, C. *The Development of Small Firearms, from 12th-century Hand Cannons to Modern-day Automatics.*
4 Fowler, W., North, A., Stronge, C. & Sweeney, P. *The Illustrated World Encyclopaedia of Guns: Pistols, Rifles, Revolvers, Machine and Submachine Guns through History in 1200 Colour Photographs.*
5 Hogg, I. *Jane's Guns Recognition Guide: Every firearm in use today.* Jane's Recognition Guides.
6 Hogg, I.V. The Greenhill Military Small Arms Data Book.
7 Greener, W.W. *The Gun and Its Development.*
8 *Jane's Infantry Weapons* (2012).
9 Mathews, *Firearms Identification* Vol. I, II & III.

2.0

Weapon Types and Their Operation

2.0.1 Introduction

In any court case, it is essential for the prosecution or the defence to be able not only to identify correctly the type of weapon being referred to, but also to have some idea as to the important component parts of its mechanism and what function they serve.

Considerable confusion exists as to what are a **pistol**, **revolver**, **self-loading pistol** and **automatic**. This is very basic firearms nomenclature, but it is so often wrongly applied. Here is an explanation of the correct usage and any alternatives which one might encounter, where they exist.

2.0.2 Handguns

There are three basic types of handgun: **single shot**, **revolving** and **self-loading** pistols. Such exotica as Double Barrelled Howdah pistols, self-loading revolvers and self-loading pistols with revolving magazines can be ignored for the purposes of this chapter.

In English nomenclature all handguns are **pistols;** some are '**single shot pistols**', others are '**revolving pistols**' and the others are '**self-loading pistols**'. American nomenclature takes a slightly less stringent approach with the terminology, using '**revolvers**' and '**pistols**'. Pistols are also referred to as '**autos**' and '**semi-automatics**'.

The term 'automatic' or 'auto' is often misused. When correctly used, the term signifies a weapon in which the action will continue to operate until the finger is removed from the trigger or the magazine is empty – hence, 'automatic'.

A true self-loading pistol will, after firing, eject the spent cartridge case and then load a fresh round of ammunition into the chamber. To fire the fresh round, the pressure on the trigger has to be released and then re-applied.

A few true automatic pistols have been commercially manufactured. Examples are the Mauser Schnell-Feuer pistol, the Astra Mod 902 and more recently the Glock Mod. 18. Fully automatic pistols have, however, never been a commercial success, due to the near impossibility of controlling such a weapon under full automatic fire. Each shot causes the barrel to rise during recoil, and the next round has fired before the firer has time to reacquire the target within the sights, causing the barrel to rise even further. Even at close range, it is unusual for more than two shots to hit a man-sized target.

Single shot pistol

The vast majority of single shot pistols are .22″ LR (Long Rifle) calibre and are intended for target use. Generally, the barrel is hinged to the frame, with some locking mechanism to keep it in place during firing. On unlocking, the barrel swings down, allowing the empty cartridge case to be removed and a fresh one inserted. Other types exist in which the barrel is firmly fixed to the frame, and there is some

---

Forensic Ballistics in Court: Interpretation and Presentation of Firearms Evidence, First Edition. Brian J. Heard.
© 2013 John Wiley & Sons, Ltd. Published 2013 by John Wiley & Sons, Ltd.

form of breech block which swings out, pulls back or slides down to expose the breech end of the barrel for loading/unloading. This type of pistol varies from the crudely made saloon pistol to highly sophisticated target pistols for competition shooting.

Following is an example of a Flobert saloon pistol (Figure 2.0.1). This type of pistol was intended for use in short distance indoor target practice using a very short BB (bulleted breech) or CB (conical breech) cartridge. These were very popular in the early part of the 20th Century.

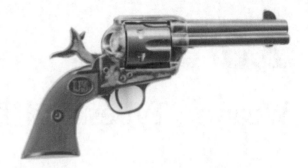

Figure 2.0.3   Colt Single Action Army revolver.

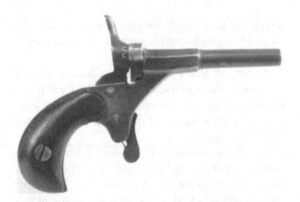

Figure 2.0.1   .22″ calibre saloon pistol.

Often wrongly classified as 'antiques', these weapons fire currently manufactured ammunition with a lethal potential.

An example of a more modern single shot pistol would be the Thompson Contender Single Shot, as pictured in Figure 2.0.2.

Revolving pistol or revolver

In a **revolving pistol**, or **revolver** as it is usually referred to, the supply of ammunition is held in a cylinder at the rear of the barrel, with each round having its own chamber. Cocking the hammer rotates the cylinder, via a ratchet mechanism, to bring a new round of ammunition in line with the barrel. Pulling the trigger then drops the hammer, thus firing the round. This is the simplest type of revolving pistol mechanism, and it is called the '**single action**' mode of operation. The earliest types of revolving pistol employed this type of mechanism. A good example of a single action revolver is the Colt Single Action Model of 1873 (Figure 2.0.3.)

The other type of revolving pistol mechanism is called '**double action**'. In this design, a long,

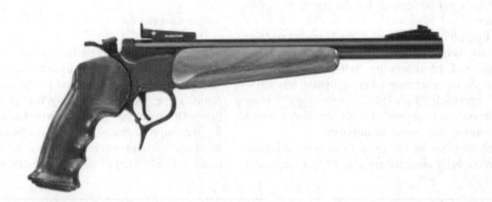

Figure 2.0.2   Thompson single shot pistol.

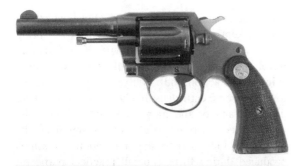

Figure 2.0.4 Colt Police Positive double action revolver.

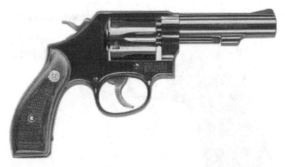

Figure 2.0.5 Smith & Wesson Mod. 10 revolver.

continuous pull on the trigger cocks the hammer, rotates the cylinder and then drops the hammer, all in one operation. Most modern revolvers employ this type of mechanism, with virtually all of them having the capability for single action mode of operation as well. An example of a double action revolver is the Colt Police Positive revolver (Figure 2.0.4).

In the past, a very few self-cocking revolving pistols have also been manufactured. These have an action which, after firing a round, automatically rotates the cylinder and re-cocks the hammer. The most successful of this type was the Webley Fosberry. This type of weapon is, however, extremely rare, and exist nowadays only as collectors' items or in museums.

Frame type

Revolvers can be sub-grouped into '**solid frame**', where the frame is made from a single forging, and '**hinged frame**', where the frame is hinged to tip either up or down for access to the cylinder.

Examples of a solid frame revolver would be the Colt Single Action Army (Figure 2.0.3), the Colt Police Positive (Figure 2.0.4) and the Smith & Wesson Mod. 10 (Figure 2.0.5).

An example of a hinged frame revolver would be the Webley and Scott revolver (Figure 2.0.6).

Access to the cylinder for loading or reloading in solid frame revolvers is generally accomplished by having the cylinder mounted on a 'crane' which can

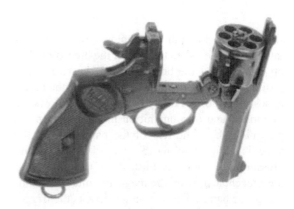

Figure 2.0.6 Webley & Scott revolver – open for loading.

be swung out from the frame. Some weapons also have the cylinder mounted on a removable axis pin which, when removed, allows the cylinder to be completely removed from the frame for loading and unloading. This type of frame is more commonly encountered in cheaper weapons. Of the two frame types, the solid frame is the most common, due to its inherent strength and ease of manufacture.

Self-loading pistol

In this type of weapon (Figure 2.0.7), the ammunition is normally contained in a removable spring-loaded magazine, usually housed within the grip frame. The barrel of the weapon is surrounded by a

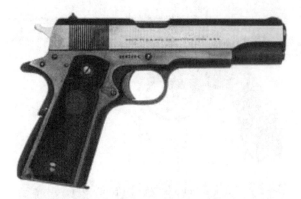

Figure 2.0.7   Colt 1911A1 self-loading pistol.

slide with an integral breechblock, which is kept into battery (i.e. when the face of the breechblock is up tight against the breech end of the barrel in a position ready for firing) with the rear of the barrel by a strong spring. Pulling back the slide allows the topmost round of ammunition in the magazine to present itself to the rear of the barrel. When the slide is allowed to move forward under spring pressure, the round is pushed by the bottom of the breechblock from the magazine into the chamber of the barrel. This action also cocks the trigger mechanism.

When the trigger is pulled, the hammer drops and the round is fired, pushing the bullet down the barrel. These gases also exert an equal and opposite force on the cartridge case, which forces the slide and breechblock to the rear. This ejects the spent cartridge case through a port in the side or occasionally, on the top of the slide. At the end of its rearward motion, the spring-loaded slide moves forward, stripping a fresh round off the top of the magazine and feeding it into the rear of the barrel, ready for firing. As the action is only self-loading, the pressure on the trigger has to be removed and then re-applied before another round can be fired.

To prevent the weapon from firing continuously, a part of the action, called a **disconnecter**, removes the trigger from contact with the rest of the mechanism. Releasing the trigger disengages the disconnecter, allowing the trigger to re-engage with the mechanism so that the fresh round can be fired.

An action such as that described above, where the slide is kept into battery with the barrel by spring action alone, is the simplest type of self-loading pistol mechanism. It is generally referred to as a **'blowback'** action and is only of any real use for lower-powered cartridges. If a blowback action were used for any of the more powerful calibres, the unsupported cartridge would, on exiting from the barrel, explode due to the tremendous pressures produced during firing. For all practical purposes, the most powerful round which can safely be fired in a blowback action weapon is a .380″ ACP (.380″ Automatic Colt Pistol, also known as the 9 mm Short) cartridge. Some blowback action weapons, such as the Astra Mod. 400 and the Dreys 1910 Military Model, have been designed to fire more powerful cartridges by having massive recoil springs. However, these are very difficult to cock, due to the strength of the recoil spring, and they generally require some method of disconnecting the spring during the cocking operation.

When more powerful ammunition is used, some other mechanism has to be employed to ensure that the pressures produced fall to a safe level before the fired cartridge case exits from the barrel. This is accomplished via a **'locked breech or delayed blowback mechanism'**. In such a weapon, the barrel is locked to the breechblock by some mechanical means during the instant of firing. With this type of action, the rearward thrust of the cartridge case against the breechblock causes the barrel and attached breechblock to move backwards together. At some point on its rearward travel, once that the bullet has exited the barrel and the barrel pressures have fallen to acceptable levels, the barrel is stopped and unlocked from the breechblock. The breechblock and slide can then continue to the rear and, in so doing, eject the empty cartridge case. On its return journey into battery with the barrel, a fresh cartridge is loaded into the chamber and the mechanism is cocked, ready to fire again.

The variety of locked-breech mechanisms is vast and outside the scope of this book. They range from the very simple Browning 'swinging link' and Luger 'toggle joint' to the more modern systems using high-pressure gas tapped from the barrel, either to keep the breech locked or to operate the unlocking mechanism.

2.0.3 Rifles

Rifle actions can be very roughly grouped into **'single shot'**, **'bolt action'**, **'self-loading'** and **'pump action'**.

Single shot

In single shot weapons, the barrel can be hinged to the frame, allowing the barrel to be dropped down for loading and unloading, or it can have some form of breech block which swings out, pulls back or slides down to expose the breech end of the barrel.

Bolt action

In bolt action weapons (Figure 2.0.8), a turning bolt slides in an extension to the barrel, which is basically the same system as in a turn bolt used to lock a door. Pushing the bolt forwards brings the bolt face into battery with the breech end of the barrel, and cocks the striker (or firing pin). Turning the bolt then locks it into place via bolt lugs engaging with slots in the barrel extension.

Other bolt action weapons cock the striker on the opening of the bolt.

Straight pull bolt actions also exist in which the rotary motion required to turn the bolt locking lugs into their recesses is applied by studs on the bolt, which slide in spiral grooves cut into the barrel extension.

Bolt action weapons are generally magazine fed, either by a tubular magazine under the barrel, through the butt stock or via a box magazine under the bolt.

Self-loading rifles

Self-loading rifles are, with the exception of the lowest power weapons, of the locked breech type. These are generally very similar to those used in locked breech pistols, but of a much stronger design to cope with the higher pressures involved. Figure 2.0.9 is an example of a self-loading rifle.

There are basically two types of self-loading rifle action:

- **Short recoil**, in which the bolt and breechblock are only locked together for about .75″ of rearward travel before unlocking. It then operates as a normal self-loading pistol would.

- **Long recoil**, in which the barrel and breechblock are locked together for the full distance of the recoil stroke. After reaching the end of its travel, the barrel is then unlocked and pushed forward by spring action, ejecting the spent cartridge during its forward motion. When the barrel is fully forward, the breechblock begins its forward motion, reloading a fresh cartridge into the chamber and cocking the action.

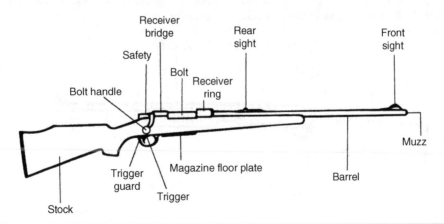

Figure 2.0.8 Bolt action rifle.

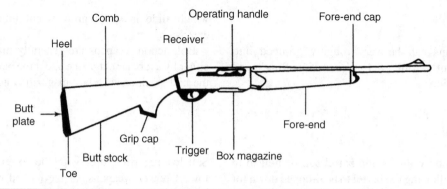

Figure 2.0.9   Self-loading rifle.

A few weapons have been produced with a **blow forward** action. These guns work in the reverse of the conventional blowback. The breech, which contains the hammer, remains stationary, while the barrel moves forward from the pressure produced during firing. The cartridge case, held stationary by the extractor, is pulled out of the chamber, and a stud on the barrel extension kicks it free. Meanwhile, a projection at the bottom of the extension pulls the next round forward out of the magazine and positions it to be chambered when the barrel returns to battery.

Pump action

In Pump Action (sometimes also referred to as **slide action**) weapons (Figure 2.0.10), the breech block is attached, via operating rods, to a moveable fore-end. On pulling back the fore-end, the mechanism locking the breechblock to the barrel is released. Pulling the fore-end to the rearmost extent of its travel, then pushing it forward, causes the empty cartridge case to be ejected, a fresh round to be loaded into the chamber and the action to be cocked.

2.0.4   Shotguns

Shotgun actions are basically the same as those found in rifles, and include single/double shot weapons with barrels hinged to the frame for loading/unloading, bolt action, self-loading and pump action. In double barrelled weapons, the barrels can be either positioned one on top of the other, 'over and under', or 'superposed' (Figure 2.0.11) or 'side by side'.

In the smaller calibres (i.e. .22″, 9 mm and .410″), double barrelled shot pistols are also occasionally encountered.

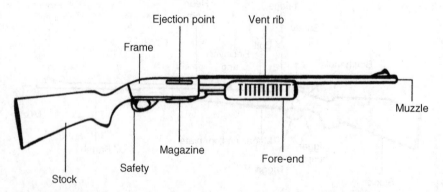

Figure 2.0.10   Pump action rifle.

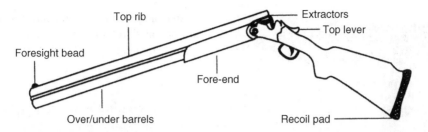

Figure 2.0.11 Over and under shotgun.

2.0.5 Combination weapons

Shotgun/rifle combinations are popular on the Continent and can consist of one shotgun barrel and one rifle barrel (**Zwilling**), two shotgun barrels with one rifle barrel (**Drilling**), two rifle barrels and one shotgun barrel (also called a **Drilling**) or, occasionally, two rifle and two shotgun barrels. Typical combination gun configurations are shown at Figure 2.0.12.

2.0.6 Sub-machine guns

Sub-machine guns were once considered outside the scope of a book such as this. In recent years, however, violent armed crime and terrorism has seen this type of weapon increasingly used.

Sub-machine guns are fully automatic weapons, usually with a single shot option, and they are generally chambered for pistol calibre ammunition.

The simplest type of action encountered is a simple blowback (Figure 2.0.13). To overcome the problems of the cartridge exiting the chamber before the pressures have dropped to safe levels, a very heavy reciprocating bolt and a large spring are employed to delay the cartridge extraction. The classic example of this type of action is the Sten gun used by the British forces in WW II (Figure 2.0.13). While this is extremely simple, is cheap to manufacture and has a reliable action, it does tend to be rather heavy and prone to accidental discharge.

More modern weapons are equipped with some form of delayed blowback action of the type used in self-loading pistols and rifle actions, for example the Uzi (Figure 2.0.14). While this does produce a much

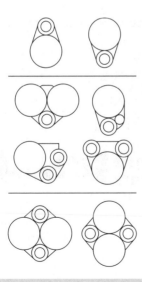

Figure 2.0.12 Typical combination gun configurations.

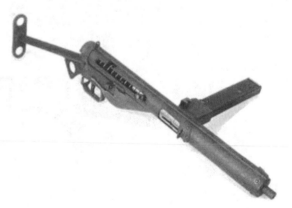

Figure 2.0.13 Sten Mk.III sub-machine gun.

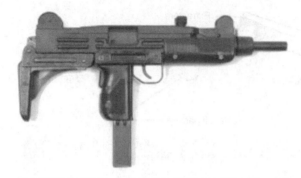

Figure 2.0.14   Uzi sub-machine gun.

lighter weapon, it is much more expensive to manufacture and, being more complicated, can be prone to malfunction.

2.0.7   Assault rifles

An assault rifle is basically a short, lightweight weapon firing a cartridge of lower power than that used in rifles, but more powerful than that used in sub-machine guns. To handle the increased pressures encountered in such cartridges, complicated systems involving gas delayed blowback or roller locking mechanisms have to be utilised to ensure that the high pressures involved have dropped to safe levels before the spent cartridge is ejected. An example of such a weapon, using a gas delayed blowback mechanism, is the Kalashnikov AK47 (Figure 2.0.15).

An example of a more modern assault rifle with a gas operated rotating bolt would be the Chinese 5.8×42 mm calibre QBZ-95-1. (Figure 2.0.16).

2.0.8   Machine guns and heavy machine guns

These are outside of the scope of this book, but basically a machine gun is a long-barrelled automatic weapon firing rifle calibre, or larger, ammunition. A heavy machine gun is very similar to a machine gun, but it is much more sturdily built, often with a water jacket around the barrel to prevent overheating and a consequential rapid rate of barrel wear. Being much heavier, they are generally mounted on a sturdy tripod and are designed for sustained high rates of fire.

2.0.9   Muzzle attachments

Rifles, pistols and revolvers can be found with six types of muzzle attachment. These are:

- Sound suppressors (often wrongly called silencers)

- Recoil reducers (also referred to as compensators)

- Flash hiders

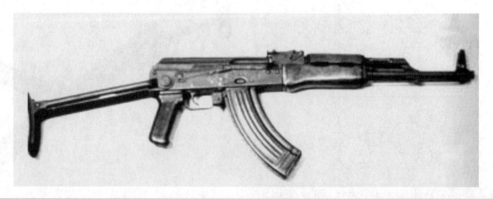

Figure 2.0.15   Kalashnikov assault rifle.

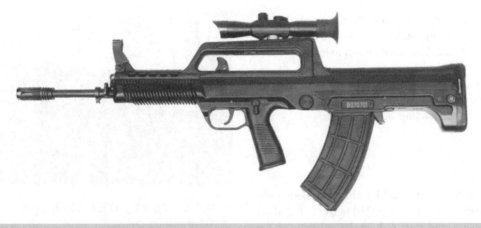

Figure 2.0.16 Chinese 5.8 × 42 mm QBZ-95-1 assault rifle.

- Muzzle counter weights (mainly for target weapons)

- Grenade dischargers

- Recoil boosters.

Shotguns can also be fitted with all of the above, although they are most likely to be found with either fixed or adjustable chokes or a recoil reducer.

Sound suppressors

There are four distinct components that together make up the noise we perceive as a gunshot. In order of loudness, these are:

1. Pressure wave from rapidly expanding propellant gases

2. Supersonic crack of bullet as it passes through the sound barrier

3. Mechanical action noise

4. Flight noise.

The pressure wave

This is produced by the rapidly expanding propellant gases. Generally, it is the only noise component that a suppressor can reduce.

As the expanding gases exit the barrel of an unsuppressed barrel, they rapidly expand, causing a loud bang, which is basically due to the gases exceeding the speed of sound (approximately 1,100 ft/sec). The suppressor reduces this noise by the slow release, through expansion and turbulence, of high-pressure propellant gases to the point where they no longer exceed this velocity.

The basic design of a sound suppressor consists of an expansion chamber (in Figure 2.0.17 below, this wraps back around the barrel to decrease the length of the suppressor) and a series of baffles to reduce the speed of the emerging gases further.

Suppressors can either be an integral part of the weapon or a muzzle attachment to be screwed on or attached via a bayonet-type fitment or with grub screws.

Integral suppressors can be designed so that the gases are bled off (ported) into the expansion chamber before the bullet reaches supersonic speeds. Example of weapons with an integral suppressor would include the High Standard HD .22″ SLP and the H&K MP5SD 9 mm PB SMG. In these

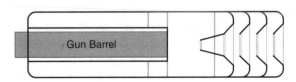

Figure 2.0.17 Typical silencer.

weapons, bleeding the gases off early reduces the final velocity of the bullet to below that of sound, thus allowing standard ammunition to be used rather than a reduced loading.

Most suppressors for supersonic cartridges can realistically be expected to reduce the noise of firing by 18–32 dB, depending on the design.

Supersonic crack

This can only be removed by either utilising subsonic ammunition, or via a ported barrel to bleed off propellant gas and thus reduce the velocity of the bullet.

Mechanical noise

This is caused by the weapons hammer, firing pin, locking mechanism, etc. This can, to a certain extent, be reduced by the use of single shot weapons with a cushioned firing pin. The WW II Special Forces Welrod is an example of such a weapon. It was made in 9 mm PB, .380 acp and .32 acp calibres, and was virtually silent in operation.

Bullet flight noise

Bullet flight noise is not loud enough to be sensed by the shooter, although it can be distinctly heard if the bullet passes close by a person. This noise resembles a distinctive high-pitched whirring sound as the bullet flies through the air. Flight noise is too quiet to be heard above the sonic crack.

Sound suppressors also function as flash suppressors and, to a certain extent, recoil reducers.

Recoil reducers

Also called **muzzle brakes** and **recoil compensators**, these are devices that are fitted to the muzzle of a firearm to redirect propellant gases upwards and to the rear. This has the effect of countering both the recoil of the gun and unwanted rising of the barrel during rapid fire. An example of a recoil

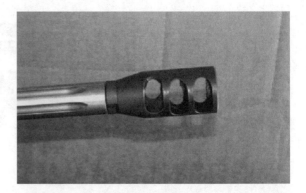

Figure 2.0.18   Recoil reducer on muzzle of a high-powered rifle.

reducer on muzzle of a high powered rifle is shown in Figure 2.0.18

Generally speaking, a muzzle brake is external to the barrel of the firearm, while a recoil compensator is typically part of the structure of the barrel proper.

A properly designed muzzle brake can significantly reduce recoil. The actual effectiveness depends to an extent on the cartridge for which the rifle is chambered, with claims of up to 60 per cent being made.

Recoil compensators are generally less efficient than muzzle brakes.

Muzzle brakes/compensators are designed to reduce what is called the '**free recoil velocity**' of the weapon. The free recoil velocity is how fast the gun comes back at the shooter. The faster a gun comes back, the more painful it is for the firer as the body has less time to absorb the recoil.

Weapons firing fast small calibre bullets generally have a smaller recoil velocity than larger calibre slow moving bullets.

There are numerous types of recoil reducer, from the simplest – a short length of tube attached at 90° to the end of the barrel to divert the gases sideways – to laser-cut slots in the muzzle end of the barrel (Magna Porting).

In conventional designs, combustion gases depart the brake at an angle to the bore and in a slightly rearwards direction. This counteracts the rearward movement of the barrel due to recoil, as well as the upward rise of the muzzle. The effect can be compared to reverse thrust systems on aircraft jet engines. The mass and velocity of the gases can be significant enough to move the firearm in the opposite direction from the recoil.

On the AKM assault rifle, the brake is angled slightly to the right to counteract the sideways movement of the gun under recoil.

A major disadvantage of recoil reducers however, is the large increase in noise levels and the gas blast which is directed back towards the firer.

One other problem with high-powered rifles, such as the Barrett .50 Browning, is the violent disruption debris from the ground, which can expose the firer's position. This is only a significant factor in military or law enforcement tactical situations.

Flash hiders

When a gun fires, only about 30 per cent of the chemical energy released from the propellant is converted into the useful kinetic energy of actually moving the projectile down the barrel. Much of the remaining energy is primarily contained in the propellant gas-particle mixture, which escapes from the muzzle of the gun in the few milliseconds before and after the bullet leaves the barrel.

This extremely hot mixture of incandescent gases and partially burnt propellant ignites on contact with the air, causing an intense 'muzzle flash'. This can be disconcerting for the firer and a distinct disadvantage under night-time military or law enforcement tactical situations. Not only does it temporarily destroy the firer's night vision, it also pinpoints his position to the enemy.

Flash hiders either physically hide the flash, by way of a cone-shaped device on the end of the barrel (e.g. Lee Enfield No.5 Jungle Carbine) or by dispersing the flash upwards or sideways via a series of fingers or a tube containing longitudinal cuts (Figure 2.0.19).

These attachments are often dual purpose items, designed not only to suppress the flash of firing but also to reduce recoil.

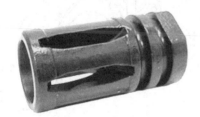

Figure 2.0.19   Flash hider for a AR15/M16 rifle.

Muzzle counter weights

These are only used on highly specialised target weapons and are designed to add stability in sighting, as well as to reduce the recoil-induced upward motion of the barrel.

Grenade dischargers

In its simplest form, a grenade discharger is a cup attached to the end of a rifle barrel, into which a grenade can be launched via a blank cartridge. Utilising this device, grenades can be propelled to much greater distances than by throwing alone.

More modern devices can be used with bulleted rounds and contain aluminium or mild steel baffles to capture the bullet.

Recoil boosters

Very few of these have been manufactured, the most notable being the muzzle attachment to the German WW II MG 34 machine gun. This attachment was intended to increase the rate of fire in this short recoiling weapon.

Some recoil operated semi-automatic pistols also have to be fitted with a recoil booster to compensate for the additional weight of the suppressor. Without a booster, short recoil pistols will not function in the self-loading mode of operation.

2.0.10   Important parts of a weapons mechanism

To delve into this subject in any great detail would involve several books, so it is, obviously, outside the scope of this book. This sub-chapter shall, therefore, concentrate mainly on handguns and those parts of the mechanism which are considered relevant to most cases that one is likely to encounter. Further in-depth information can be accessed via the list of books in the 'Further reading' section at the end of this chapter.

To simplify matters as far as possible, Figure 2.0.20 is a generic view of a modern double action revolver, illustrating the major parts of a revolver and where they are located.

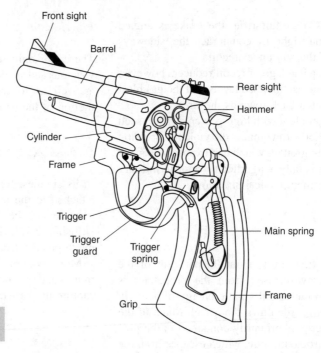

Front sight

Barrel

Rear sight

Hammer

Cylinder

Frame

Trigger

Trigger
guard

Trigger
spring

Main spring

Frame

Grip

Figure 2.0.20 Generic diagram of a modern double action revolver.

Following are a series of diagrams illustrating the various components of a revolver and a brief description of their function.

2.0.11 Bent and sear

Single action revolvers

All trigger mechanism have a bent (Figure 2.0.21) and a sear (Figure 2.0.22) of some description, whether it be in a single action revolver, as illustrated, a single shot weapon, a self-loading pistol, a rifle or a sub-machine gun. It is part of the mechanism by which a firing mechanism is held in the cocked position and then released by pulling the trigger to fire the weapon.

The angle at which the sear and bent interact is crucial to the correct operation and safety of a weapon when it is cocked. If the angle of interaction is too steep, then the pressure required on the trigger to fire the weapon will be excessive to the point of it

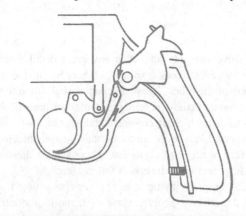

Figure 2.0.21 Bent.

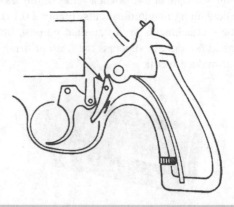

Figure 2.0.22 Sear.

being impossible to fire. If it is too shallow, the opposite could be true and the trigger pressure could be excessively light, rendering the weapon prone to accidental discharge. In extreme cases, it may even be that the weapon cannot even be cocked.

During manufacture, these parts are either case-hardened or heat treated to ensure that, during the normal operational life of the weapon, they do not become worn to the point of becoming dangerous.

Attempts are often made by 'amateur gunsmiths' to reduce the trigger pressure required on the trigger to fire the weapon by removing metal from either the bent or sear. This is usually done to give the weapon a 'hair trigger' – something which it rarely does. The angle at which these two components interact is absolutely crucial. Any such attempt to modify them by anyone other than a trained gunsmith is rarely successful, and usually ends up ruining the trigger mechanism.

Half cock safety

In most single action revolvers, as well as some self-loading pistols, there is a **half cock safety**, which

exists as a second, deeper bent below the normal one. When the hammer of a single action weapon is gently pulled back to about half its normal travel, the sear will drop into what is called the 'half cock or safety bent'. As this is much deeper than the normal bent, the hammer cannot be released by simply pulling the trigger and the weapon is in a safe mode. To fire the weapon, the hammer must first be pulled all the way back so that the sear engages with the full cock bent. The weapon can then be fired in the normal way.

Double action revolvers

Double action revolvers are somewhat more complicated, in that they be fired either by a long pull on the trigger, which cocks and drops the hammer, or by manually cocking the hammer as in a single action revolver.

Figure 2.0.23 is a simplified diagram showing the major parts.

During single action operation, the tail of the hammer rests on the tail of the trigger. However, during double action operation, the tail of the trigger

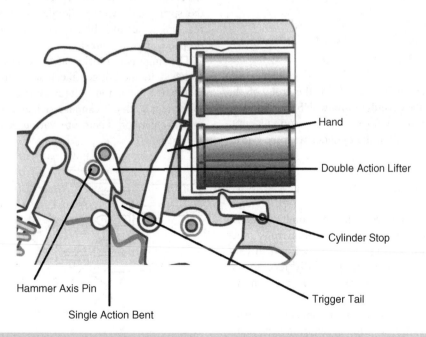

Figure 2.0.23 Double action revolver mechanism.

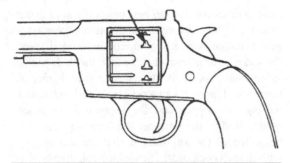

Figure 2.0.24   Cylinder stop notch.

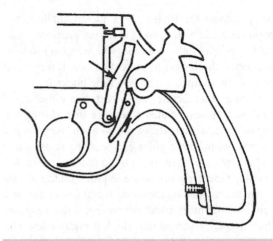

Figure 2.0.25   Transfer bar safety.

acts on the hammer lifter which is situated above the hammer's axis pin. As the trigger is pulled, the hammer is cammed back until the point is reached where the trigger tail disengages from the lifter. At this point, the hammer is released, allowing the firing pin to fall onto a cartridge.

Also shown in Figure 2.0.23 is the 'hand' which is attached to the tail of the trigger. This engages with the 'ratchet' at the rear of the cylinder and is the method by which the cylinder is rotated on pulling the trigger, bringing a fresh cartridge in line with the firing pin for firing.

2.0.12   Other important parts of a revolver mechanism

As can be seen in Figure 2.0.23, the front of the trigger acts on the **cylinder stop**, which engages with the cylinder stop notch (or cylinder stop cut out – Figure 2.0.24), to align the cylinder with the barrel.

Safety mechanisms in revolvers

Apart from the half cock notch found mainly in single action revolvers, there are numerous other safety mechanisms that have been used in revolvers. Modern revolvers, however, generally tend to use either a transfer bar (Figure 2.0.25) or a hammer block (Figure 2.0.26).

With the transfer bar safety mechanism, the firing pin is 'floating'. It is situated in the frame and is not part of the hammer. The hammer is prevented from

reaching the firing pin by the design of the frame and hammer. When the trigger is pulled, the transfer bar moves up into a position where it is in between the hammer face and the firing pin. Energy can then be transferred to the firing pin to fire a cartridge in the weapons chamber.

Usually, the firing pin is spring loaded away from the cartridge and it will, depending on the strength of the spring, negate any likelihood of the firing pin reaching a cartridge by inertia alone if the weapon is dropped onto its muzzle.

The hammer block safety consists of a bar attached to the trigger mechanism in such a way that, when the action is at rest, it pushes the hammer to the rear so that it cannot reach and fire a cartridge in the chamber. There are various designs of this

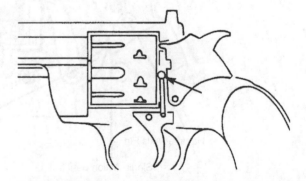

Figure 2.0.26   Hammer block safety.

safety mechanism, some of which are better than others.

2.0.13 Hand and ratchet

The **hand** (also known as the **cylinder pawl**) is a lever, attached to the trigger (Figure 2.0.27), which acts on the **ratchet** (Figure 2.0.28) to rotate the cylinder. The number of teeth on the ratchet correspond to the number of chambers in the cylinder. The cylinder is locked into a position where the chamber is exactly lined up with the bore of the barrel by the **cylinder stop** locking into the **cylinder stop notch**.

Any wear on the ratchet, hand or cylinder stop notch will prevent the chamber lining up with the bore of the weapon during firing. Such a misalignment will cause the bullet to emerge from the muzzle of the weapon with material shaved off due to contact with the breech end of the barrel. In one case, this misalignment was

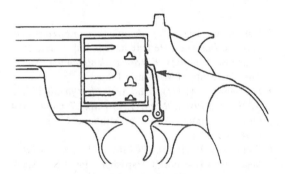

Figure 2.0.27 Hand.

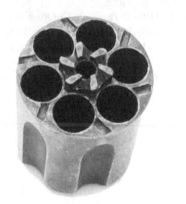

Figure 2.0.28 Cylinder ratchet.

such that the deceased appeared to have been shot by two bullets. Such extreme cases are rare, however, because once the alignment becomes too great, the firing pin will not align with the centre of the primer and the gun will fail to fire.

Self-loading pistols

The general working principle of a self-loading pistol has been explained earlier in this chapter. However, to reiterate: a self-loading or semi-automatic pistol is a type of handgun which uses a single chamber and barrel and a mechanism powered by the previous shot to load a fresh cartridge into the chamber from the magazine. In a self-loading pistol, the magazine is usually housed within the grip frame. Each time the trigger of a semi-automatic pistol is pulled, a single shot is fired, after which the energy of the shot is used to eject the fired cartridge case and to reload the chamber from the magazine for the next shot.

Self-loading pistols can be divided into 'blowback' and 'locked breech' categories, according to their principle of operation. The blowback operating principle is suitable for smaller, low-powered calibres such as the .22″ LR, 7.65 mm Browning (also known as .32 ACP) and the 9 mm Browning Short (also known as .380 ACP).

In blowback actions, the resistance of the recoil spring and the mass of the slide are sufficient to retard the opening of the breech until the projectile has left the barrel and breech pressure has dropped to a safe level.

For more powerful calibres, such as the 9×19 mm Parabellum and .45 ACP, some form of locked breech is needed to retard breech opening until the barrel pressures have dropped to a safe level. Otherwise, the cartridge would explode violently if left unsupported by the barrel.

Some blowback pistols have been produced for higher energy cartridges, but these require a very heavy slide and stiff spring, making them bulky, heavy and difficult to operate.

There are numerous types of action, safety and trigger mechanisms employed in self-loading pistols. As with revolvers, self-loading pistols can be either single action or double action. However, all have a bent and sear arrangement for capture and release of the firing pin, as utilised in revolvers.

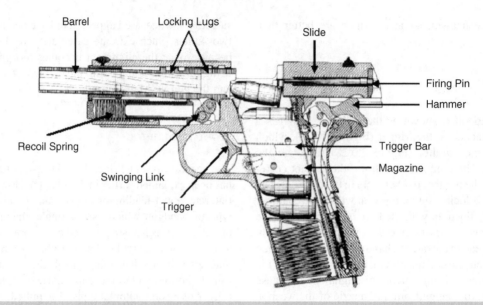

Figure 2.0.29   Generic diagram of a self-loading pistol.

For further information on the types of action and safety mechanisms employed in self-loading pistols, the references in the Further reading section at the end of this chapter would constitute a good starting point.

The diagram in Figure 2.0.29, is a good generic example of a swinging link, locked breech self-loading pistol.

Further reading

1 Hatcher, J., Jury, F. & Weller, J. (1957). *Firearms Investigation, Identification and Evidence*, 2nd Edition. The Stackpole Company.

2 Gunther, J. & Gunther, C. (1935). *The Identification of Firearms – From Ammunition Fired therein with an Analysis of Legal Authorities*. John Wiley & Sons.

3 Burrard, G. (1934). *The Identification of Firearms and Forensic Ballistics*. Herbert Jenkins Ltd.

4 Mathews, J. (1962). *Firearms Identification*, Vol. 1. The University of Wisconsin Press.

5 Skennerton, I. (1997). *Small Arms Identification Series No. 9: .455 Pistol, Revolver No 1 Mk VI*. Gold Coast, QLD, Australia: Arms & Militaria Press. ISBN 0-949749-30-3.

6 Smith, W.H.B. (1979). *1943 Basic Manual of Military Small Arms* (facsimile). Harrisburg, PA, USA: Stackpole Books. ISBN 0-8117-1699-6.

7 The War Office (UK) (1929). *Textbook of Small Arms*. HM Stationery Office.

8 Cary, L. (1961). *The Colt GunBook* (Fawcett Book 447). Greenwich, CT, USA, Fawcett Publications.

9 http://www.hallowellco.com/abbrevia.htm

10 Mathews, J.H. (1962–1973). *Firearms identification*, Vols I, II & III. Springfield, IL, USA, Thomas.

2.1

Gas and Air Powered Weapons

2.1.1 Introduction

Anyone who presents forensic evidence in court with respect to air, gas and other types of non-cartridge powered weapons must know the difference between the various types, their operation, their power and the types of missiles they are capable of firing. This chapter will, with illustrative cases, explain in some detail how each and every type of commercially available weapon of this type works and the ammunition it fires.

Whether air weapons fit within the general definition of a firearm, i.e. 'a lethal barrelled weapon' can be a very controversial issue. There are, obviously, high-powered air weapons that will easily kill a human being. At the other end of the scale, there are those low-powered air guns which, when firing a soft lead pellet, would have insufficient energy to penetrate skin. However, the same low-powered air gun could fire a steel dart with sufficient energy to penetrate a major artery (see Figure 2.1.7 for the construction of an air gun dart). When firing a lead pellet or a steel ball bearing, such low-powered air guns would, once again, be incapable of causing more than a large bruise. However, the ball bearing could seriously damage an eye, the shock of which could lead to death in an elderly person.

The legislation pertaining to these weapons is quite complex, and to delve into it in any great detail would be outside the scope of this book. However, an insight into how countries deal with this type of weapon, and a brief outline of their legislation, can be found at Appendix 11.

2.1.2 Weapon types

Gas and air weapons can be rifles or pistols, but they all utilise compressed air or some type of gas to propel the missile. Most fire a lead projectile, usually of .22″ (5.5 mm), .177″ (4.5 mm) or .25″ (6.25 mm) calibre. Steel darts, plastic pellets or large soft plastic balls filled with paint are also used in certain weapons.

Air weapons have a very long history, dating back to about 1850, and their use in warfare has been regularly recorded. One notable instance was their use by the Austrian army against the French during the Napoleonic wars from 1799 to 1809.

Modern air weapons are typically of much lower power than cartridge weapons, and they are designed for casual target use, vermin control or target shooting. The cheaper weapons tend to be smooth-bored and are intended for use with either steel balls ('BBs') or darts with cotton flights.

Spring air weapons

The most basic form of an air weapon is one in which the compressed air for discharging the missile is obtained by means of a spring-loaded piston contained within a compression chamber

Forensic Ballistics in Court: Interpretation and Presentation of Firearms Evidence, First Edition. Brian J. Heard.
© 2013 John Wiley & Sons, Ltd. Published 2013 by John Wiley & Sons, Ltd.

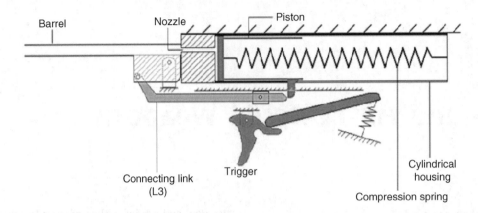

Figure 2.1.1   Internal mechanism of a spring air weapon.

(see Figure 2.1.1). Cocking the gun causes the piston assembly to compress the spring until a bent at the rear of the piston engages the sear. Pulling the trigger releases the sear and allows the spring to decompress, pushing the piston forward and compressing the air in the chamber directly behind the pellet.

By nature, most spring piston guns are single-shot breech-loaders, but weapons with a tubular or cylinder magazine are also available.

Spring guns are typically cocked by a mechanism requiring the gun to be hinged at the mid-point (called a break barrel), with the barrel serving as a cocking lever, or by use of a side lever, under-barrel lever or motorised cocking powered by a rechargeable battery.

Spring-piston guns have a practical upper limit of 1,250 ft/s (380 m/s) for .177″ calibre (4.5 mm) pellets. Higher velocities cause unstable pellet flight and loss of accuracy. However, most .177″ (4.5 mm) and .22″ (5.5 mm) calibre weapons tend to be kept below this level to circumvent air and gas weapon legislation, which places a limit on the power of air weapons.

Gas spring weapons

Some makes and model of air rifle (e.g. Weihrauch, Theoben) incorporate a gas spring instead of a mechanical spring. Pressurised air or nitrogen is held in a chamber built into the piston, and this air is further pressurised when the gun is cocked. It is, in effect, a 'gas spring', also referred to as a 'gas ram' or 'gas strut'. Gas spring units require higher precision to build, since they require a low friction sliding seal that can withstand the high pressures when cocked.

Pneumatic or pump-up weapons

Pneumatic air guns utilise pre-compressed air as the source of energy to propel the projectile. Weapons which use an onboard pump to pressurise the air in their reservoir can be single-stroke and multi-stroke.

Multi-stroke pneumatic air guns require 2 to 10 pumps of an onboard lever to store compressed air within the air gun. Variable power can be achieved through this process, as the user can adapt the power level for long or short-range shooting.

There are two types of such multi-stroke air weapons:

- those with a 'knock-open valve' where only a certain amount of the air is released with each pull of the trigger;

- those with a 'knock-off' valve, where all the air is released with a single pull of the trigger.

Knock-open valve weapons give a number of shots of consistent velocity, depending upon the pressure contained in the reservoir. With a knock-off valve, all the air is released at once, giving a single shot of much higher velocity.

Single-stroke pneumatic air weapons, as the name implies, are pressurised by a single stroke of the lever. The single-pump system is usually found in target rifles and pistols, where the higher muzzle energy of a multi-stroke pumping system is not required.

Pre-charged pneumatic guns have their gas reservoirs filled using either by a high-pressure hand pump (often capable of attaining pressures of 30 MPa) or by decanting the necessary volume/-pressure of air from a diving cylinder. Because of this design, these weapons can be of very high power.

Carbon dioxide (CO_2) powered weapons

Most CO_2 guns use a disposable cylinder such as a 'Powerlet or 'Sparklet' that is purchased pre-filled with 12 or more grams of pressurised carbon dioxide (CO_2). Some weapons, usually the more expensive models, use larger refillable CO_2 reservoirs, such as those used in paintball guns.

Carbon dioxide-powered guns have two significant advantages over pre-charged pneumatic air guns:

1. They have a simpler system for compact storage of energy as a small volume of liquid converts to a large volume of pressurised gas.

2. No pressure regulator is necessary, as the vapour pressure of pressurised carbon dioxide is dependent only on temperature, not tank size. Thus, each shot will provide exactly the same pressure of gas.

One disadvantage of using carbon dioxide as a propellant is that the pressure of gaseous CO_2 at ordinary ambient temperatures is only around 850–1,000 psi (6 to 7 MPa), which is only a third of the safe working pressure of a typical full pneumatic powered weapon (20 MPa or 2,900 psi). The

effect of this is that, generally speaking, CO_2 guns are lower powered than pneumatic weapons.

Airsoft weapons

Airsoft guns are replica firearms that fire lightweight plastic pellets using a compressed gas such as green gas (propane and silicone mix). These weapons are designed to be non-lethal and to provide realistic replicas for combat simulations. Due to the low pressures available with the Freon type gases used, airsoft weapons are quite low powered.

Paintball guns

A paintball gun, is the main piece of equipment in the sport of 'paintball'. The guns use an expanding gas, such as carbon dioxide (CO_2), compressed air or electronically ignited propane to propel paintballs through the barrel. The paintball guns can take on virtually any form, including self-loading pistols, rifles and even sub-machine guns. The muzzle velocity of these guns is purposely kept around 300 ft/sec (91 m/s) to reduce the risk of serious injury.

The paintballs comprise a soft plastic shell filled with various coloured water-based paints. These can be obtained in various calibres, with 0.68″ (17 mm) and 0.5″ (12.5 cm) being the most popular.

Automatic electric guns (AEG)

This type of gun can take any form, from a pistol to heavy machine gun. AEGs use a rechargeable battery or batteries to drive an electric motor which cycles an internal piston/spring assembly in order to fire the pellets (Figure 2.1.2). Automatic, three-round burst, semi-automatic and fully automatic operation are all possible, which gives these guns the popular name 'automatic electric guns' or AEGs.

These guns are quite low-powered, due to the battery-operated method of compressing the air. They can, in the fully automatic versions produce high rates of fire which can be between 100 and 1,500 rounds per minute. They generally fire lightweight plastic pellets or balls.

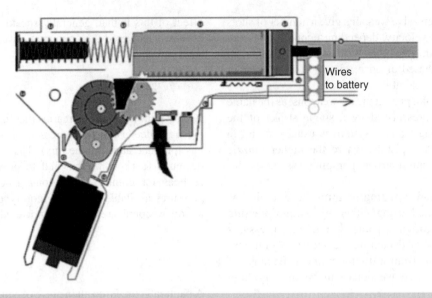

Wires
to battery

Figure 2.1.2   Mechanism in an automatic electric gun (AEG).

Spring-powered weapons

These are really no more than toys and work on a principle similar to a billiard cue and ball. They generally fire steel BBs, which are held at the breech end of the barrel by a magnet. A spring-powered rod strikes the ball and propels it out of the smooth-bored barrel. They are, consequentially, of very low power and accuracy.

2.1.3   Ammunition

Air gun pellets

The variety of air guns pellets is very large indeed, ranging from simple straight-sided cylinders with a flat head to complex pellets with hard metal or plastic inserts to aid penetration. The head of the pellet can be flat, round, hollow or may have a pointed tip. The most common, however, is the simple round-headed wasted pellet, often referred to as a 'Diablo' (Figure 2.1.3). It is generally constructed from soft lead.

For target shooting, a flat-nosed design is preferred in order to cut a sharp hole in the target (Figure 2.1.4).

Sheridan, the American air gun manufacturer, manufactures pump-up rifles and pistols in 0.20″ (5 mm) caliber. The pellets for these guns are unusual in that they are straight-sided, with a

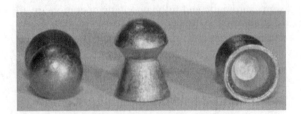

Figure 2.1.3   Typical lead air gun pellet.

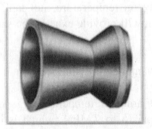

Figure 2.1.4   Flat-nosed pellet for target shooting.

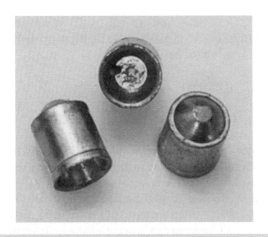

Figure 2.1.5 .20″ (5 mm) Sheridan pellet.

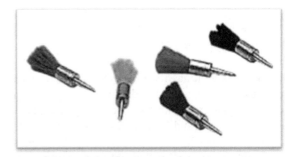

Figure 2.1.6 Air gun darts.

driving band at the base and a blunt conical nose (see Figure 2.1.5).

Calibre

For target shooting, the .177″ (4.5 mm) calibre pellet is preferred, as the trajectory for a given gun is flatter than that for a .22″ (5.5 mm) calibre.

The most common calibre of all is the .22″. Being heavier than the .177″ (4.5 mm) calibre pellet, it is far superior for hunting purposes.

The .20″ (5.0 mm) calibre is found in some European air guns and those manufactured by the American air gun manufacturer Sheridan. This is generally considered to be a 'compromise' calibre, having a flatter trajectory than the .22″ (5.5 mm) but more energy transfer for hunting than the .177' (4.5 mm). See Figure 2.1.5.

The .25″ (6.35 mm) calibre is the largest commonly available calibre. This calibre is renowned for its impact, having the most energy retention of all calibres. It does have a highly parabolic trajectory at low energy levels, and is thus more suited for higher-powered rifles.

Air gun darts

As the steel shank of these darts can seriously damage rifling, they are really only suitable for use in smooth-bored guns. The dart's tail also causes a huge amount of drag, which restricts the range (Figure 2.1.6).

Steel BBs

As with air gun darts, these are only intended for use in smooth-bored guns. This is not just due to the propensity for damaging the rifling, but as they are steel they cannot expand and seal the bore against loss of pressure during firing. They are generally of .173″ (4.4 mm) calibre to allow their use in .177″ (4.5 mm) barrels (Figure 2.1.7).

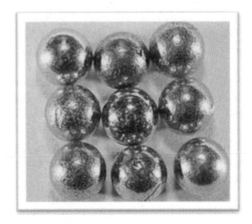

Figure 2.1.7 Steel BBs.

2.1.4   Considerations

Air gun legislation

Each jurisdiction has its own definition as to what constitutes an air gun. In addition, there are often different classes of air guns based upon bore or muzzle energy, and sometimes based upon the type of missile the gun is designed to fire. Guns designed to fire metal pellets are more tightly controlled than airsoft or paintball guns.

There may be minimum ages for possession, and sales of both air guns and ammunition may be restricted. Some areas may require permits and background checks similar to those required for firearms possession.

On top of the requirement of what constitutes an 'air gun' is the consideration as to whether an air gun is a 'firearm'. There will obviously be those instances where an air gun has been used to commit a crime, but the gun is not covered by the energy or other restrictions which require the possession of a firearms license. The question is then, what constitutes a 'firearm'? Generally it is considered to be something with a barrel capable of discharging a missile with sufficient force as to be capable of causing an injury of sufficient magnitude that death may result – that is, a 'lethal barrelled weapon'. Appendix 11 gives the legislation pertaining to air weapons for a number of countries. Below is also a list of the penetration capabilities of various missiles at various velocities, which gives an indication as to the injuries which may result.

Penetration potential of air weapon ammunition

Following is a short list of the penetrative power of various types of air weapon ammunition. These are the results of unpublished work by the author.

- .22″ (5.5 mm) lead air gun pellet requires a minimum of 250 ft/sec (76.2 m/sec) to penetrate unsupported fresh human skin.

- .177″ (4.5 mm) lead air gun pellet requires a minimum of 300 ft/sec (91.5 m/sec) to penetrate unsupported fresh human skin.

- .22″ (5.5 mm) lead air gun pellet at 450 ft/sec (137.2 m/sec) to make a hole in, but not penetrate, .25 inch (0.61 cm) plate glass.

- .22″ (5.5 mm) lead air gun pellet at 600 ft/sec (183 m/sec) will penetrate .25 inch (0.61 cm) plate glass.

- Steel BB at 200 ft/sec (61 m/sec) will make a hole but not penetrate .25 inch (0.61 cm) plate glass.

- Steel BB or .177″ (4.5 mm) lead pellet at 200 ft/sec (61 m/sec) will detach part of the coloured portion (iris) of a human eye, leaving what appears to be a second pupil.

- Steel BB or .177″ (4.5 mm) lead pellet at 400 ft/sec (122 m/sec) will burst a human eye.

- .177″ (4.45 mm) steel dart at 120 ft/sec (36.6 m/sec) will penetrate to the shank in human skin.

Air gun injuries

There is a general misconception that air weapons are no more than toys and that they are unlikely to cause more than a trivial injury. Nothing could be further from the truth, as the statistics show:

- Air guns of one sort or another have been implicated in cases of manslaughter, wounding, robbery, criminal damage, rape, domestic violence and animal cruelty.

- In 2009, at least four people were killed in Great Britain alone. In one case, a woman committed suicide using an air gun.

- In 2008, at least four people were killed in Great Britain, including a teenage girl who was shot at a party by a man with an air rifle, a toddler who died after being accidentally shot by his sister with their father's gun and two cases of men who took their own life with an air weapon.

- The total number of recorded air gun injuries is nearly two and a half times the number of injuries caused by cartridge-powered handguns, rifles and shotguns combined.

One notable case in the early 1970s involved a young criminal who, while attempting to avoid arrest, fired at a police officer with a Harrington Gat air pistol. The Gat is a poor-quality smooth-bored air pistol which is cocked by pushing the barrel, against the main spring, into the barrel housing. This type of mechanism results in a very low-powered weapon discharging missiles right on the threshold of skin penetration.

During the trial for resisting arrest with a firearm, his defence barrister claimed that the pistol was of such low power that he would have no hesitation in firing the weapon at his new born baby's fontanel. This was a somewhat silly statement to make and to which the judge took umbrage. He instructed the firearms examiner in the case (Mr J. McCafferty) to confirm (or otherwise) the validity of this statement.

Two aborted foetuses were obtained from the mortuary and shot as instructed with steel BBs fired from the Gat pistol in the case. The missiles easily penetrated the fontanel and went on a further two inches (5 cm) into the brains of both foetuses. The case was, not unexpectedly, reported by the press in the most lurid of terms with 'Ballistics experts shoots new born babies' being just one headline! The defence's argument was rejected and the youth was convicted of attempted murder.

Not all cases involving air gun deaths involve death by shooting. There have been several instances where people cocking under-lever air rifles with the butt on the ground have let go of the cocking lever. The resultant and violent return of the lever struck the person under the sternum, resulting in almost instant death.

Further reading

1 Hoff, A. (1972). *Airguns and Other Pneumatic Arms*. London, Arms & Armour Series.
2 Wesley, L. (1955). *Air Guns and Air Pistols*. London.
3 Blackmore, H.L. (1971). *Hunting Weapons*. London.
4 Saltzman, B. *The Three Basic Types of Airguns*. American Airguns. Retrieved 2007-09-14.
5 Smith, W.H.B. (2009) *Gas, Air and Spring Guns of the World* (Classic Gun Books). Stackpole Classic Gun Books.
6 *Pneumatic Weapons, Including: Air Gun, BB Gun, Blowgun, Pneumatic Weapon, Airsoft Gun, 10 Metre Air Rifle, 10 Metre Air Pistol, Paintball Marker*. Hephaestus Books, 2011.
7 Wesley, L. (1971) *Air Guns and Air Pistols*.
8 Gaylord, T. 1998. The State of Big Bore Air Rifles in the US. *Airgun Revue* **3**, pp. 26–37. Ellicott City, MD, GAPP Inc.
9 Beeman, R. (1977). Four Centuries of Air Guns. *Air Guns Digest*, pp. 14–25. Northfield, IL, DBI Books.
10 Wolff, E. (1958). *Air Guns*. WI, Milwaukee Public Museum.
11 Adler, D. & Fjestad, S. (1998). Beeman Precision Airguns dedication. *Blue Book of Gun Values*, 19th Edition, pp. 1272–1273. Minneapolis, MN.
12 Beeman, R.D. (2000). Proceeding on to the Lewis & Clark airgun. *Airgun Revue* **6**, pp. 13–33. Ellicott City, MD, GAPP Inc.

2.2

Rifling Types and Their Identification

2.2.1 Introduction

Rifles, revolvers, self-loading pistols and most single-shot pistols have rifled barrels.

Shotguns are generally smooth-bored, although some older weapons were provided with a short length of rifling at the muzzle for use when firing solid slugs. This system of rifling was called **'paradox rifling'**.

Rifling consists of a series of spiral grooves cut into the inside surface of the bore of the barrel, and these are there to impart a spin to the bullet through its longitudinal axis. This gyroscopic effect stabilises the bullet during its flight, preventing it from tumbling end over end and losing its accuracy.

Identification of the type of rifling used in a barrel, and knowledge as to how it is produced, can be highly significant for the investigation of a case and an interpretation of the results.

As will be seen later on in this chapter, it is the lands in a barrel which impart the stria used in the comparison process, *not* the grooves. Where difficulties can arise is in the understanding that it is the *lands in a barrel* which produce the *grooves in a fired bullet* and these are, obviously, the areas used for comparison with fired bullets from a scene. During the qualification process for an expert witness, he/she should be rigorously examined on the knowledge of this vital aspect of the comparison process. Misidentifications can easily be made if only the lands on the fired bullet are used for comparison purposes. If there is any hesitation on this aspect, or if the video or photographs show that the comparison has been carried out using only the bullet lands, then there is more than adequate reason to have the evidence excluded.

Stria on the lands of a bullet are often used as a reference point to line up the correct orientation between two bullets, but these are never used as the final arbiter as to whether two bullets have been fired from the same weapon.

It is not unknown for comparison microscopists to use such reference points as part of the identification point itself, leading to a misidentification.

It is of note that it does not matter which end of the barrel the rifling is viewed from – the direction of twist is the same.

Illustrative Case 1

During the investigation of a murder case which occurred on a small island in the tropics, all of the legally owned weapons were called into the laboratory for comparison purposes. Eventually, a revolver was identified as being the one used in the shooting; the owner was arrested, tried, found to be guilty of the crime and was jailed for a substantial period of time.

Forensic Ballistics in Court: Interpretation and Presentation of Firearms Evidence, First Edition. Brian J. Heard.
© 2013 John Wiley & Sons, Ltd. Published 2013 by John Wiley & Sons, Ltd.

During an appeal, however, it was found that the positive comparison between the crime scene bullet and the revolver had been wrongly made. A search through the island's firearms records revealed that when the revolver under question had been purchased, a second revolver, with a consecutive serial number to the first, had been mistakenly delivered by the manufacturer. When, eventually, this second revolver was located, it was found to produce near identical bullet land stria to the first. The groove stria were, however, completely different.

When the manufacturers were contacted, they confirmed that to cut costs, a length of tubing sufficient to make three barrels had been rifled in one operation using a broach rifling tool. The barrel was then cut into the required lengths and the weapons sequentially numbered. It was the use of a single broaching tool to manufacture three barrels in one operation which produced near identical rifling grooves in all three barrels. However, as the lands in the barrel were produced by a rotating drill which left continuingly changing rotational stria, the land surfaces in the three barrels were completely different from one another.

2.2.2 Basics

Rifling in a barrel consists of '**lands**' and '**grooves**'. The grooves are the depressions cut away by the rifling cutter. The lands are the portions of the barrel not touched by the rifling cutter and are, therefore, left standing proud.

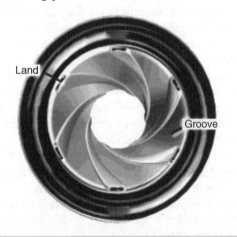

Figure 2.2.1 View of right hand twist rifling, showing lands and grooves.

History

Some writers assign the invention of spiral grooved barrels to Gaspard Kollner, a gunsmith of Vienna, in the 15th century. Others fix the date at 1520 and attribute it to Augustus Kotter of Nuremburg. German weapons bearing the coat of arms of the Emperor Maximilian I and made between 1450 and 1500 have spiral grooved barrels and are, in fact the earliest identifiable rifled weapons.

Both straight and spiral forms of rifling are encountered in early weapons, although it is generally accepted that the straight form of rifling was to accommodate the fouling produced in these early black-powdered weapons.

The number of grooves encountered can be anything from a single deeply cut rifling, up to twelve or more in micro-grooved rifling. The form of groove also varies, with square, round, triangular, ratchet or even comma-shaped grooves. The actual number of rifling grooves appears to have little influence on the stabilising effect of the rifling (Figure 2.2.1).

One of the problems encountered with muzzle-loading weapons was the difficulty experienced in

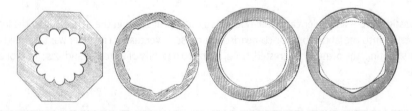

Figure 2.2.2 Different rifling forms.

forcing the projectile down the bore. If the bore was of sufficient diameter to take up the rifling, a large mallet was required to force it down the bore. If, on the other hand, it was of reduced diameter to assist in its insertion, the gases produced on firing would escape past the bullet, leading to reduced velocity. In addition, the bullet would take up little of the rifling and thus become unstable in flight. The Brunswick rifle overcame this problem by having a belted bullet and a barrel with two grooves to match exactly the rib on the bullet.

Several other designs were tried, in which the bullet was rammed down onto various projections inside the breech end of the barrel. These projections deformed the bullet, thus filling out the bore. Unfortunately, the deformation was irregular and led to erratic behaviour of the bullet.

Greener, in 1835, produced the first expansive bullet, the rear of which contained a steel plug. On firing, this was forced up into the bullet, deforming it uniformly.

In 1852, Minie, a Frenchman, was awarded a British government contract for the production of an expanding bullet with a steel plug in the base almost exactly the same as the Greener bullet. This resulted in some acrimonious legal action by Greener, who was awarded a sum of money, recognising his as the earliest form of expanding bullet.

At about the same time that Minie invented his expanding bullet, Lancaster produced a rifle with a spiral oval bore. This provided easy loading of the bullet, did not require any mechanism to expand the base of the bullet and, as there were no sharp corners in the rifling, it did not suffer the same problems with fouling as had been encountered with conventional rifling.

In 1854, Whitworth patented the first polygonal rifling system, which overcame most of the problems and proved to be extremely accurate as well. Unfortunately, Whitworth did not have practical experience in the manufacture of weapons and was unable to produce guns with the consistency required. As a result, his invention was soon overtaken by others.

The invention of the breech-loading weapon eliminated the problems of having to expand the bullet to fill the bore. The bullet could be made of the correct diameter to fill the bore and could be inserted into the rifling at the breech end of the barrel. In addition, instead of the deep grooving and a long, soft bullet necessary for easy loading and expansion at the breech of a muzzle-loader, shallow rifling and harder bullets could be used. This configuration resulted in more uniform bullets, higher velocities, better accuracy and improved trajectory.

Rifling rate of twist

This is a subject unlikely ever to be encountered during court proceedings. However, see Illustrative Case 2 below.

Illustrative Case 2

The subject of rifling twist calculations did appear during a murder trial, where I was questioned at some length on this subject. The case involved questions regarding the rate of rifling twist and the revolutions per minute that a bullet would go through during its passage over a set distance. It centred round a gutter wound in a deceased person's arm. A gutter wound is where the bullet does not penetrate, but simply carves a groove through the muscle during its passage.

Photographs of the wound (Figure 2.2.3) showed it to be black in colour, and the question was 'could this be due to close range gun powder residues or was it due to cauterisation of the wound due to the friction caused by the rotation of the bullet?'

The wound was approximately three inches (7.5 cm) in length and, as the rate of twist of the rifling was one rotation in ten inches (one revolution in 25 cm), the bullet would have made less than one third of a rotation during its passage across the arm. The speed of the bullet could have cauterised the wound, but it was more probable that what was seen on the photographs was simply congealed blood. The lack of discharge residues on either side of the wound ruled out the possibility of a close-range shot.

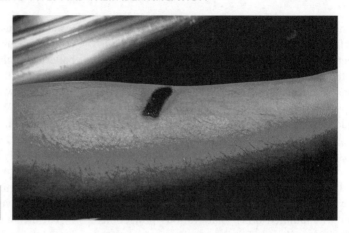

Figure 2.2.3 Gutter wound in arm of deceased.

Rate of twist calculation

The number of inches of the barrel required for the rifling to prescribe one complete spiral is called the '**twist**'. For most modern weapons, this is consistent throughout the barrel's length.

The actual degree of twist cut into a barrel will be carefully calculated with relation to the bore of the weapon, the velocity, the length of the intended projectile, its density and its weight.

One of the first persons to try to develop a formula for calculating the correct rate of twist for firearms' was George Greenhill, a mathematics lecturer at Emmanuel College, Cambridge. His formula is based on the rule that the twist required in calibres equals 150 divided by the length of the bullet in calibres. This can be simplified to:

$$\text{Twist} = 150 \times D^2/L$$

Where: D = bullet diameter in inches; L = bullet length in inches

This formula had limitations, but it worked well up to and in the vicinity of about 1,800 f/s (550 m/s). For higher velocities, most ballistic experts suggest substituting 180 for 150 in the formula.

The Greenhill formula is simple and easy to apply, and it gives a useful approximation of the desired twist. It was based on a bullet with a specific gravity of 10.9, which is approximately correct for a jacketed lead-cored bullet. In this equation, bullet weight does not directly enter into the equation. For a given

calibre, the heavier the bullet, the longer it will be. See Table 2.2.1 below.

The actual degree of twist is critical. Too high a degree of twist and the bullet will be unstable, as a

Table 2.2.1 The twist necessary to stabilise various calibres

Cartridge	Rate of twist
.22″ Short	1 in 24″
.22″ Long Rifle	1 in 16″
.223″ Remington	1 in 12″
.22-250″ Remington	1 in 14″
.243″ Winchester	1 in 10″
6 mm Remington	1 in 9″
.25-06″ Remington	1 in 10″
.257″ Wetherby Magnum	1 in 10″
6.5 × 55 Swedish Mauser	1 in 7.5″
.260″ Remington	1 in 9″
.270″ Winchester	1 in 10″
7 mm-08 Remington	1 in 9.25″
7 mm Remington Magnum	1 in 9.25″
.30″ Carbine	1 in 6″
.30-30 Winchester	1 in 12″
.308″ Winchester	1 in 12″
.30-06″ Springfield	1 in 10″
.300″ Winchester Magnum	1 in 10″
.300″ Wetherby Magnum	1 in 10″
.303″ British	1 in 10″
.32″ Winchester Special	1 in 16″
.35″ Remington	1 in 16″
.357″ Magnum	1 in 16″
.380″ ACP	1 in 10″

top is when first spun, with a consequential loss of accuracy. Too little spin and the bullet will lose stability and start to tumble end over end.

Older weapons often had a '**gain twist**', in which the rate of twist increased from breech to muzzle. This was to assist in the soft lead bullet gripping the rifling with the high rate of acceleration given by black powder propellants.

Rifling can be right or left hand twist, with neither appearing to have any advantage over the other. Also, neither is affected by whether it is fired in the Northern or Southern hemisphere.

The number of grooves cut into a barrel can range from one to 24, or even more in what are called '**micro grooved**' barrels. Once again, the difference between having five grooves or 24 grooves seems to be more academic than practical.

The main interest of rifling as far as the forensic firearms examiner is concerned is the **micro stria** (microscopic scratch marks) it contains. The micro stria are produced as part of the manufacturing process and are totally random in their distribution, shape and size. As such, they are individual to a particular weapon and form an identification system which can be unique.

A general overview of the characteristics of rifling, their form and manufacturing processes follows.

2.2.3 Class characteristics

When dealing with rifling, each weapon will possess a series of family resemblances which will be present in all weapons of the same make and model. Correctly called '**class characteristics**', these relate to the number of lands and grooves, their direction of twist, their inclination of twist, their width and their depth.

Class characteristics have been measured and technical information obtained for literally thousands of different firearms. These measurements have been compiled into vast databases and are commercially available for use either in table form or on a PC [1,2].

[1] Crime Laboratory Information System (CLIS), General Rifling Characteristics File, US Department of Justice, Federal Bureau of Investigation, Washington, DC.
[2] Mathews, J.H. (1962). *Firearms Identification* Vols I, II & III. Madison, WI, University of Wisconsin Press.

By simply measuring the number, width and degree of rotation of the rifling grooves on a bullet, it is possible, with a fairly high degree of accuracy, to determine which make and model of weapon it was fired from. This, however, is little more than of academic interest, as it usually has no bearing on case investigations.

The spiral grooves that constitute the rifling in a barrel are there to impart a rapid spin on the bullet's longitudinal axis. The gyroscopic effect of this spin stabilises the bullet, preventing it from tumbling or yawing during its flight, and thus improving its accuracy.

In the past, barrels were often rifled with a '**gain twist**', where the rate of twist increases from breech to muzzle. This is also referred to as '**progressive rifling**'. The purpose of gain rifling was to allow lead bullets to build up the rate of spin gradually along the length of the barrel. The sudden acceleration of the bullet at the breech end of the barrel could cause the soft lead to strip through the rifling and thus not acquire the correct degree of stabilisation on leaving the barrel. This effect is called '**skidding**'.

With modern lead alloys, jacketed bullets and progressive burning propellants, this is not such a problem, so gain twist rifling is hardly ever encountered.

One class of weapon in which the phenomenon of skidding is very prominent, however, is revolvers. In a revolver, the chambers of the cylinder are smooth-bored and possess no rifling. During the bullet's progress from the chamber to the beginning of the rifling in the barrel, considerable linear velocity is built up. At this point, however, the bullet has no rotational velocity at all. As the bullet enters the rifling, there is a very short period during which the bullet is attempting to catch up with the rifling, i.e. travelling along the rifling but with little or no rotational velocity. The result is an observed short length of rifling engraved on the bullet, which appears to be parallel with its longitudinal axis. As these marks are more pronounced at the nose end of the bullet, they have the appearance of a widening of the land impression at this point. The marks so produced are called '**skid marks**' and are a very useful, and simple, identifier for bullets which have been fired in a revolver (Figure 2.2.4).

This skidding is really a by-product of a problem with revolvers concerning the gap between the barrel and cylinder. This gap not only causes skidding of the bullet, but also allows the escape of high pressure

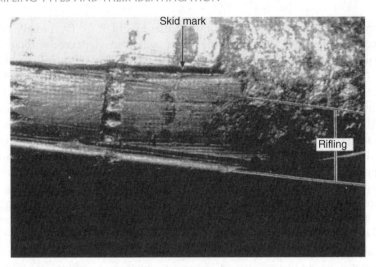

Figure 2.2.4 Rifling on a bullet fired from a revolver, showing 'skid marks'.

gases, thus losing some of the potential energy of the propellant.

Attempts have been made to overcome both problems, the most notable of which was the Russian 7.62 mm Nagant revolver used during the Second World War. This weapon fired a round of ammunition which had a bullet seated entirely within the cartridge case, and with the case mouth tapering to a smaller diameter than the bullet. When the hammer was cocked, the mechanism moved the whole of the cylinder forward so that the breech end of the barrel actually entered the chamber to be fired. In so doing, the case mouth of the cartridge entered the rear of the barrel, engaging the bullet into the beginning of the rifling. This was not particularly good at preventing either the skidding or the leakage of gases. It was also a very complex and expensive mechanism to place in what was a service issue revolver.

In self-loading pistols, skidding is not exhibited to any significant degree, as the chamber is the same length as the cartridge case. As a result, the bullet virtually touches the rifling and has very little, if any, opportunity to build up longitudinal velocity without rotational velocity.

2.2.4   General introduction to rifling

There are a number of different methods by which the rifling may be cut into the barrel of a weapon. A competent forensic firearms examiner should not only be aware of the various methods, but should also be able to identify which method has been used in a particular weapon.

The ability to identify correctly the type of rifling is, in fact, of little or no use to the examiner when carrying out a micro stria comparison. It is, however, one of those questions that are frequently encountered during the qualification of an expert in court, and it can reveal weaknesses in his or her training and experience.

Rifling process

The actual rifling of a weapon is carried out in a number of stages. First, the weapon is rough-bored using a simple drill. It is them reamed in order to smooth out the roughest of the spiral scratches produced during the drilling.

The barrel is then rifled using one of the methods as listed later in this chapter under the heading 'Rifling methods'.

After rifling, the barrel is then given a final smoothing. The most frequently used methods for this are '**lead lapping**' and '**ball burnishing**'.

In lead lapping, a lead plug of the same diameter as the bore is repeatedly pulled through the rifling while being washed through with a fine abrasive. As the barrel becomes progressively smoother, the fineness of the abrasive is increased. This is the most commonly used method and gives a finish satisfactory for most uses.

Ball burnishing is generally only carried out on high-quality rifles and consists of repeatedly pushing a steel ball bearing of the same size as the barrel lands through the bore. This flattens out any irregularities in the bore, leaving a mirror-like finish.

Very high quality weapons and military rifles, in which the bore is subjected to extremely high temperatures, can also have the bore of the barrel chromium-plated. This results in an extremely hard, mirror-like surface which is very resistant to corrosion, metal fouling and bore wear.

Rifling methods

Hook cutter rifling

The most simple method of cutting the grooves is by use of a 'single hook cutter'. In this, a hardened steel cutter, in the shape of a crochet hook, is set into a recess in a steel rod of slightly smaller diameter than the bore of the barrel being rifled (Figure 2.2.5). As the cutter is dragged through the bore, the barrel is rotated at a fixed rate to impart the spiral of the rifling. Each pass of the tool only cuts one groove, so the barrel must be re-positioned and the process repeated for the number of grooves required. As each pass of the cutter only removes a few thousands of an inch of metal, the height of the 'hook' must be raised and the grooves all cut again, with up to 80 passes being made for each groove. This is very time-consuming and, as the hooks rapidly wear, it is an expensive method of rifling.

Hook rifling can be identified by;

- the presence of longitudinal striations in the cut grooves;

- the similarity (as the same tool is used for every groove) between the micro stria in all of the grooves.

Scrape cutter rifling

The 'scrape cutter' method of rifling uses a bar with curved and hardened steel scrapers set into it. The number of these scrapers corresponds to the number of grooves required. As a result, all grooves are cut with one pass, after which the height of the scrapers is increased and further passes made. This method produces extremely fine rifling and is used on some of the best weapons.

Scrape cutter rifling is very similar to hook cutter except that, because a different scraper is used for each groove, there will be no underlying similarity between the grooves.

Broach rifling

The most commonly used rifling method is called 'broach rifling'. This, in a very simplified form, can

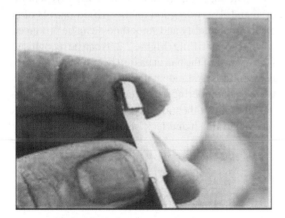

Figure 2.2.5 Hook cutter.

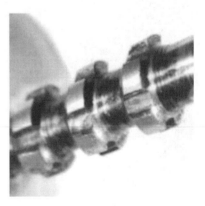

Figure 2.2.6 Part of a broach rifling cutter.

be thought of as a series of 20–30 steel discs on a rod, with each disc being slightly larger than the one preceding it (Figure 2.2.6). Into each disc is cut the profile and number of grooves required, with the last disc possessing the final calibre and dimension required. A broach cutter can thus cut all the grooves to the final dimensions in a single pass.

Broach cutter rifling can be recognised by the longitudinal striations in the grooves of the weapons bore.

Button rifling

This is a very commonly used method, but generally only on cheaper weapons, particularly those of .22″ calibre.

In this type of rifling, the barrel is bored slightly smaller than the final required diameter. A 'button' (Figure 2.2.7) on the end of a long rod, containing an exact negative of the rifling required, is then pushed or pulled through the bore, forcing the metal to expand into the final shape required. This is a single operation and is very cheap way of rifling a weapon.

Button rifling is, especially in cheaper weapons, very easy to identify, as the circular marks produced during the reaming of the bore are not eliminated during the rifling. These marks are simply pressed into the metal and are visible on both the lands and the grooves.

Figure 2.2.8 clearly shows the reaming marks which have been impressed into the lands and grooves by the button rifling tool.

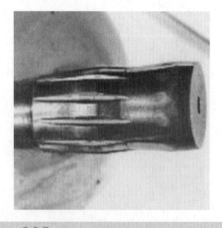

Figure 2.2.7   Button rifling tool.

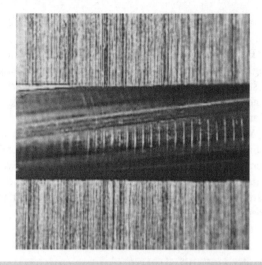

Figure 2.2.8   Section through a button rifled barrel.

Swage or hammer rifling

Another method, which is similar to button rifling but which produced a very much higher quality of rifling, is called 'swaging' or 'hammer rifling'. In this method, the bore is reamed slightly larger than the required final diameter. A mandrill (an extremely hard steel plug tapered at both ends) containing an exact negative of the rifling profile required is then passed through the bore, while the outside of the barrel is either hammered or hydraulically squeezed onto it. This method causes the metal not only to work harden, but also increase in density. Assuming the mandrill is of a good quality, rifled barrels of an exceptional quality and smoothness can be produced.

This type of rifling (Figure 2.2.9) can be recognised, if the outside of the barrel has not been turned down, by the peculiar spiral indentations on the outside surface due to the hammering or squeezing process. Other than that, the only other identifying characteristic is the mirror-like finish and lack of striations in the rifling.

Other methods of rifling

Other methods of rifling, such as electrolytic and gas cutting, do exist and are used, but only to a very limited extent.

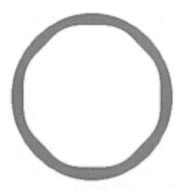

Figure 2.2.9 Swaged rifling.

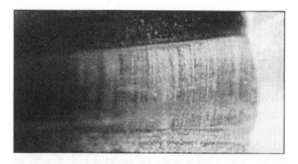

Figure 2.2.10 Reaming marks on lands of an electrochemically etched barrel.

A report on the use of 'electrochemical machining' for the production of rifling in barrels appeared in the journal of the Association of Firearms and Toolmark Examiners in 1988[3]. The barrels reviewed in said article were being made by Cation Co., a small company in Rochester, New York, USA, for an arms manufacturing company called Coonan Arms.

Electrochemical machining is not exactly a new method of rifling barrels, as it was reportedly used by Krupp, the famous German arms making company, to manufacture their cannon barrels as early as 1920.

Since 1993, Smith & Wesson has also been using an electrochemical machining technique to rifle most of their revolver barrels. The only revolver barrels that S&W still broach rifle are their .22 calibre barrels and ported barrels.

In the modern process, a mandrill is made slightly smaller than the bore size of the drilled barrel blank. Strips of plastic are glued to the mandrill in a spiral pattern corresponding to the desired shape of the rifling. The mandrill is then inserted into the barrel blank and an electrolytic fluid is circulated down the gaps left between the plastic strips and the bore.

A direct current is then applied between the barrel blank and the mandrill, with the mandrill being made the cathode. The current strips away metal from the exposed areas of the barrel between the plastic strips, forming the grooves.

Electrochemical rifling is more similar in shape to button and broach rifled barrels, but the shoulders

between lands and grooves are not as sharp as in machine cut rifling. This is apparent upon examination of test fired bullets.

While it would appear that striation matching on fired bullets fired from electrochemically machined barrels could be problematical due to the non-machine tool method of manufacturing the rifling, this has not been found to be the case.

This results from two distinct factors:

1. As the barrel lands are not etched during the rifling process, the reaming marks are still present (Figure 2.2.10).

2. The stripping away of metal during the etching process leaves a totally random stippled effect on the barrel grooves. Hence, both lands and grooves bear individual matchable characteristics.

Current rifling forms

When black powder was used as a propellant, the extremely heavy fouling produced was a major problem. After a few rounds, the bore became so heavily fouled that subsequent rounds would hardly touch the rifling, leading to a subsequent fall-off in the weapon's accuracy.

In an attempt to counter this problem, a whole variety of rifling profiles were designed, with each claiming to have distinctive advantages over the rest. Every shape imaginable was tried at one time or another, including square, round, triangular, ratchet,

[3] Pike (1988). Electrochemical Machining, A New Barrel Making Process. *AFTE Journal*, January 1988.

comma and polygroove rifling, which looked like the petals on a flower. Whitworth and Lancaster, both very prolific arms inventors, were very successful with their oval-bored (Whitworth) and square-bored (Lancaster) rifling.

With the advent of smokeless propellants, the necessity for these complicated rifling profiles, and their expensive production costs, virtually disappeared.

Modern rifling tends to be either a square or '**polygonal**'. Polygonal rifling has no sharp edges and consists of a rounded profile, which can be difficult to discern when looking down the barrel. This type of rifling is almost exclusively manufactured using the hammer or swage process.

The advantages of polygonal include:

- no sharp edges to wear,

- no corners for fouling to build up,

- less metal fouling on driving surfaces of the rifling and

- lower friction between bullet and rifling resulting in higher velocity.

It is interesting to compare the profile of the Lancaster oval rifling with polygonal rifling and see how little the science of rifling has advanced since the early 1850s (Figure 2.2.11).

Additional reading

1 Greener, *The Gun*. New York, Bonanza Books (reprint).

2 *Association of Firearms and Toolmark Examiners Glossary*.

3 Mathews, (1962). *Firearms Identification* Vol I. Madison, WI, Wisconsin Press.

4 Burdock, J.E. (1981). A General Discussion of Gun Barrel Individuality and an Empirical Assessment of the Individuality of Consecutively Button Rifled .22 Caliber Rifle Barrels. *AFTE Journal* 13 (2), 84–95.

5 Batty, W. (1985). A Comparison of Three Individual Barrels Produced from One Button Rifled Barrel Blank. *AFTE Journal* 17 (3), 64–69.

6 Hall, E. (1983). Bullet Markings From Consecutively Rifled Shilen DGA Barrels. *AFTE Journal* 15 (1), 33–53.

7 Davygdow, A.D. & Kozak, J. (1990). *High rate electrochemical shaping*. Nauka. Moscow (in Russian).

8 Domanowski, P. & Kozak, J. (2001). Inverse problem of shaping by electrochemical generating machining. *Journal of Material Processing Technology* 109, 347–353.

9 Kozak, J., Dabrowski, L., Lubkowski, K., Rozenek, M. & Slawinski, R. (2000). CAE-ECM system for electrochemical technology of parts and tools. *Journal of Materials Processing Technology* 107, 293–299.

10 Clifton, D., Mount, A.R., Alder, G.M. & Jardine, D. (2002). Ultrasonic measurement of the inter-electrode gap in electrochemical machining. *International Journal of Machine Tools & Manufacture* 42, 1259–1267.

11 Kozak, J., Budzynski, A.F. & Domanowski, P. (1998). Computer simulation electrochemical shaping (ECMCNC) with using universal tool electrode. *Journal of Materials Processing Technology* 76, 1–3.

12 Hall, E. (1983). Bullet Markings from Consecutively Rifled Shilen DGA Barrels. *AFTE Journal* 15 (1), 33–53.

13 DeFrance, C.S. & Van Arsdale, M.D. (2003). Validation Study of Electrochemical Rifling. *AFTE Journal* 35 (1).

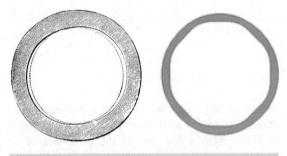

Figure 2.2.11 Lancaster oval-bored rifling, cf polygonal (swaged) rifling.

2.3

Home-made, Improvised and Converted Firearms

2.3.1 Introduction

Most countries have strict laws regarding the manufacture of home-made guns and the converting of toys and replica weapons into missile-firing weapons. Generally, it is also immaterial as to whether the weapon so formed is capable of firing a missile with lethal potential. In these cases, it is the act of attempting to or actually modifying something that has the potential to discharge a missile that carries the offence. The UK Firearms Act states:

'If an imitation weapon has the appearance of being a firearm to which section 1 of the 1968 Act applies and the imitation firearm is not capable of discharging a missile **but** can be readily converted into a firearm then section 1(1) Firearms Act 1982 states that the weapon is to be considered a firearm for the purposes of the Act. The Act defines "readily convertible" when "it can be so converted without any special skill on the part of the person converting it **and** the work involved in converting it does not require equipment or tools other than such as are in common use by persons carrying out works of construction and maintenance in their own homes." Section 1(6) Firearms Act 1982.

The Forensic Science Provider will be required to test the weapon to ascertain whether it is readily convertible.'

The onus, however, lies on the defence to show that accused did not know and had no reason to suspect that the imitation firearm was so constructed or adapted as to be readily convertible into a firearm. In this respect 'readily convertible' is an extremely open-ended statement and it would be for the defence to argue that, for example, the requirement for a special diamond-tipped drill to remove hard steel inclusions places the gun outside of the definition of being readily convertible.

At the other end of the scale, in the USA, home-made guns are legal and any person can make a gun for his own use, provided it is not of a type specially regulated by the Bureau of Alcohol, Tobacco and Firearms. Guns made for sale to others, machine guns, 'destructive devices', short-barrel rifles and short-barrel shotguns would require either a licence or a tax stamp from the Alcohol, Tobacco and Firearms Bureau.

2.3.2 Improvised firearms

An **improvised firearm** is a firearm manufactured by someone who is not a regular maker of firearms (i.e. a firearms manufacturer or a gunsmith), and is typically constructed by adapting existing materials to the purpose. Called by many names, these improvised

Forensic Ballistics in Court: Interpretation and Presentation of Firearms Evidence, First Edition. Brian J. Heard.
© 2013 John Wiley & Sons, Ltd. Published 2013 by John Wiley & Sons, Ltd.

firearms range from crude weapons that are as much a danger to the user as the target, to high-quality arms produced by cottage industries made completely from new materials or using salvaged materials.

Improvised firearms are more commonly found where legal and commercially produced firearms are unaffordable or strictly controlled. If commercial ammunition is obtainable, then improvised arms will generally be built to fit that ammunition. If commercial ammunition is not available, then muzzle-loading designs may still be produced.

Most countries have controls in place that regulate the production, sales and possession of firearms and ammunition. This means that improvised firearms are, for the most part, illegally produced, which makes their possession and use criminal as well. Improvised firearms are commonly used as tools by criminals and insurgents, and are therefore often associated with such groups.

The essential part of any improvised firearm is the barrel and chamber. For small, low-pressure cartridges such as the common .22 calibre (5.5 mm) rimfire cartridges, even very thin walled tubing will suffice. Author Harlan Ellison describes the zip guns used by gangs in 1950s New York City as 'being made from tubing used in coffee percolators or car radio aerials strapped to a block of wood to serve as a handle. A rubber band provides the power for the firing pin, which is pulled back and released to fire. The use of such weak barrel tubing results in a firearm that can be more dangerous to the shooter than the target; the poorly fitting smoothbore barrel provides little accuracy and is liable to burst upon firing.'

2.3.3 Converting air weapons

Converting an air pistol or rifle into a weapon capable of firing .22″ (5.56 mm) rimfire ammunition (provided it is of the break barrel type, of good quality and not one of the plastic guns designed to fire light weight plastic pellets) can be a relatively simple operation. All that is required is for the breech end of the barrel to be slightly counter-bored to accommodate the cartridge rim and a floating firing pin to be inserted into the air transfer port. Such convertible air weapons do not, however, satisfy the definition of being 'readily convertible'.

The number of weapons considered to be readily convertible by the police and forensic science services is huge, but a couple of examples follow.

The Brocock Air Cartridge System (BAC)

The Brocock Air Cartridge System is a type of weapon which falls readily into the 'readily convertible' category.

The Brocock Air Cartridge System uses a self-contained 'cartridge', roughly the size of a .38″ special cartridge, which contains an air reservoir, a valve and a .22″ calibre (5.5 mm) pellet. The weapon is basically an 'Uberti' firearm that has been modified at source to fire these 'air cartridges'. Converting the air gun back into a cartridge-firing weapon capable of firing .22″ or .38″ calibre ammunition is relatively simple and, as a result, they have been used in numerous crimes. In the UK, an attempt to stop this ready supply of easily convertible

---

Illustrative Case 1

A man had been planning the demise of his wife some time and decided to carry out the deed with a home-made firearm. As the cartridge of choice was a 12 bore shotgun cartridge, he naturally assumed that only one shot would be required. He found that a 12 bore cartridge would fit, albeit loosely, into $\frac{3}{4}$″ (1.83 cm) cast iron gas piping, and this could serve both as chamber and barrel. To hold the cartridge in position, a cast iron gas pipe end cap was screwed into place. A hole was drilled through the cap and a nail inserted, which acted as a firing pin. No hammer, trigger mechanism or grip was provided – just a domestic hammer to hit the nail with. Not unexpectedly, when the gun was fired, it blew up in the man's hand, removing most of it in the process. The shot did, however, exit the 'barrel' with sufficient force to kill the woman almost instantly.

This case illustrates the fact that although a home-made weapon can explode on firing, the missile will often still exit the barrel with sufficient force to be potentially lethal.

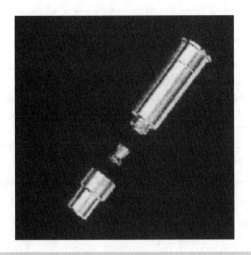

Figure 2.3.1   Brocock Air Cartridge.

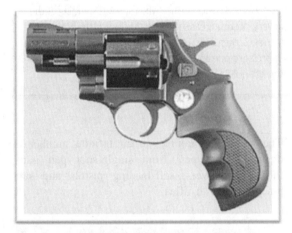

Figure 2.3.2   Brocock Air Cartridge revolver.

air weapons was made via the Anti-Social Behaviour Act of 2003. This is a piece of legislation that basically outlaws 'any air rifle, air gun or air pistol which uses, or is designed or adapted for use with, a self-contained gas cartridge system'. Brocock still make various air cartridge rifles but, in the UK, a firearms certificate is required for their possession.

Olympic .380 blank firing revolver

This blank-firing gun is widely used in the commercial world for the starting of races and dog training.

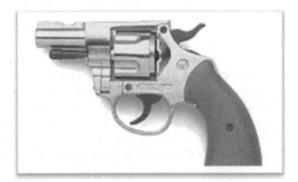

Figure 2.3.3   Olympic .380 blank firing revolver.

However, a significant number of converted Olympic .380″ BBMs have been recovered by the police after having been used in criminal activity, and the decision was made to declare them 'illegal weapons' under British firearms legislation. The bright red pistol could be bought legally over the counter in sporting shops and on the internet for around £90. However, once it has been converted and painted black, it could be sold to the underworld for more than £500.

2.3.4   Home-made and converted toys and replica weapons

Blank and flare guns are also regularly converted into cartridge-firing firearms. In flare guns, this may be accomplished by replacing the (often plastic) barrel with a metal pipe strong enough to chamber a shotgun shell, or by inserting a smaller bore barrel into the existing barrel to chamber a firearm cartridge, such as a .22″ long rifle.

Toy guns are a much more difficult proposition to convert into lethal barrelled weapons. The problem here is that toy guns are made from very cheap quality zinc alloy casting, with no structural strength. This type of construction necessitates the barrel and chambers to be lined with steel tubing of sufficient thickness to cope with the pressures produced on firing conventional ammunition. These conversions are of such complexity that it would often be just as easy to start from scratch. Not only that, but the soft alloys used in the trigger mechanism result in a working life of just a few rounds before the bearing surfaces wear out.

Illustrative Case 2

A retired army major thought that what elderly golfers required was a way of assisting them with the shot from the tee to the green. Taking a standard 1.5″ (3.7 cm) flare gun, he substituted the barrel with one made of steel of sufficient size to take a golf ball. The chamber was reduced to take a .38″ calibre blank cartridge of the type used in nail-driving guns. By selecting the relevant strength cartridge and the correct elevation, one could, with this device, propel a golf ball from the tee and onto the green. From there, the major assumed, the golfer would be able to putt the ball into the cup. Unfortunately, any weapon capable of firing a 1.62 ounce (45.9 g) golf ball several hundred yards would be more than capable of inflicting a lethal injury. As such, his 'invention' was rejected.

Illustrative Case 3

This is another case involving a married man plotting the demise of his wife, but this time the weapon of choice was a First World War Webley 1″ (2.45 cm) flare pistol. This weapon originally had a brass barrel and frame, but the enterprising husband had replaced the barrel with one made of steel. The barrel was chambered for a .410″ shotgun cartridge, and a 2.5″ (6.125 cm) long cartridge was chosen for the deed. The woman was shot twice – once when she was standing at the top of the stairs, at a range of about 20 feet (6 metres), and then at very close range as she lay on the floor at the bottom of the stairs. Initially, I test fired the weapon with 2″ (4.9 cm) long cartridges, then 2.75″ (6.7 cm) cartridges and eventually 3″ (7.35 cm) cartridges. The 3″ long cartridge is an extremely high-pressure one and, while the barrel was very thick and extremely strong, the frame could not take the strain and I was left holding just part of the grip!

Replica guns are likewise a difficult proposition for conversion, but for reasons other than thin-walled casting. As they are designed to work and look like a real weapon, the castings are much more robust. In an attempt to prevent them being converted into lethal barrel weapons, hard steel inclusions are cast off-centre in the barrel and, in revolvers, in the chambers. While specialist drills can be purchased that will penetrate such hard steels, the hard steel inserts being cast off-centre causes the drill to skid off onto the softer metal. However, by using a lathe to hold the parts rigidly in line, this problem can, with considerable difficulty, be overcome. It is debatable whether the necessity for such specialised equipment to convert such a replica places it within the 'readily convertible' category.

Home-made and improvised weapons

With only moderate engineering experience it is quite feasible to construct a home-made weapon. They come, of course, in an infinite number of designs and types, from single-shot pen guns, through revolvers, self-loading pistols and sub-machine guns to rifles.

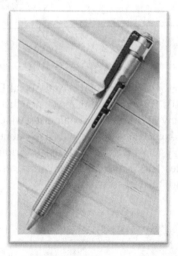

Figure 2.3.4   Home-made .22″ calibre pen gun.

North Western Frontier weapons

Located in between Kohat and Peshawar, Darra Adam Khel is a town in the Khyber Pakhtunkhwa province of Pakistan where a wide variety of hand made copy firearms are produced. These range from anti-aircraft guns to pen guns. Weapons are hand made by individual craftsmen using traditional manufacturing techniques, usually handed down from father to son. The quality of the guns is generally high and the craftsman are able to produce replicas of almost any gun.

Weapons made in the Philippines

Danao City, in the Cebu province of the Philippines, has been making improvised firearms so long that the makers have become legitimate and are manufacturing firearms for commercial sale. The Danao City makers manufacture .38″ and .45″ calibre revolvers, and also semi-automatic copies of the Ingram MAC-10 and Intratec TEC-DC9 submachine guns. These weapons are generally referred to as 'Paltek guns'.

Australian home-made weapons

In 2004, an 'underground weapons factory' was seized in Melbourne, Australia, yielding, among other things, a number of silenced copies of the Owen sub-machine gun, suspected to have been built for sale to local gangs involved in the illegal drug trade.

Many improvised firearms have also been used in other countries such as India, Russia, China and Hong Kong, where they have been used in domestic homicides, armed robberies and terrorism. Some examples follow:

Home-made sub-machine guns

Many different type of weapons have been made and converted by terrorists. In Northern Ireland, a large number of sub-machine guns were made, both from ex-military decommissioned sub-machine guns and also completely home-made weapons.

Figures 2.3.8 and 2.3.9 illustrate some examples of home-made sub-machine guns utilising standard square and round section tubing. Information indicates that these were retrieved by police while

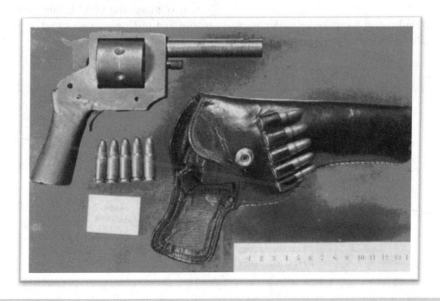

Figure 2.3.5 Home-made 7.62 × 25 mm calibre 'revolver' from the Far East.

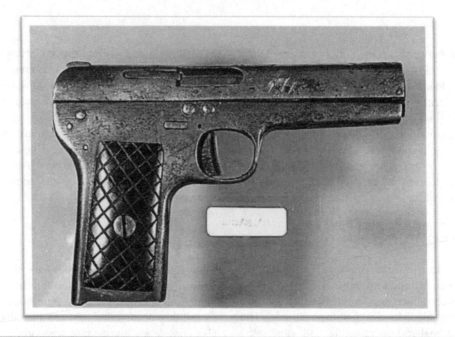

Figure 2.3.6   7.62 × 25 mm calibre home-made self-loading pistol.

investigating loyalist paramilitary groups in North-ern Ireland.

2.3.5   Home-made ammunition

Apart from muzzle-loading with black powder, wad-ding and missile, constructing ammunition from

scratch is a very difficult proposition. The major problems include:

- the **cartridge case** must be made of a material that will obturate the bore during firing, while being thin and pliable enough to retain its original size for extraction;

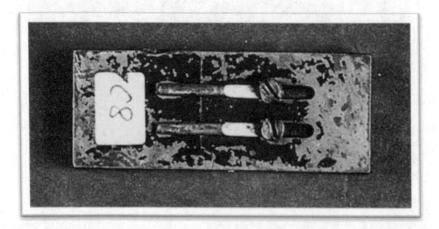

Figure 2.3.7   Paltex two-shot .22″ Magnum calibre palm pistol.

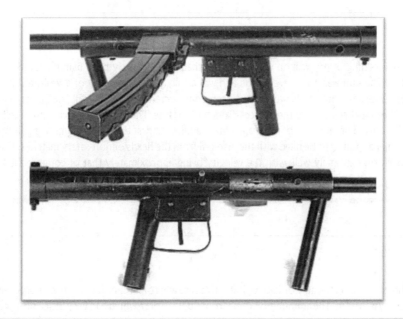

Figure 2.3.8   Home-made sub-machine gun.

- the **priming compound** must be sensitive enough to fire on being struck by the firing pin, but not so overly sensitive that it might detonate by rough handling;

- the **propellant** must have a temperature of ignition sufficiently low that it can be ignited by the primer, have progressive burning qualities such that the

bullet exits the muzzle but does not blow up the gun, and must be sufficiently consumed that there is little residue left in the bore.

These, as well as a number of others, are all difficult obstacles to overcome. The author has dealt with numerous cases involving home-made ammunition, none of which has been entirely successful.

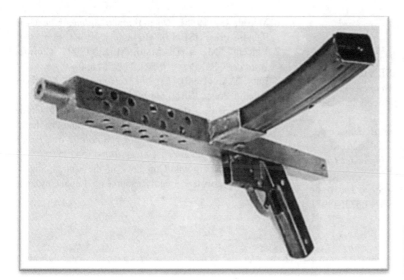

Figure 2.3.9   Home-made sub-machine gun utilising square section tubing.

Illustrative Case 4

A home-made self-loading pistol weapon was submitted that had obviously been manufactured in the North Western Frontier. The gun was a very well made and was a fully functional copy of a Walther PPK in .25″ ACP (6.35 mm) calibre. The ammunition, however, had been constructed from .32″ ACP (7.65 mm) calibre cartridge cases, which had been turned down to the correct diameter in a lathe. The propellant was nitrated cellulose of some description and consisted of a mixture of white and pink granules. At first this was thought to be nitrated desiccated coconut! The primer appeared to be filled with the material from the heads of non-safety matches. The ammunition did, however, perform extremely well, with the velocity being approximately that of commercial .25″ ACP ammunition.

Illustrative Case 5

At the other end of the scale, the author had to deal with a case where ammunition had been purposely modified to destroy the gun it was fired in. The ammunition came from a police force which had very little gun crime, but wanted those weapons that were in the hands of the criminal element to be removed from circulation. The firearms examiner for the force involved suggested that ammunition which had been modified to give excessive pressures should be covertly released onto the streets. The theory was that any weapon using this modified ammunition would explode on firing and be destroyed.

Unfortunately, the firearms examiner had not realised that, even if the gun did blow up, the missile would still leave the barrel at extremely high velocity. While destroyed weapons, along with several fingers belonging to the robbers, were found at armed crime scenes, there was also a fatality due to an innocent bystander being shot with a very high velocity bullet. Extremely large amounts of money had to be expended to 'buy back' this modified ammunition before further innocent bystanders were injured.

Further reading

1 Trub, J. (1993) *Zips, Pipes, And Pens: Arsenal Of Improvised Weapons*. Paladin Press. ISBN 0873647025

2 Anonymous (1983). *Improvised Weapons of the American Underground*. Desert Publications. ISBN 0879471107

3 Brown, R. (1999). *Homemade Guns & Homemade Ammo*. Breakout Productions. ISBN 1893626113

4 McLean, D. (1992). *Do-It-Yourself Gunpowder Cookbook*. Paladin Press. ISBN 0873646754

5 Hollenback, G. (1996). *Workbench Silencers: The Art Of Improvised Designs*. Paladin Press. ISBN 0873648951

6 Métral, G. (1985). *Do-It-Yourself Submachine Gun*. Paladin Press. ISBN 0873648404

7 Vincent J.M. & Di Maio, M.D. (1999). *Gunshot Wounds*. CRC Press. ISBN 0849381630

8 Luty, P.A. (1998). *Expedient Homemade Firearms*. Paladin Press. ISBN 9780873649834

9 Koffler, B.B. (March 1970). Zip Guns and Crude Conversions. Identifying Characteristics and Problems. *The Journal of Criminal Law, Criminology, and Police Science (Northwestern University)*, 115–125

10 en.wikipedia.org/wiki/Gun_laws_in_the_United_States

11 www.cps.gov.uk < Legal Resources > Legal Guidance

2.4

Antique Weapons

2.4.1 Introduction

The subject pertaining to antiques and their exemption from the provisions of the relevant firearms legislation is extremely complicated. Each country has its own ideas as to what should be classified as an 'antique' and, even within a country's legislation, there can be anomalies. For example, the UK legislation states that a 1995 Pedersoli 12-bore muzzle-loader is not considered 'obsolete' under Section 58, but an 1840 Manton is – and they are exactly the same weapon!

In the UK, "*Section 58(2) of the 1968 Firearms Act exempts from the provisions of the Act – including certificate controls under sections 1 and 2 and prohibition under section 5 – all antique firearms which are sold, transferred, purchased, acquired or possessed as curiosities or ornaments.*"

The term 'antique firearm' is, as yet, undefined in UK law but the guidance makes it clear that if the firearm is 'used', then the exemption cannot be claimed and the item must be certificated.

There is a rebuttal presumption that ammunition should not be held, which creates a problem for the collector of both firearms and ammunition. The Home Office provides a list of 'obsolete chamberings' to assist the collector and the police.

Although the letter of the law does not prohibit the possession of the component of ammunition for S.58(2) firearms, or equipment to assemble such ammunition, such possession puts at risk the whole concept.

In the USA, the situation is probably even more complex, with a vast number of weapons being listed as 'antiques' and more being added to the list on an almost monthly basis.

Under the United States Federal Gun Control Act of 1968, antique firearms and replicas are largely exempted from restrictions. Antique firearms are defined as: '*any firearm with a frame or receiver manufactured in or before 1898 regardless of ignition system, or any firearm with a matchlock, flintlock, percussion cap, or similar type of ignition system, and any replica of an antique firearm if the replica is not designed or redesigned for using rimfire or conventional centre fire ammunition, or uses fixed ammunition, which is no longer manufactured in the United States and which is not readily available in the ordinary channels or commercial trade, any muzzle loading rifle, muzzle loading shotgun, or muzzle loading pistol, which is designed to use black powder, or a black powder substitute, and which cannot use fixed ammunition*'.

It should be noted, however, that antique firearms exemptions vary considerably under state laws.

2.4.2 Background

A **reproduction** is a copy of an original weapon (some are exact copies and some are manufactured with a certain amount of licence) which has the capability of discharging a missile with potentially lethal force. These reproductions are generally copies of older weapons, flintlocks, percussion cap weapons and weapons such as the Colt Single Action Army.

Forensic Ballistics in Court: Interpretation and Presentation of Firearms Evidence, First Edition. Brian J. Heard.
© 2013 John Wiley & Sons, Ltd. Published 2013 by John Wiley & Sons, Ltd.

Generally, these reproductions are only intended for use with black powder propellant, although most of the cartridge weapons can fire ammunition loaded with modern nitrocellulose-based propellants.

2.4.3 Defining 'antique'

The legislation is, to say the least, complicated. An overview of some of the current legislation follows:

Under UK legislation

Section 58(2) of the 1968 Act exempts from the provisions of the Act all antique firearms which are sold, transferred, purchased, acquired or possessed as curiosities or ornaments. The word '*antique*' is not defined in the Act, but Home Office guidance on the subject can be summarised briefly as follows:

- If modern ready-made ammunition can be bought and fired using the weapon, it cannot be classed as an antique.

- A muzzle-loading firearm is antique.

- A breech-loading firearm using a rimfire cartridge exceeding .23″ (but not 9 mm) is antique.

- A breech-loading firearm using an ignition system other than rimfire or centre is antique.

- A breech-loading centre fire firearm originally chambered for cartridges which are now obsolete and retains that original chambering is antique.

In addition to the above, the Home Office has a list of 'obsolete calibre' rifles, shotguns and pistols. These may be bought, sold and possessed without a licence of any kind, provided that they are owned as curios only. These weapons may not be fired and to possess ammunition for them is likely to invalidate any claim that they are not for use. No ammunition is considered 'obsolete'.

Among the 'obsolete calibres' are pinfires, muzzle-loaders, rimfires (not including .22″ and 9 mm) and large bore shotguns including 4-bore and 8-bore.

The rules only apply to pre-1939 manufactured weapons.

Pre-1939 rifles, shotguns and punt guns chambered for the following cartridges – 32-bore 24-bore, 14-bore, 10- bore ($2\frac{5}{8}″$ and $2\frac{7}{8}″$ chambers only), 8-bore, 4-bore, 3-bore, 2-bore, $1\frac{1}{8}$ bore, $1\frac{1}{4}$ bore and $1\frac{1}{2}$ bore – are all considered 'obsolete'.

A list of 'obsolete calibres' can be found at www.david-squires.org.uk/antiques.htm.

United States of America

Under the United States Gun Control Act of 1968, antique firearms and replicas are largely exempted from licensing restrictions.

Antique firearms are defined as: *any firearm with a frame or receiver manufactured in or before 1898 regardless of ignition system, or any firearm with a matchlock, flintlock, percussion cap, or similar type of ignition system, and any replica of an antique firearm if the replica is not designed or redesigned for using rimfire or conventional centre fire ammunition, or uses fixed ammunition, which is no longer manufactured in the United States and which is not readily available in the ordinary channels or commercial trade, any muzzle loading rifle, muzzle loading shotgun, or muzzle loading pistol, which is designed to use black powder, or a black powder substitute, and which cannot use fixed ammunition.*

Note: antique firearms exemptions vary considerably under state laws.

Canada

The law regarding antiques is as follows. The *Criminal Code* defines antique firearms as:

- firearms manufactured before 1898 that were not designed or have been redesigned to discharge rimfire or centre-fire ammunition; or

- firearms prescribed as antique firearms in the *Criminal Code* regulations. These are:

  - black powder reproductions of flintlock, wheel-lock or matchlock firearms, other than handguns, manufactured after 1897 (all other reproductions must be registered and owners must have a firearm licence to possess them; for example, reproductions of percussion cap muzzle-loading firearms like American Civil War Enfield and Springfield rifles will be considered firearms and not antiques);

- rifles manufactured before 1898 that can discharge only rimfire cartridges, other than .22″ calibre short, .22″ calibre long or .22″ calibre long rifle cartridges;

- rifles manufactured before 1898 that can discharge centre-fire cartridges (whether with a smooth or rifled bore), have a bore diameter of 8.3 mm or greater, measured from land to land in the case of a rifled bore, with the exception of a repeating firearm fed by any type of cartridge magazine;

- shotguns manufactured before 1898 that can discharge only rimfire cartridges, other than .22″ calibre short, .22″ calibre long or .22″ calibre long rifle cartridges;

- shotguns manufactured before 1898 that can discharge centre-fire cartridges, other than 10-, 12-, 16-, 20-, 28-, or 410-gauge cartridges;

- handguns manufactured before 1898 that can discharge only rimfire cartridges, other than .22″ calibre short, .22″ calibre long or .22″ calibre long rifle cartridges;

- handguns manufactured before 1898 that can discharge centre-fire cartridges, other than a handgun designed or adapted to discharge .32″ Short Colt, .32″ Long Colt, .32″ Smith and Wesson, .32 Smith and Wesson Long, .32–20″ Winchester, .38″ Smith and Wesson; .38″ Short Colt, .38″ Long Colt, .38–40″ Winchester, .44–40″ Winchester, or .45″ Colt cartridges

Australia

All single-shot or double-barrel muzzle-loading firearms manufactured before January 1, 1901 are considered antique firearms in all states of Australia and can be legally purchased and owned (and, in some states, used) without licences.

Cartridge-loading firearms manufactured prior to January 1, 1901 may or may not be considered 'antique', depending on the commercial availability of ammunition.

Finland

All black powder firearms made before 1890 are exempt from licence requirements.

Norway

In 2008 a new Norwegian firearms law redefined an 'antique' as any gun produced before 1891, or that is chambered in a calibre the Crown (Norwegian Department of Justice) considers obsolete.

Poland

Any firearm manufactured before 1885 that uses only black powder as a propellant and is separately charged (meaning not utilising fixed cartridges), and replicas of such weapons, do not require a licence.

Spain

Guns manufactured before 1870 are considered exempt antiques under Article 107 of the Regulations on Arms.

Sweden

Guns manufactured before 1890, and that do not support 'gas tight' cartridges (gastät enhetspatron), are considered antique and do not require a licence under Sweden's 1996 gun law (1996:67).

Switzerland

Guns manufactured before 1870 are considered exempt antiques under Article 2, alinea 3 of the Federal Gunlaw (amendment 2008-12-12).

As can be seen from the above few countries, the legislation pertaining to 'antiques' is far from standard and, in many cases, is flawed and confusing. The following may assist in determining the relevant legislation:

- The Pre-1899 Antique Guns FAQ by James Wesley Rawles.

- UK Home Office Guidance to the Police on Antique Guns.

- NRA (UK) White Paper on Controls on Firearms.

- UK Home Office Obsolete Calibres List.

- Regulations Prescribing Antique Firearms, Canada Gazette Part II, Vol. 132, No. 20.

- Canadian National Firearms Association Web Page on Antique Firearms Laws.

3.0

Proof Marks

3.0.1 Introduction

The identification of proof marks may seem a little esoteric, but such marks can reveal a substantial amount of information about the background of a weapon – for example, where and when it was made, has it been imported or exported, has it been modified or substantially repaired and where and when this took place. All of this may have a substantial influence on the case at hand.

The Gun Barrel Proof Acts were really the first examples of consumer protection in the UK. Any firearms which are offered for sale or transfer must be 'of proof', i.e. they have been tested for safety with a higher than normal pressure cartridge and they have been stamped with the relevant '**proof marks**' accordingly. At one time, the two Proof Houses (London and Birmingham) used to permit 'Certificates in lieu of marks' for valuable or collectible guns and 'Certificates of inability to prove' for those for which proof ammunition was not available. Strictly speaking, this was *ultra vires* (beyond the powers granted under the Gun Barrel Proof Acts), and nowadays this is not possible.

The laws of proof are entirely separate from the laws regarding possession of firearms. Logically, an 18th Century musket or a Colt Model 1851 'Navy' revolver are both still firearms under the Firearms Acts (although such a weapon might be possessed without a certificate as a 'curio or ornament' under S.58(2)) and thus it should be 'of proof'. It has to be said, however, that custom and practice in the antiques trade for the last 150 years has been to sell antique firearms without regard to their proof status.

3.0.2 Proof marks

Proof marks are stamps applied to various parts of a weapon, during and after manufacture, to show that the weapon is safe for use with the ammunition for which it was designed.

In England, the London and Birmingham Proof Houses were established (in 1637 and 1813 respectively) by Royal Charter to protect the public from the sale of unsafe weapons. In 1914, the director of the Liège Proof House in Liège, Mr. Joseph, created the Permanent International Commission for Firearms Testing (CIP.).

The CIP has progressively established a set of uniform rules for the proofing of firearms and ammunitions to ensure the reciprocal recognition of the proof marks of each of its member states.

A convention between the 14 member states was signed in 1969, ratified and converted into law in each signing state, so that the rules can be enforced to assure that every firearm and cartridge on the market has successfully passed the compulsory proofing and approval.

The CIP safeguards that every civil firearm and all ammunition sold in CIP member states are safe for the users. To achieve this, the firearms are all

Forensic Ballistics in Court: Interpretation and Presentation of Firearms Evidence, First Edition. Brian J. Heard.
© 2013 John Wiley & Sons, Ltd. Published 2013 by John Wiley & Sons, Ltd.

professionally proofed at CIP-accredited proof houses before they can be sold to consumers.

At present, these member states include the UK, Austria, Belgium, Chile, the Czech Republic, Finland, France, Germany, Hungary, Italy, Russia, Slovakia, Spain and the United Arab Emirates.

A number of other countries have their own forms of proof, either in-house or centrally run. For various reasons, these have not been acceptable to the European proof houses and the weapons have to be fully proofed before they are legally saleable in those countries.

There are also a number of countries which have a separate military proofing system for service weapons. These, once again, are not accepted by the European commercial proof houses. Weapons bearing military proof marks have thus to be commercially proofed before they can be legally sold in Europe.

The USA does not have a proofing system – merely acceptance marks stamped by the various manufacturers to say that they have been fired and found to function. These marks include inspectors' marks, factory marks and, in the case of military weapons, proof marks. None of these marks are accepted by CIP member states.

3.0.3   Types of proof

There are basically three types of proof: **provisional proof, definitive proof and reproof**.

- Provisional proof is only for shotgun barrels in the early stages of manufacture. This type of proof is designed to prevent the manufacturer from continuing work on barrel blanks which may have hidden defects.

- Definitive proof applies to all weapons and shows that the weapon has been tested with an over-charge of propellant and missile. Generally this calls for between a 30–50 per cent

increase in pressure over the standard round of ammunition.

- Reproof is an additional test which may be applied after a weapon has been repaired or altered in some way.

3.0.4   Proof marks and the examiner

Proof marks can be a very valuable aid to the forensic firearms investigator, as they can give information as to the age, history and country of origin of a weapon.

Many countries have specific exemption from their firearms legislation for weapons which are 'antique'. At one time, the situation was simple, with an antique being considered to be anything over 100 years old. This, however, no longer holds true, as many weapons (e.g. the Colt Single Action Army Model of 1873) are well over this age and can fire modern centre fire ammunition.

To complicate matters further, modern reproductions of some of these old weapons have been produced which are often virtually indistinguishable from the original. In these cases, the original proof mark could prove to be the only method of dating a weapon accurately.

This is, however, a very complex subject and requires much research and experience in the interpretation of the marks before accurate information can be obtained.

Many papers and books have been written on this subject, but probably the most authoritative is *The Standard Directory of Proof Marks* by Wirnsberger (see Further reading list below).

3.0.5   Examples of proof marks

To list the proof marks of just the countries that make up the 14 member states of the CIP would take far too many pages for this book to accommodate. However, the following gives an example of the types of mark impressed by various countries.

British proof marks (Figure 3.0.1)

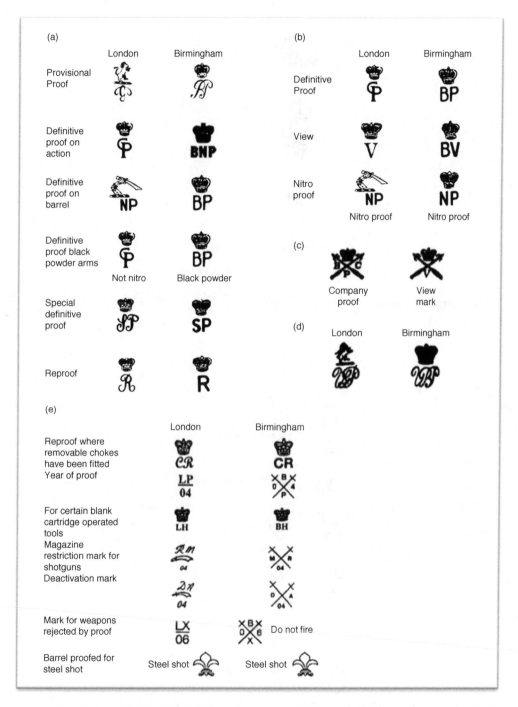

Figure 3.0.1 British Proof Marks. (a) under 1954 Rules of Proof; (b) under 1925 Rules of Proof; (c) Birmingham proof marks 1813–1904; (d) proof marks used between 1887 and 1925; (e) under 1988 Rules of Proof.

British military (Figure 3.0.2)

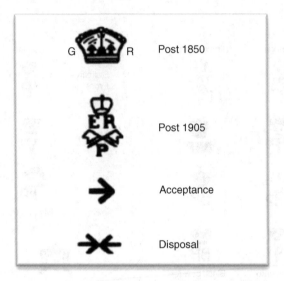

Figure 3.0.2 British military proof marks.

Spanish proof marks (Figure 3.0.3)

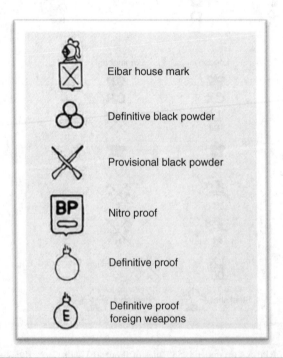

Figure 3.0.3 Spanish proof marks.

Belgian proof marks (Figure 3.0.4)

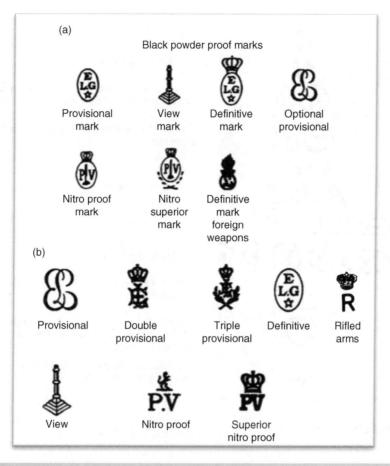

Figure 3.0.4   Belgian proof marks: (a) since 1968; (b) before 1968.

Russian proof marks (Figure 3.0.5)

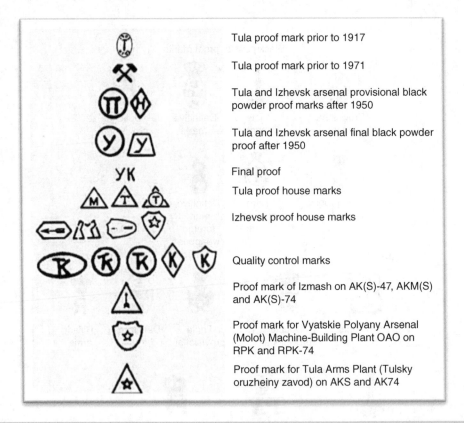

Tula proof mark prior to 1917

Tula proof mark prior to 1971

Tula and Izhevsk arsenal provisional black powder proof marks after 1950

Tula and Izhevsk arsenal final black powder proof after 1950

Final proof
Tula proof house marks

Izhevsk proof house marks

Quality control marks

Proof mark of Izmash on AK(S)-47, AKM(S) and AK(S)-74

Proof mark for Vyatskie Polyany Arsenal (Molot) Machine-Building Plant OAO on RPK and RPK-74

Proof mark for Tula Arms Plant (Tulsky oruzheiny zavod) on AKS and AK74

Figure 3.0.5   Russian proof marks.

Russian Federation proof marks (Figure 3.0.6)

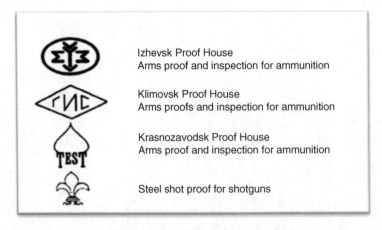

Izhevsk Proof House
Arms proof and inspection for ammunition

Klimovsk Proof House
Arms proofs and inspection for ammunition

Krasnozavodsk Proof House
Arms proof and inspection for ammunition

Steel shot proof for shotguns

Figure 3.0.6   Russian Federation proof marks.

Japanese proof marks – military (Figure 3.0.7)

Symbol	Arsenal/subcontractor	Period of operation
⊛	Koishikawa arsenal (Tokyo) on rifles	1870–1935
⊛	Kokura arsenal on rifles	1935–1945
⊗	Nagoya arsenal on rifles	1923–1945
✪	Jinsen arsenal (Korea) on rifles	1923–1945
⊛	Mukden arsenal (Manchuria) on rifles	1931–1945
⊛ ⊖	Toyo Kogyo on rifles	1939–1945
⊗ ◇	Tokyo Juki Kogyo on rifles	1940–1945
⊛ ◇	Tokyo Juki Kogyo on rifles	1940–1945
⊗ △	Howa Jyuko on rifles	1940–1945
⊗ ◆	Izawa Jyuko on rifles	1940–1945
⚓	Toyokawa arsenal on handguns	1940–1945
⚓	Sasebo arsenal on handguns	1940–1945
⚓	Yokosura arsenal on handguns	1940–1945
⚓	Kure arsenal on handguns	1940–1945
⚓	Maisuru arsenal on handguns	1940–45
⊕	Current proof mark	

Figure 3.0.7 Japanese proof marks – mainly WWII military.

American military proof mark (Figure 3.0.8)

Figure 3.0.8 American military 'flaming ball' proof mark.

American inspector's marks

All USA arms and Navy small arms carry initials which are called inspector's marks. These marks appear on stocks, grips or metal parts. Some arms, especially older ones, have more than one inspector's initial or initials. The barrel is inspected before the rest of the arm is produced, so thus there may be one inspector's mark on the barrel and another on the rest of the parts.

The army and navy purchase arms from commercial outlets and also contract directly with the manufacturers. The navy also purchase some arms from the army. From the early days of 1831, most small arms contract inspectors have been civilians or Springfield Armory employees. Officers who served as inspectors were from the Army Ordnance Department or the Navy Bureau of Ordnance. There were also sub-inspectors who had regular jobs at Springfield Armory, and small arms inspection was in addition to their regular duties.

The good thing about these marks is that they give a very accurate date for the manufacture of the weapon and where it was made. There are far too many inspectors' initials to list here, but the following links provide excellent details of the marks, who they referred to and when they were applied.

- http://www.mikescivilwar.com/inspectors.htm

- http://proofhouse.com/cm/us_inspector.htm

Further reading

1 Wirnsberger, G. *The Standard Directory of Proof Marks*. Distributed by Blacksmith Co., Southport, CT. ISBN-13: 9780891490067.
2 *Notes on the Proof of Shotguns and Other Small Arms*. Issued by the Worshipful Company of Guardians of the Birmingham Proof House
3 https://store.bluebookinc.com/info/pdf/firearm/proof marks.pdf

4.0

A Brief History of Ammunition

4.0.1 Introduction

A history of ammunition could fill several volumes all by itself. The following will, however, give a brief primer on the subject, which can be expanded if required via reference to the books listed under 'Further reading' at the end of this chapter.

To know how ammunition developed, it is important to have an understanding of why the various components are constructed and how they fit together. This is especially so when dealing with the difficult subject of what constitutes an 'antique' and why. For example, knowing what a pinfire round of ammunition is, how it is constructed and why the weapon is classified as an antique can be of considerable importance in a case of this type.

4.0.2 Basics

The first forms of ammunition consisted of loose powder, carried in a flask or horn, and various projectiles which were loaded into the barrel from the muzzle end. These early projectiles were often irregularly shaped stone balls or arrow-like objects.

By the 15th Century, ammunition had become fairly standardised and consisted of 'black powder' propellant (a mixture of charcoal, sulphur and potassium nitrate), followed by some wading, a spherical lead ball and further wading to retain it all in place. Materials other than lead had been used for the projectile, and it was recognised from an early period that the lighter the material the higher the velocity. However, due to its ballistic properties and the ease of casting it into spheres or bullet-shaped projectiles, lead remained the preferred material.

Elongated bullets with a hollow base (to move their centre of gravity towards the nose of the bullet) and a pointed nose had been experimented with for some time, but they did not receive any real favour until the mid-1800s.

During the latter part of the 16th Century, as a result of the need for rapid reloading, pre-measured powder charges were introduced. These were contained in small paper bags, which were torn open and the contents poured down the barrel. The paper bag followed this, as did the wadding. The bullet, which was carried separately, was hammered into place last of all.

Towards the end of the 1600s, the bullet was tied into the top of the powder bag, resulting in the first 'self-contained' cartridge.

These early 'self-contained' cartridges still required an external priming method to provide a flash to ignite the main propellant charge. It was not until the introduction of the breech-loader, where the ammunition is loaded from the rear of the barrel, that true self-contained ammunition appeared.

Early attempts at including the priming charge within the cartridge include the volcanic, lip, cup, teat, annular rim, needle, pin and rim fire systems. Most of these had a very short life span and, with the exception of the rimfire, only the pinfire attained any degree of popularity.

Forensic Ballistics in Court: Interpretation and Presentation of Firearms Evidence, First Edition. Brian J. Heard.
© 2013 John Wiley & Sons, Ltd. Published 2013 by John Wiley & Sons, Ltd.

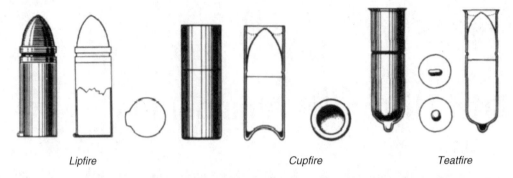

Lipfire   *Cupfire*   *Teatfire*

Figure 4.0.1   Some obsolete cartridge configurations.

Early 'self-contained' systems

The **Dreyse needle fire** rifle was invented by the gunsmith Johann Nikolaus von Dreyse (1787–1867) and was first produced as a fully working rifle in 1836 (see Figure 4.0.2). From 1848 onwards, this weapon was gradually introduced into the Prussian service, then later into the military forces of many German states.

The name 'needle gun' comes from its needle-like firing pin, which passed through the cartridge case to impact on a percussion cup glued to the base of the bullet.

The cartridge was a self-contained paper case containing the bullet, priming cup and black powder charge. The bullet, which was glued into the paper case, had the priming cup glued to its base. The upper end of the case was rolled up and tied together. Before the needle could strike the primer, its point had to pass through the paper case, then through the powder charge, before striking the primer cup on the base of the bullet. The theory was that this would give a more complete ignition and, thus, combustion of the charge of propellant. Unfortunately, this led to severe corrosion of the needle, which then either stuck in the bolt or broke off, rendering the rifle useless. It was, however, a major step forward in the production of a modern rifle firing a self-contained cartridge.

The **pinfire** was at its most popular between 1890 and 1910 and was still readily available on the Continent until 1940. It had, however, fallen out

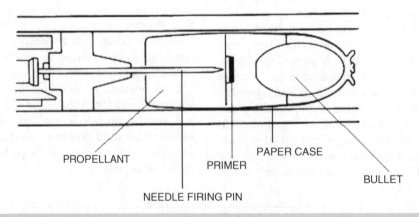

PROPELLANT   PRIMER   PAPER CASE

NEEDLE FIRING PIN   BULLET

Figure 4.0.2   Dreyse needle fire.

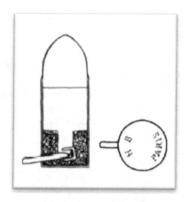

Figure 4.0.3   Pinfire ammunition.

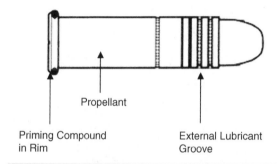

Propellant

Priming Compound
in Rim

External Lubricant
Groove

Figure 4.0.4   Rimfire ammunition.

calibres were also available (Figure 4.0.3). It can still be obtained in shooting quantities from specialised ammunition dealers.

Of the early ignition systems, only the **rimfire** has survived, and this only in .22″ calibre.

In rimfire ammunition (Figure 4.0.4) the primer composition is spun into the hollow rim of the cartridge case. As a consequence, the propellant is in intimate contact with the priming composition. On firing, the weapon's firing pin crushes the thin rim of the cartridge case, compressing the priming composition and so initiating its detonation.

Calibres of rimfire ammunition up to .44″ rifle were available around the 1850s, but it was not possible, given the technology available at that time, to produce a cartridge case strong enough to withstand reliably the pressures produced.

The **centre fire cartridge** removed this limitation by providing a relatively soft cup containing the priming compound (the priming cap or 'primer'), which is set into the centre of the base of a much stronger cartridge case (see Figure 4.0.5). Although practical centre fire cartridges were available as early as 1852 in England, the final forms were not perfected until 1866 by Colonel Berdan (an American) and 1867 by Colonel Boxer (an Englishman). These primer cap designs have never really been improved upon and are still in use today. Interestingly, Boxer primed cartridge cases are normally used in American ammunition and Berdan in European ammunition.

A list of the dates of introduction for some of the more popular calibres of ammunition can be found in Appendix 5.

of favour in England by 1914 and it was virtually unobtainable by 1935.

Calibres available for use in pinfire revolvers were 5 mm, 7 mm, 9 mm, 12 mm and 15 mm, and shotgun ammunition in 9 mm, 12-bore and various other

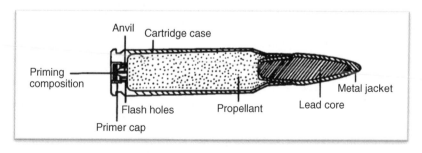

Figure 4.0.5   Centre fire cartridge.

Further reading

1 Hogg, I.V. *The Illustrated History of Ammunition*. Chartwell Books. ISBN-10: 0890099510

2 McConaughy, M. (1920). *History of small-arms ammunition*. United States Army Ordnance Dept.

3 Barnes. F.C. (2006). *Cartridges Of The World*.

4 Harding, C.W. *Eley Cartridges: A History Of The Silversmiths And Ammunition Manufacturers*.

5 Harding, C.W. (2009). *The Birmingham Cartridge Manufacturers*.

6 Hackley, F.W., Hackley, F.W., Woodin, W.H. & Scranton, E.L. *A History of Modern U.S. Small Arms Ammunition*. ISBN-10: 1577470338.

7 Hoyem, G.A. *History & Development Of Small Arms Ammunition, Vol. 1: Martial Long Arms: Flintlock through Rimfire*. ISBN: 0960498281.

4.1

Ammunition Components

4.1.1 Introduction

It never ceases to amaze how often **a round of ammunition** is called a 'bullet' or a 'cartridge'. Such basic nomenclature can make one appear unprepared when examining in chief or cross-examining. This is such basic nomenclature that it should never be misused.

Likewise centre fire and rimfire ammunition should never be confused or calibre (can also be spelled 'caliber'). However, when dealing with Berdan and Boxer primed ammunition, even the experienced can become unstuck.

The following will not only enable the correct terminology to be used, but also to ascertain the depth of knowledge possessed by the expert.

4.1.2 Basics

A round of ammunition (*not* a cartridge or bullet) is composed of four parts:

1. The **cartridge case.** This holds all the components together.

2. The **bullet or projectile.** This is inserted into the cartridge case mouth and is the part of the round that is discharged from the firearm.

3. The **propellant**. In modern ammunition this is nitrocellulose, together with small amounts of other chemicals to stabilise and modify its burning characteristics.

4. The **primer**. This is a highly sensitive mixture of chemicals which explodes violently on being struck. When the priming mixture explodes, it sends an extremely hot jet of flame into the propellant, igniting it in the process.

The following should clarify exactly what each component is, what it does and what it is made of.

'A round of ammunition' generally refers to a single, live, unfired, cartridge comprising the missile, cartridge case, propellant and some form of primer. The term is also applied to live blank and tear gas ammunition – hence, a **round of live blank ammunition** or a **round of live tear gas ammunition**.

The **primer** is basically the means for igniting the propellant:

- In **rimfire** ammunition, the explosive priming compound is spun into the hollow rim of the cartridge case.

- In **centre fire** ammunition there is a small cup, called a **primer cap** (also called a cup) containing the priming compound. This primer cap is inserted into a recess in the centre of the cartridge case.

Once the primer has been struck by the hammer, the priming compound explodes with great violence, sending a flame into the propellant and thus igniting it.

Forensic Ballistics in Court: Interpretation and Presentation of Firearms Evidence, First Edition. Brian J. Heard.
© 2013 John Wiley & Sons, Ltd. Published 2013 by John Wiley & Sons, Ltd.

The **propellant** is a chemical or mixture of chemicals which, when ignited, produces a very large quantity of gas. These gases, when confined within a barrel and behind a missile, provide the propulsion to drive the missile down the bore and out of the barrel. The propellant, whether it be a single-based nitrocellulose propellant or a double-based nitrocellulose/nitro-glycerine propellant, does not explode – it simply burns extremely quickly, producing a large volume of gas.

A **cartridge case** refers to the ammunition case and primer and does not include the bullet. It can be either a 'fired cartridge case' or a 'live cartridge case'. A 'live cartridge case' has a live, unfired primer, but there is no propellant or bullet present.

A **bullet** refers to the missile alone. It can be either a 'fired bullet' or an 'unfired bullet'.

Pellets can be either the individual lead, steel or non-toxic missiles in the form of spherical balls found in shotgun ammunition, or the lead pellets for use in air weapons. The term 'lead slug' is also sometimes used to describe air gun pellets, but this not the correct term for this type of missile.

Shot is another term for the lead, steel or non-toxic spherical balls in shotgun ammunition, i.e. 'lead shot'. This is an acceptable alternative to 'pellet'.

4.1.3   Ammunition types

Small arms ammunition basically consists of a cartridge case, primer, propellant and some form of missile. There are really only three types of small arms ammunition in current production: 'rimfire', 'centre fire' and 'caseless'.

Rimfire ammunition consists of a short brass tube, generally .22″ in diameter, closed at one end. The tube contains a charge of propellant and has a bullet at the open end. The closed end of the tube is formed into a flat head, with a hollow rim which contains the priming compound. The round is fired when the firing pin strikes the rim, crushing and thus exploding the priming compound. The flame produced by this explosion ignites the propellant, thus driving the bullet from the cartridge case.

Centre fire ammunition is also generally made from brass, but the head is thick and heavy, with a central recess or pocket for the primer cap. A hole leading from the primer pocket into the cartridge allows the flash from the priming compound to reach the propellant, thus igniting it.

Caseless ammunition consists of a bullet with the propellant formed around the bullet as a single solid piece. There is no cartridge case. The primer is generally located at the rear of the propellant and is not enclosed in any metallic cup. This type of ammunition has not found any real favour, due to problems in making the propellant strong enough to stand rough treatment.

Blank ammunition is exactly the same as bulleted ammunition, except for the omission of the missile. In blank ammunition, the case mouth is sealed, either by crimping the metal or by inserting a wax plug or paper disc. The wax or paper is usually coloured white, or sometimes black. These cartridges are only used for military training, starting races or theatrical purposes, and they are only intended to produce a sharp crack on firing. Blank ammunition is available in all calibres.

Tear gas cartridges are the same as blank ammunition, except they contain a small quantity of a lachrymatory/sternutatory (makes the eyes run and causes sneezing) substance. This is generally one of the following compounds:

- CN gas (chloracetophenone),

- CS gas (o-chlorobenzalmalonitrile),

- phenyacylchloride,

- nonivamide,

- bromoacetone,

- xylyl bromide,

- syn-propanethial-S-oxide (from onions)or

- oleoresin capsicum (from Chili peppers).

In tear gas ammunition, the case mouth is never crimped, but is closed either with a card disc, a wax plug or a plastic cover; these are invariably red or yellow in colour.

The most common calibre of tear gas ammunition encountered is 8 mm. This is intended for use in small self-loading pistols specifically designed for the discharge of this type of ammunition. Tear gas ammunition in .22″ calibre is also quite common, but this is generally intended for use in revolvers. Cartridges for use in 8 mm 'gas guns' have also been encountered, loaded with talcum powder of various colours (for theatrical purposes), scent (for room freshening) and even fly killer!

Power tool, nail-driving or stud gun cartridges are very similar to blank and tear gas ammunition, and it is quite easy to mistake one for the other. In general, these are .22″, .25″, .32″ or occasionally .38″ calibre. The mouth of the cartridge case is either rolled over onto a card disc or crimped. A colour coding system, either coloured lacquer over the crimp or a coloured disc, is used to designate the strength of the cartridge. Care should be taken not to confuse a power tool cartridge using a red coloured card disc with a tear gas cartridge. The only real way of distinguishing between the two is by disassembling the cartridge.

Grenade launcher cartridges are only encountered in military rifle calibres and, as the name indicates, they are designed for the discharge of a grenade from a normal service rifle. The case mouth is invariably crimped, and some colour code (e.g. the case painted black) distinguishes this type of cartridge from standard blank ammunition.

Flare cartridges are designed for signalling purposes and come in many calibres. They usually contain a solid pellet of a chemical or metal that will burn extremely brightly when ignited. This is usually magnesium metal dust, with some oxidising agent to make it burn more brightly.

Dummy cartridges have neither primer nor powder, and they are only used for weapon functioning tests or for practising the safe loading and unloading of weapons. These cartridges are normally chromium-plated or painted a silver colour.

Snap caps are for the practice of firing a weapon without damaging the firing pin and lock mechanism, by firing it without a cartridge in place. This is generally called 'dry firing'. Snap caps usually have a piece of rubber or hard plastic in place of the primer, and the case is chromium or nickel plated for identification purposes. Although snap caps are available in all calibres, the most commonly encountered are in shotgun calibres.

4.1.4 Primer cap types

In **rimfire** ammunition, the firing pin crushes the soft hollow rim of the cartridge against the rear of the barrel to explode the priming compound.

In **centre fire** ammunition, the priming compound is held in a cup in the base of the cartridge case. Merely striking the base of the cup with a firing pin would do little more than dislodge the priming compound from the cup. An **anvil** has to be provided for the priming compound to be crushed against by the impact of the firing pin. In modern ammunition, there are basically three ways in which this is achieved. These are called the **Boxer**, **Berdan** and **battery cup** priming systems.

The **Berdan primer** was designed in 1967 by Colonel Berdan of the US Army Ordinance Department (see Figure 4.1.1). In this system, the anvil is actually part of the cartridge case in the form of a small peg in the primer pocket. Around the anvil are a number of small flash holes to permit the passage of the ignition flame from the primer to the propellant. Due to the ease and low cost of manufacture, Berdan primers are used mainly in military ammunition.

The **Boxer primer** was developed in 1866 by Colonel Boxer of the Royal Laboratory at Woolwich Arsenal, England (see Figure 4.1.2). In this type of primer, the anvil is a small bent disc of steel which fits into the cup, making the primer completely self-contained. The flash hole in the cartridge case is centrally located and as it is of a relatively large diameter (approximately 1.5 mm in pistol ammunition). It is thus quite easy to push out the fired cup with a thin rod for reloading purposes. Boxer primed ammunition is almost exclusively used in commercial ammunition.

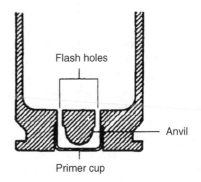

Figure 4.1.1   Berdan primer.

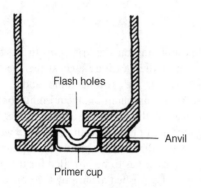

Flash holes

Anvil

Primer cup

Figure 4.1.2   Boxer primer.

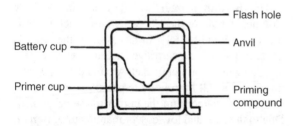

Flash hole

Battery cup

Anvil

Primer cup

Priming compound

Figure 4.1.3   Battery cup primer.

The **battery cup** system consists of a plain, anvil-less cup, which fits into a slightly larger inverted flanged cup containing its own anvil (see Figure 4.1.3). The flanged cup provides a rigid support for the primer cup and anvil. This self-contained assembly fits into a recessed pocket in the base of the cartridge case. Battery cup primers are used exclusively in shotgun ammunition.

4.1.5   Cartridge cases

In the Western world, cartridge cases are almost invariably made of brass, with a 75 : 25 copper/zinc alloy. Other materials have been used, including steel and plastic, but not on any commercial basis.

Aluminium-cased pistol ammunition has recently acquired some commercial success, due to the cost saving of aluminium over brass. There are, however, a number of disadvantages, including their being non-reloadable and less robust than their brass counterparts. however, for large-scale users who do not wish to reload their empty cartridge cases,

or who are firing for purely training purposes, the savings can be very considerable and far outweigh the disadvantages.

In modern ammunition from Russia, Warsaw Pact countries and China, the cartridge cases are invariably made of steel. In China the steel is coated with copper to prevent rusting, while elsewhere it has a heavy green/grey coat of lacquer for the same reason. In World War II, due to a shortage of raw materials, a number of countries, notably Germany and Russia, used lacquered steel cartridge cases as well. These are still sometimes encountered.

Shotgun cartridges generally have a brass base with a plastic, or sometimes paper, case. All-plastic shotgun cartridges have been produced, but they have not proved to be a commercial success.

The main purpose of the cartridge case, other than for holding the components together, is to expand and seal the chamber during firing. This is called '**obturation**', and it prevents the explosive escape of high-pressure gases through the breech. During manufacture, the brass is annealed to give the case the correct degree of hardness. If this is correct, the brass will regain its original shape after the pressure has subsided and the case will be easy to extract from the chamber. If it is too hard, the case will crack, and if too soft it will cling to the chamber walls and be extremely difficult to remove.

Cartridge case types (Figure 4.1.4)

Cartridge cases generally come in one of three shapes:

- **Straight cased**, where the case diameter is approximately the same along its length.

- **Bottle-necked**, where a wide bodied case is, just before the case mouth, reduced in diameter to that of the bullet. This permits a very much larger volume of propellant to be used, and consequently higher velocities to be obtained, than in straight-sided cases.

- **Tapered case**, where a wide-based cartridge case is gradually reduced in diameter along its length. These tend to be in old European sporting rifle calibres and are seldom encountered nowadays.

The cartridge case can be sub-divided into a further five categories, according to the configuration of its base.

1. **Rimmed**: these have a flange at the base which is larger than the diameter of the body of the cartridge case. This flange is to enable the cartridge to be extracted from the weapon in which it is used. When describing rifle ammunition and the metric method of designating the ammunition is used, these are often identified by an 'R' after the case length measurement, i.e. $7 \times 57\,$mmR. The vast majority of revolvers are designed for use with rimmed ammunition.

2. **Semi-rimmed**: these have a flange which is slightly larger than the diameter of the cartridge case and a groove around the case body just in front of the flange. When describing rifle ammunition and the metric system is used, these are identified by 'SR' in the cartridge designation.

3. **Rimless**: in these, the flange diameter is the same as the case body and there is, for extraction purposes, a groove around the case body just in front of the flange. There is generally no letter system to designate this cartridge base type. Self-loading pistols are almost invariably designed for use with semi-rimmed or rimless ammunition.

4. **Rebated**: this has an extractor flange which is smaller than the diameter of the cartridge case. The designation used in the metric system is 'RB'. This type of cartridge case configuration tends to be reserved for high-powered cannon ammunition.

5. **Belted case**: these have a pronounced raised belt encircling the base of the cartridge. This belt is for additional strength in high pressure cartridges. The metric designation is 'B'. This type of cartridge case is generally only found in very high-power rifle cartridges or military cannon ammunition.

At this juncture, it would be appropriate to clarify what each part of a cartridge case is called. This, once again, is a confusing subject. The diagram in Figure 4.1.5 should, however, clarify this subject matter.

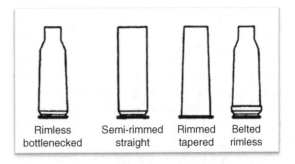

Figure 4.1.4 Cartridge case types.

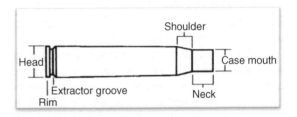

Figure 4.1.5 Correct nomenclature for the various parts of a cartridge case.

Cartridge calibre nomenclature

A basic understanding of this subject is essential, as it is area where the inexperienced can really show lack of knowledge. Knowing the difference between a $9 \times 18\,$mm and a $9 \times 19\,$mm cartridge, for example, may seem a little insignificant, but it is an area where the unwary can easily be tripped up and made to look very foolish. Having said that, it is a vastly complicated subject and there are very few set rules.

The first identifier is whether the cartridge in question is referred to in metric or imperial measurements. This generally indicates whether it is of British/American or European origin. Where British or American cartridges are concerned, the designation is always in inches and the zero in front of the decimal point is always omitted – for example, a cartridge with a bullet measuring $0.32''$ in diameter would be referred to as a $.32''$.

Where European cartridges are concerned, the measurement is always quoted in millimetres, e.g. $9\,$mm.

Even this apparently simple identifier is confusing, as a number of cartridges are identified by both systems, e.g. 9 mm Short is also .380″ Auto, and 7.65 mm is also .32″ ACP.

Probably the most confusing part of cartridge nomenclature is the calibre. This is basically a numerical approximation of the diameter of the bullet. It very frequently bears little relationship to the actual bullet measurement; for example, the .455″ Webley revolver cartridge has a bullet measuring .450″ and a .38″ Special bullet measures .357″. This discrepancy is, however, much more of a problem with older English cartridge nomenclature than it is with modern metric designations: a 9 mm Parabellum bullet is 9 mm in diameter, and a 5.56 mm does have a bullet measuring 5.56 mm.

The nominal calibre is often further identified by a name which can identify it among groups of the same calibre, e.g. 9 mm Parabellum, 9 mm Bayard, 9 mm Short, 9 mm Makarov, 9 mm Steyr, etc. The addition of a name often identifies the weapon for which the cartridge was originally designed; for example, the 9 mm Mauser was designed for the 9 mm 'broom handled' Mauser, 5.75 mm Velo-Dog for the 5.75 mm Velo-Dog revolver (designed, as its name implies for early cyclists and motor cyclists to protect themselves against attack by dogs!) and a .32″ ACP (Automatic Colt Pistol) for the Colt self-loading pistol.

In the Continental system, it is usual, especially in rifle calibres, to add the cartridge case length to further identify the cartridge i.e. 5.56 × 54 mm, 6.5 × 57 mm. Pistol ammunition can also take this form, although it is not always referred to, i.e. 9 × 19 mm is 9 mm Parabellum, 9 × 18 mm is the 9 mm Makarov and 7.62 × 25 mm is the Russian Tokarev pistol round.

As explained earlier, the case length can also be given a letter to indicate the type of case, e.g. 6.5 × 57R is a cartridge with a rimmed case, while 7.92 × 61RB is a cartridge with a rebated head. This can become even more confusing when a bullet type is appended to the suffix, e.g. the 6.5 × 57RS is a rimmed cartridge with a 'Spitzer', or pointed, bullet.

Another suffix appended to the designation of self-loading pistol ammunition is 'ACP'. This merely indicates that it was originally designed for use in Colt self-loading pistols, e.g. .32″ ACP and .380″ ACP.

The letters ACP stand for Automatic Colt Pistol, which is somewhat confusing in itself. An automatic weapon is one in which the weapon will continue to fire 'automatically' until the finger is released from the trigger or the magazine is empty. The correct designation for the pistols for which the .380″ and .32″ ammunition were designed is a self-loading or semi-automatic pistol.

In American ammunition, there is often a set of figures that can indicate the year of introduction for that particular calibre of ammunition, e.g. .30-06″ is a .30″ calibre rifle round introduced in 1906, while a .30-03″ is the same calibre, but introduced in 1903.

Where it really becomes confusing is when the weight of 'black powder' for which the cartridge was originally designed is included; for instance, a .30-30″ is a .30″ calibre rifle bullet originally designed to be driven by 30 grains of black powder propellant.

Even more confusing (if that is possible) is the system of including the bullet weight into the title, e.g. .45-70-500, which is a .45″ calibre rifle bullet propelled by 70 grains of black powder with a 500 grain bullet. What makes this system particularly difficult to deal with is that the majority of these cartridges no longer use black powder, but instead use a much smaller charge of modern smokeless propellant.

In old British sporting and military cartridges, the term 'Express cartridge' is often used. This originated with the introduction of a high velocity rifle and cartridge by the gun makers Purdy, who designated it the 'Express Train' model. The 'Train' part was eventually dropped and 'Express' was reserved for any large capacity cartridge with a high velocity. For cartridges with even higher velocities, the term 'Super Express' was also pressed into service. These cartridges were, however, all loaded with black powder, and when 'smokeless' propellants came into being, these 'Express' cartridges were re-designated 'Nitro Express'. Realising that even more power could be extracted from smokeless cartridges, the gun makers increased the case length and called these new super rounds 'Magnum Nitro Express'.

In recent years the term 'Magnum' has crept into the terminology for pistol ammunition and a 'Magnum' suffix, e.g. .22″ Magnum, .32″ Magnum, .357″ Magnum, etc. is now used to designate a round of much higher than standard velocity.

One other piece of information which can be included in the designation is the nominal velocity, e.g. .25-3000, which is a .25″ bullet at a velocity of 3000 feet/second. This is, however, unusual, and in the stated case was only used as an advertising gimmick.

4.1.6 Shotgun ammunition

Shotgun ammunition is once again a confusing subject, with the smaller calibres being referred to by the approximate bore diameter, e.g. .22″, 9 mm, .410″. Once past .410″, the calibre changes to a 'bore' (or, if using the American nomenclature 'gauge') size, where the 'bore' is the number of lead balls of the same diameter as the inside of the barrel which weigh one pound. Thus, a 12-bore shotgun has a barrel diameter of .729″ and 12 round lead balls of .729″ diameter weigh exactly one pound.

It should be pointed out here that the 'bore' size, when dealing with shotguns, is different from the bore size of rifled weapons. In rifled weapons, the bore size is the diameter measured across the tops of the rifling lands.

Size of pellets in shotgun ammunition

The missiles used in shotgun cartridges can vary from a single ball or cylinder of lead of the same diameter as the bore, down to pellets so small they are referred to as 'dust shot'. As each country has its own method of nomenclature for these shot sizes, the matter can be quite confusing. A table giving the shot sizes, weights and equivalent sizes for a number of countries follows:

The pellets used in shotgun cartridges have traditionally been made of lead, with a small amount of antimony to increase their hardness. Lead accumulation in wildfowl has prompted the use of other materials. Of these, the most common are:

- Soft steel, usually with a copper coating.

- Bismuth, a heavy metal often alloyed with iron.

- Tungsten, a very heavy metal often alloyed with iron.

Table 4.1.1 Table Showing Bore Size and the Weight of the Lead Ball That Fits the Bore

Bore (gauge)	Diameter of Bore		Weight of Lead Ball		
	(in)	(mm)	(oz)	(grains)	(grams)
$1\frac{1}{2}$*	1.459	37.05	10.667	4661	302.30
2*	1.325	34.34	8.000	3496	226.80
3*	1.158	29.41	5.333	2329	151.20
8	.835	21.21	2.000	874	56.70
10	.775	19.69	1.600	699.3	45.36
12	.729	18.516	1.333	581	37.80
13	.710	18.04	1.231	538	34.89
14	.693	16.23	1.143	500	32.40
16	.663	16.83	1.000	437	28.34
20	.615	15.63	0.800	349.6	22.67
24	.579	14.71	0.667	291.45	18.90
28	.550	13.97	0.571	249.5	16.20
32	.526	13.36	0.500	219	14.17
$67\frac{1}{2}$	.410	10.41	0.237	103.5	6.71

N.B. The bores marked * are found only in punt guns and other rare weapons. The .410 shotgun is never referred to as a $67\frac{1}{2}$ bore, only as .410″. Similarly, 9 mm and .22″ calibre shotguns are only referred to as 9 mm and .22″. The bore diameter for these two calibres is 9 mm and .22″ respectively.

Conversion factors: inch/mm 25.4
                 oz/grain 437
                 oz/grams 28.34

Table 4.1.2 Shotgun Pellet Sizes

Number Shot/oz	diameter (inches)	diameter (mm)	English	American	French	Belgian	Italian	Spanish
6	0.36″	9.1 mm	LG					
8	0.33″	8.4 mm	SG	00 buck		9G	11/0	
11	0.30″	7.6 mm	Special SG	1 buck	C2	12G	9/0	
15	0.27″	6.8 mm	SSG	3 buck	C3			
35	0.20″	5.2 mm	AAA	4 buck	0			
70	0.16″	4.1 mm	BB	Air rifle	1	00	00	1
100	0.14″	3.6 mm	1	2	3		1 or 2	3
140	0.13″	3.3 mm	3	4	4		3	4
170	0.12″	3.1 mm	4	5	5		4	5
220	0.11″	2.8 mm	5	6	6	5	5	6
270	0.10″	2.6 mm	6			6	6	
340	0.095″	2.4 mm	7	$7\frac{1}{2}$	7	7	$7\frac{1}{2}$	7
400	0.09″	2.3 mm	$7\frac{1}{2}$	8	$7\frac{1}{2}$	$7\frac{1}{2}$	8	$7\frac{1}{2}$
450	0.085″	2.2 mm	8		8	8		8
580	0.08″	2.0 mm	9	9	9	9	$9\frac{1}{2}$	9

Sizes and weights given are for lead shot. The abbreviations used in this table are as follows:

LG	Large Goose
SG	Small Goose
Special SG	Special Small Goose
SSG	Small Small Goose

The subject of non-toxic shot is discussed in much greater detail in Chapter 4.6.

It should also be noted that cartridges for clay pigeon shooting are often loaded with lead shot which has been copper-coated to increase its hardness. This could be confused with copper-coated steel shot, but a simple test with a magnet will differentiate between the two.

Shotgun slugs

A shotgun slug is a single projectile primarily designed to be fired from a smooth-bored shotgun. Shotgun slug ammunition is available in most of the common shotgun calibres.

The simplest form of slug is a round ball (sometimes referred to in the USA as a pumpkin ball or pumpkin shot). Since it is a symmetrical projectile, it will not significantly deviate from its intended path if it begins to spin due to air pressure. However, a smooth-bored shotgun firing a round ball is essentially a musket, with its inherent short range and accuracy problems.

To enhance a slug's performance, both externally and terminally, requires it to be elongated and to have its centre of mass moved forwards. Being elongated, it is also preferable for the missile to be spin-stabilised to prevent it tumbling.

The original Brenneke slug (Figure 4.1.6) overcame these problems via the use of a solid lead, pre-rifled projectile with an attached plastic, felt or cellulose fibre wad. The wad provides drag stabilisation by moving the centre of mass forwards. The cast rifling has little or no effect in spinning the projectile as it passes through the air.

Another early design was the *Foster slug* (Figure 4.1.7). This was basically a short, round-nosed bullet with a deep cup in the base. Foster slugs are also made with 'rifling' type grooves cast into the outside of the missile. These do not have any effect in spinning the projectile as it passes through the air. The cupped base expands on firing producing a seal (or obturating) with the bore.

While it is generally accepted that shotgun slugs do not have to be fired through a cylinder barrel, it is not recommended that full choke barrels be used. This is due to the fact that the pressure required to compress the slug through the choke will eventually flare the end of the barrel, thus reducing the degree of choke.

Saboted slugs are sub-calibre missiles which have a discarding plastic collar surrounding the missile to bring it up to standard calibre. They are generally designed to be fired from a special rifled shotgun barrel to spin-stabilise the missile. Originally, these were called 'Paradox' weapons and had a short length of rifling at the muzzle end of the barrel. More modern weapons can have rifling at the end of the barrel or along its full length.

Due to the reduced drag and high initial velocity, saboted slugs have significant advantages in external ballistics over a normal shotgun slug. Some saboted slugs use fins or a lightweight plastic portion at the rear of the missile to provide stability from smooth bores.

The Brenneke shotgun slug

The Brenneke slug was developed by the German gun and ammunition designer Wilhelm Brenneke (1865–1951) in 1898. The original Brenneke slug was a solid lead projectile with fins cast onto the outside, much like a modern rifled Foster slug (see below). It has a plastic, felt or cellulose fibre wad screwed to the base that remains attached after firing. This wad serves both as a gas seal and as a form of drag stabilisation, much like the mass-forward design of the Foster slug.

The fins or rifling are easily deformed to pass through choked shotgun barrels. Extensive tests have shown that these fins do not impart any significant stabilising spin on the projectile.

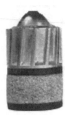

Since the Brenneke slug is solid, rather than hollow like the Foster slug, the Brenneke will generally deform less on impact and provide deeper penetration. The sharp shoulder and flat front of the Brenneke mean that its external ballistics restrict it to short range use, as it does not retain its velocity well.

The Brenneke slug is available in a number of normal shotgun calibres, but 12-bore and .410″ calibre are probably the most popular.

The Foster shotgun slug

The Foster slug was developed by Karl Foster in 1931. The defining characteristic of a Foster slug is the deep depression in the base, which places the centre of mass very near the tip of the slug – much like a shuttlecock. If the slug begins to tumble in flight, drag will tend to push it back into straight flight. This gives the Foster slug stability and allows for accurate shooting out to ranges of about 50–70 yards.

Foster slugs may also have rifling, which consists of 11–12 fins, either cast or swaged on the outside of the slug. Contrary to popular belief, these fins impart little or no spin to the slug as it travels through the air.

The actual purpose of the fins is to allow the slug to be safely swaged down when fired through a choked shotgun barrel, although accuracy will suffer when such a slug is fired through chokes tighter than improved cylinder. Cylinder choke is the one recommended for best use.

As with all shotgun slugs, it is possible to fire Foster slugs through a shotgun-slug[1] (i.e. rifled) barrel. It

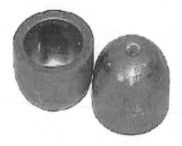

---

[1] A shotgun with rifling at the muzzle end of the barrel.

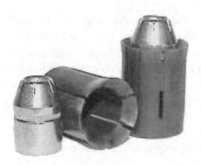

Figure 4.1.8   Saboted shotgun slug.

should be noted, however, that as the slug is not lubricated, leading of the rifled portion of the barrel becomes a great problem, necessitating regular cleaning to maintain any degree of accuracy.

The sabot slug (Figure 4.1.8)

The main characteristic of a sabot slug is the plastic carrier or sabot, which is of bore size, or sometimes a little larger, to enable the sabot to engage the rifling found in modern slug barrels.

The slugs contained in sabots can be anything up to .50″ calibre and are usually hollow pointed. Those for police use are usually of a solid hard metal alloy material for barricade penetration or door lock and hinge removal.

Although the sabot slug is used primarily in rifled barrels, some designs of sabot slugs can be fired in smooth-bore shotguns, most notably the Brenneke Rubin Sabot, a sub-calibre slug utilising the familiar Brenneke attached wad system.

The smaller projectile held within sabots will have a much flatter trajectory and will travel at much higher velocities than the more traditional Foster or rifled slug. When fired from a rifled barrel, saboted slugs will produce near-rifle type accuracy.

Another advantage of the sabot type of shotgun slug is that no lead comes into contact with the barrel, thus preventing lead fouling.

Penetration of Foster and sabot slugs

The following table gives an indication of the penetration potential of shotgun slugs. Penetration figures for normal shot are for comparison purposes. It is generally accepted by those involved in the wound ballistics field that a minimum penetration of 12 inches of ten per cent ordnance gelatine is one of the criteria needed to provide reliable incapacitation of a human assailant. When used in a police or Military situation, shotgun slugs are often used against hard targets.

To illustrate the penetration potential of shotgun slugs, tests were carried out using standard NATO 0.138″ steel test plates. The results are shown in Table 4.1.4. Buckshot loads are also shown for comparison purposes.

It is a common misconception that shotgun slugs have an extremely short range as well as a very poor trajectory. This is not quite true, although past 125 yards (114 m), the velocity and hence kinetic energy does drop off quite considerably

Currently there is a huge range of shotgun slugs available and more are being produced every day (see Figure 4.1.9).

Table 4.1.3   12-Gauge Penetration Tests in 10 per cent Gelatine

Load	Number of Pellets	Penetration at 7 Yards (6.4 m)
000 buck	8	14″–16″ (35–40 cm)
00 buck	9	13″–15″ (33–38 cm)
1 buck	16	12″–14″ (30–35 cm)
#4 buck	27	9″–11″ (23–28 cm)
#6 shot (copper-plated hard shot)	280	4″–6″ (10–15 cm)
1 oz Foster slug	–	18″ (46 cm)
450 g sabot slug	–	21″ (53 cm)

Table 4.1.4 12-Bore Penetration Tests Against SAE 1010 0.138″ NATO Steel Plate

Load	7 yd (6.4 m)	25 yd (23 m)
000 buck	N	N
00 buck	N	N
1 buck	N	N
4 buck	N	N
1 oz Foster slug	P	D
450 g sabot slug	P	P

P = Penetrated
D = Dented
N = No effect

Table 4.1.5 12g Foster Type Rifled Slug (20″ Barrelled Shotgun)

Range (Yards)	Velocity (ft/sec)	Zero = 75 Yards (Drop in Inches)	Zero = 100 Yards (Drop in Inches)
0	1440	−1.0	−1.0
25	1320	0.7	1.4
50	1200	1.1	2.5
75	1120	0	2.1
100	1050	−2.8	0
125	1000	−7.5	−4.0
150	960	−14.4	−10.2

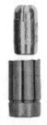
Remington Copper Solid Black Magic

Federal Barnes Expander

Lightfield Hybrid

Remington Buckhammer

Winchester Platinum Tip

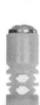
Hastings Magnum

Federal TrueBall

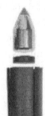
Hornady SST

Standard Brenneke with Felt Wad

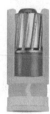
Brenneke Slug in Plastic Wad wth Plastic Base Wad

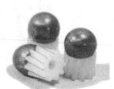
Round Ball with Rifled Plastic Base Wad

Figure 4.1.9 Different types of shotgun slugs.

Other types of specialised single-missile shotgun ammunition

These include the breaching or **Hatton** cartridge and tear gas rounds.

The Hatton round (Figure 4.1.10)

The Hatton round is made specifically for police or military use and is designed for the breaching of doorways. It is typically fired at a range of 4–6 inches, aimed between the doorknob and door jamb, with the intent of destroying the locking mechanism. It can also be used to remove the hinges in a similar way.

The missile is a single 12-bore, frangible slug weighing 770 grains (1.6 oz). The round is made of compressed zinc or lead powder bonded with hard wax. When fired, the full force of the round is delivered to the target, minimising the risk of injury to persons behind the door being opened. On impact, the missile breaks up into powder, thus removing any chance of ricochet.

These rounds will penetrate vehicle tyres, fire doors clad on both sides with metal plate, cell-type doors, 12 mm thick Makralon and bullet-proof glass from a range of 1.5 metres. Hatton ammunition can only be used in Magnum shotguns with three-inch chambers and unchoked barrels.

Steel slugs

There are also a number of all-steel sub-calibre saboted slugs. Examples include Russian 'Tandem' Wadcutter-type slug (the name is historical, as early versions consisted of two spherical steel balls), ogive 'UDAR' ('Strike') slugs and French spool-like 'Balle Blondeau' and 'Balle fleche Sauvestre' ('Sauvestre flechette') with steel sabot inside expanding copper body and plastic rear empennage. Made of non-deforming steel, said slugs are suitable for shooting in heavy undergrowth, but they may produce over-penetration. They also may be used for disabling vehicles by firing into the engine compartment, or for defeating hard body armour.

Plumbata slugs (Figure 4.1.11)

A plumbata slug is really a variation on a saboted slug and has a plastic stabiliser attached to the projectile. The stabiliser may be fitted into a cavity in the bottom of the slug, or it may fit over the slug and into external notches on the slug. With the first method, discarding sabots may be added. With the second, the stabiliser may act as a sabot, but it remains attached to the projectile and is commonly known as an 'Impact Discarding Sabot' (IDS).

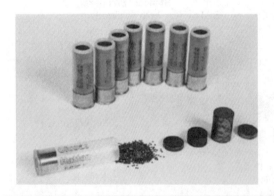

Figure 4.1.10 The Hatton breaching round.

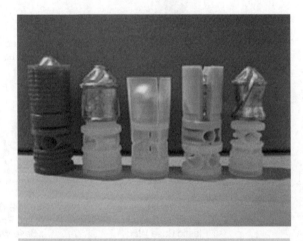

Figure 4.1.11 Examples of plumbata slugs.

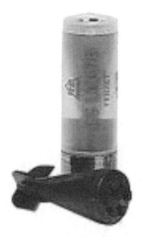

Figure 4.1.12 Ferret tear gas round 12-bore.

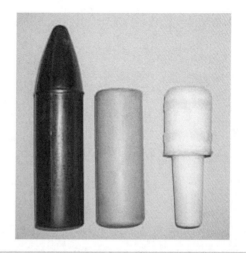

Figure 4.1.13 Various plastic and rubber baton missiles.

Tear gas ammunition – the ferret round (Figure 4.1.12)

This usually contains a finned, plastic bomblet-type missile filled with CS gas. The plastic comes in various grades, depending on the material being penetrated. These are only for police and military use.

Dragon's Breath

This is another highly specialised shotgun round, which contains a zirconium-based pyrotechnic material. When the round is fired, a huge flame erupts from the gun's barrel that can extend up to 300 feet. This is only for extremely specialised military use, as the effect it produces is similar to that of a short-ranged flamethrower.

Bean bag ammunition

Basically a nylon or Kevlar bag containing lead shot. For extremely short range, non-lethal, anti-personnel use.

Baton round (Figure 4.1.13)

A plastic or rubber missile designed to be ricocheted from the ground for crowd control.

Further reading

1 Hogg, I.V. (1985). *The Illustrated Encyclopedia of Ammunition*. London: The Apple Press. ISBN 1-85076-043-8.
2 *Small arms ammunition identification guide*. Revised edition (1971). Normount Technical Publications. ISBN-10: 0879471751
3 Hogg, I.V. (1982) *The Small Arms Ammunition Identification Manual*. Arms & Armour Press. ISBN-10: 0853684685.
4 Defense Intelligence Agency. *Small Calibre Ammunition Identification Guide. Volume 1: Small-Arms Cartridges Up to 15 mm*. Washington DCDirectorate For Scientific And Technical Intelligence.
5 Barnes, F.C. *Cartridges of the World: A Complete and Illustrated Reference*. Holt Bodinson.
6 http://smallboreshotgun.org/2009/01/26/shotgun-slugs-what-are-they-and-how-do-they-work/
7 http://www.chuckhawks.com/shotgun_slugs.htm

4.2

Bullet Types

4.2.1   Introduction

Despite it being a fairly simple topic to understand, there is a terrible amount of misunderstanding surrounding the subject of bullets, their designation and construction. For example, people often refer to hollow point bullets as 'dum-dum' bullets (which they are not) and talk about how they are banned for police use by the Hague Conventions of 1899 and 1907 (only related to military use, not civilian) and the Geneva Protocol of 1925 (which relates to the amelioration of prisoners and the use of chemical agents in time of war). The following will give an insight into this subject matter and, hopefully, dispel the majority of these misconstrued 'facts'.

4.2.2   Basics

Originally, a bullet was a simple lead sphere, and this worked well with the smooth-bored muzzle-loading early firearms. The sphere, however, is a very poor ballistic shape and it rapidly loses velocity. With the introduction of rifling came the ogival-shaped bullet (basically the profile of a pointed arch), which had a length in excess of twice its diameter. This provided an easily stabilised bullet with excellent accuracy and was a good shape for penetrating the air (i.e. a good ballistic profile).

4.2.3   Bullet materials

Modern ammunition comes with a bewildering variety of bullet profiles, materials and construction to cater for every conceivable circumstance. To attempt to cover all the available varieties is beyond the scope of this book. The following, however, covers the basic types of bullet which may be encountered.

In small arms ammunition, bullets are either jacketed or unjacketed. While unjacketed bullets can be made from all manner of materials, the most common by far is lead. The lead will be alloyed with varying quantities of antimony, to give it hardness, and tin (if it is a cast bullet) to assist in the moulding process. Molten lead-tin alloys expand on cooling, thus filling the mould in which they are made.

Plain lead bullets can be manufactured either by casting from molten metal or by being swaged from lead wire. In swaging, lead wire is cut into the appropriate length, then cold-forged with hydraulic pressure into a die with the correct dimensions and shape of the finished bullet. Nowadays, virtually all commercially manufactured lead bullets are swaged.

Jacketed bullets have a plain lead core covered with a thin layer of a much harder material. This can be a copper/zinc alloy (gilding metal), a copper/nickel alloy (cupronickel), or plain steel coated with either a copper wash or a thick coat of lacquer to

Forensic Ballistics in Court: Interpretation and Presentation of Firearms Evidence, First Edition. Brian J. Heard.
© 2013 John Wiley & Sons, Ltd. Published 2013 by John Wiley & Sons, Ltd.

prevent corrosion. Jacketed bullet are used for a variety of reasons: for better engagement with the rifling in high velocity bullets; to prevent bullet damage and feeding jams in weapons with a self-loading mechanism; and to prevent bullet break-up in hunting ammunition when used on heavy or thick-skinned game.

A variation on the jacketed bullet theme is to coat plain lead bullets with a thick layer of black nylon. This ammunition, called 'Nyclad', prevents lead fouling in the bore of the weapon, reduces lead contamination in ranges and is said to reduce friction with the bore thus enhancing velocity.

Ammunition with a wash of copper over the lead, known as 'luballoy' or 'golden bullets', is also available. This coating is intended to reduce the deposition of lead on the inside surface of the barrel. Lead deposition in the weapon's bore effectively reduces the internal diameter, giving rise to an increase in internal pressures and a loss of accuracy due to a drop in the efficiency of the rifling.

At one time, copper-washed bullets were quite popular, but nowadays this construction is unlikely to be found in calibres other than .22″ rimfire. This is probably due to the fact that the copper coating has been found to be no more effective than the much cheaper standard bullet lubricant made from paraffin wax and graphite.

To reduce lead contamination in ranges, ammunition is also manufactured with a thick coating of

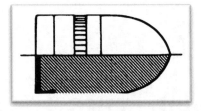

Figure 4.2.1   Round-nosed lead bullet with gas check.

copper electro-deposited over a plain lead core. As the surface coating is electro-deposited the jacket material extends over the whole surface of the bullet. This ammunition is very popular for training purposes, as there is no exposed lead surface on the bullet from which volatilisation can take place. As lead volatilised from the bullets base is the major source of lead contamination in ranges, this type of bullet construction can significantly reduce the health hazard due to lead contamination in heavily used ranges. This electro-plated deposition tends to be much harder than conventional copper/zinc jacket materials.

Gas checks are used when plain lead non-jacketed bullets are used in high velocity cartridges. This is to prevent the rifling from stripping the lead from the bullet, leading to a build-up of lead in the barrel that will decrease accuracy. These gas checks use small copper or gilding metal cups which are pressed onto the base of the bullet (Figure 4.2.1).

Illustrative Case 1

The author was asked for assistance in determining why the scores returned from the police force's twice-yearly range courses suddenly dropped from around a normal 85 per cent pass rate to 23 per cent. The force had recently changed from a normal copper/zinc jacketed bullet to one with an electroplated jacket. Tests carried out in the firearms laboratory showed there to be no difference between the accuracy of both types of bullet but, when the revolvers used for the range courses were examined, it was found that the rifling was appreciably shallower than would normally be expected.

It transpired that the revolvers had been used for range courses for many years and had fired tens, if not hundreds, of thousands of rounds of ammunition. This had virtually worn out the rifling. While bullets with a normally constructed jacket gripped the rifling perfectly well, the much harder electroplated jacketed bullets simply skidded down the bore and were not rotationally stabilised. This was graphically illustrated on the targets, with the holes caused by the electroplated bullets being elongated (keyholed), showing that the bullets were tumbling in flight. By simply rotating the revolvers used for the range courses on a regular basis, the problem was completely eliminated.

Alternatives to lead

Almost every imaginable material has been used at one time or another to replace lead. For example:

- Wood or compressed paper for bulleted blanks.

- Phosphor bronze or aluminium for lightweight, extremely high velocity bullets.

- Teflon-coated tungsten for metal-penetrating bullets.

- Compressed lead or iron dust for fairground gallery ranges.

- Plastic for short-range training.

- Magnesium for use as a signalling flare.

In addition to the above are the very many plain metals and alloys used for the production of 'nontoxic' bullets. These are dealt with in more detail in Chapter 4.5.

4.2.4 Other bullet types

Exploding bullets are available in most small arms calibres. These have a very large cavity in the nose, into which is placed a small amount of explosive material. A primer cup, with a small ball bearing to act as an anvil, is inserted backwards and used as a detonator.

Although they are more commonly encountered in military ammunition, **tracer bullets** are also available commercially. The bullets in these rounds have a very brightly burning chemical compound in the base, which permits observation of the bullet during its flight. Virtually all calibres are available, including 12-bore shotgun.

Military ammunition, especially in the larger calibres, can also be loaded with bullets containing **tear gas**, **incendiary** or **explosive** compounds. These can be identified by the coloured varnish round the case mouth.

4.2.5 Bullet nose configuration

Apart from the normal **round-nosed** configuration (Figure 4.2.1), properly called 'ogival', the list of bullet shapes is almost endless.

Some of the more common shapes include:

- **Wadcutter**: flat-nosed bullet with a sharp shoulder. Generally used by target shooters and designed to produce a clear cut punched out hole in the paper target (see Figure 4.2.2).

- **Spitzer**: a German term applied to an elongated ogival bullet with a sharp point.

Illustrative Case 2

The 1982 assassination attempt on the American President, Ronald Reagan, was made using .22″ calibre explosive bullets. While the bullets did not explode, they did cause considerable tissue damage to the President and the explosive material in the nose of the bullet caused serious poisoning-type symptoms.

Illustrative Case 3

A case to illustrate the dangers of tracer ammunition involved a husband who vented his frustrations with his wife by shooting his bedroom wardrobe (!) with a 12-bore shotgun. Unfortunately, the round he fired contained a tracer pellet, which set light to the wardrobe and then the house. His only comment when being questioned by the police in front of the wreckage of his home was, "But I only shot the door once!"

- **Soft-point or semi-jacketed**: a jacketed bullet with the jacket cut back at the nose to reveal the lead core.

- **Hollow point**: generally a semi-jacketed bullet, the nose of which has a cavity. This is designed to expand on impact with soft targets, thus increasing the wounding effect of the bullet (see Figure 4.2.3).

- **Dum-dum**: a .303″ rifle bullet design developed in the Indian arsenal of Dum-Dum in 1894. This initially consisted of a standard .303″ rifle bullet which had the front of the metal jacket trimmed back to expose the lead core. It was designed to expand rapidly on impact, causing a massive wound, and it was first used against the 'savage tribesmen' at the battle of Omdurman in 1898. Although it was very effective, it did have one major drawback: as the modified bullet was a standard .303″ bullet with the lead core exposed at the base, there was a tendency for the lead core to be blown out of the jacket, making it all but impossible to load the next round. This was rectified by the Mk. III bullet, which had a jacket completely covering the base of the bullet. A hole was bored in the nose of the bullet and a short metal tube was inserted into this to increase expansion. In 1899, the Hague Convention outlawed this type of bullet in military service. However, it should be noted here that the Hague Convention is not applicable to civilian applications, and police forces are not restricted by any military conventions in the type of bullets they can use. The term 'dum-dum' is often misused to denote hollow point bullets.

- **Rifled slug**: a generally plain lead (but can also be steel and lead or plain steel) projectile for use in smooth-bored shotguns. To impart spin (and therefore stability) to the projectile, wing-like helical ribs are formed on the outside surface. It is generally intended for use against large, soft-skinned game, such as deer, but it is also used by police and security forces against cars and for taking the locks from doors.

- **Saboted bullet**: a sub-calibre (i.e. smaller than the bore of the weapon) bullet surrounded by a lightweight sheath, generally of plastic, which is discarded as soon as the missile leaves the barrel. By using a smaller, much lighter, bullet in a larger barrel, exceedingly high velocities can be obtained. While most calibres have been manufactured, only the larger rifle calibres have ever become popular, and these are generally referred to by the trade name 'Accelerator'. Solid steel saboted missiles are available in 12-bore shotgun calibre for penetrating cars, but this type of ammunition is generally restricted to police and security forces.

- **Flechette**: a thin, nail-like missile, stabilised by fins. Originally designed as extremely high velocity single projectile saboted loadings for rifles developed by the US military in the 1950s, they proved to be rather inaccurate and unreliable. Multiple missile loadings in 12-bore shotgun cartridges proved to be much more satisfactory, and this version is in general use with the US Army as the 12-bore Close Assault Weapon.

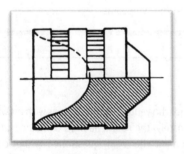

Figure 4.2.2   Wadcutter bullet.

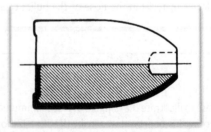

Figure 4.2.3   Round-nosed jacketed hollow point bullet.

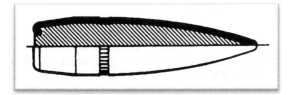

Figure 4.2.4 Boat-tailed or streamlined bullet.

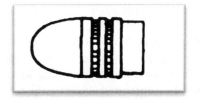

Figure 4.2.5 Heeled bullet with outside lubrication.

4.2.6 Bullet base configuration

While most small arms bullets have a base which is the same diameter as the body, long-range rifle bullets have the rear section of the bullet tapered. This is to reduce base drag and is referred to either as a '**boat-tailed bullet**' (US nomenclature) or a '**streamlined bullet**' (British nomenclature). (see Figure 4.2.4) These bullets are generally military, but can also be encountered in commercial long-range hunting ammunition.

A '**heeled bullet**' is one in which the rear portion of the bullet, which fits into the cartridge case, is reduced so that the case diameter is the same as the driving surface of the bullet (see Figure 4.2.5). This type of bullet is now only encountered in .22″ rimfire ammunition, but in the past virtually all revolver ammunition was of this type.

4.2.7 Bullet lubrication

Plain lead bullets must have some type of lubrication on their outside surface to reduce friction with the bore. Jacketed bullets do not generally require any form of lubrication.

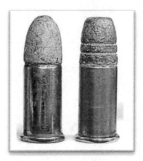

Figure 4.2.6 Inside lubricated bullet compared with an outside lubricated bullet.

Lead bullet lubricant generally contains a mixture of Vaseline, beeswax and graphite, although modern silicone-based waxes are being used to a certain extent.

In modern ammunition, the lubricant is held in a plain or knurled groove round the bullet, called a cannelure, which is generally located on the portion of the bullet inside the cartridge case. This is called an '**inside lubricated bullet**'; it makes the round cleaner to handle and it prevents the grease from picking up pieces of grit and

---

Illustrative Case 4

One example of how important bullet lubrication is involved the purchase of 10,000,000 rounds of revolver ammunition by a police force. The brand chosen was not one of the most well known, but they did advertise their bullets as having 'a state of the art lubricant'.

Unfortunately, it was found that after the first ten or so rounds through a weapon, it became increasingly difficult to hit the target, and after 50 rounds, the bullets were not even coming out of the barrel at all. The so-called 'state of the art lubricant' was an exceedingly thin smear of varnish which had next to no lubrication value. With each round fired, lead was being stripped from the bullet and was welding itself to the inside of the bore. After 50 rounds, there was so little of the bore open that the bullets stuck in the barrel.

other material which might damage to the bore of the weapon.

In older ammunition, the grease is either in a cannelure outside of the case or is applied to the whole exposed area of the bullet. This is called an **'outside lubricated bullet'** (Figure 4.2.6). Apart from .22″ rimfire ammunition, this type of lubrication system is hardly ever encountered nowadays.

Further reading

1 Hogg, I.V. (1982). *The Cartridge Guide*. London/Melbourne, Arms and Armour Press. ISBN 13:9780853684688.
2 Labbett, P. (1980). *Military Small Arms Ammunition of the World*. London/Melbourne, Arms and Armour Press.
3 Brandt, J. & Erlmeier, H. (1967). *Manual of Pistol and Revolver Cartridges*. Verlag Wiesbaden, Germany.

4.3

Headstamps and Other Identifying Features on Ammunition

4.3.1 Introduction

Headstamps are a series of letters, numerals and symbols stamped into the head of a cartridge case during its manufacture. The examination and interpretation of these marks is, potentially, a very important subject, as it enables the determination of the ammunition's country of origin, whether it is of commercial or military manufacture and, if military, the date of manufacture. In some cases, the marking will reveal what type of priming compound, propellant and missile is present, and what material the cartridge case has been fashioned from. While this may seem to be of minor importance, such information can be vital in cases involving terrorism.

In certain cases, it can also assist in eliminating a suspect, as the following illustrates.

Illustrative Case 1

A man and a wife were found dead in a cabin far off the beaten track. Both had been killed by a single .22″ shot to the head at a distance greater than three feet (1 m). No suspect, fired cartridge cases or weapon could be located. However, several years later, two fired and corroded cartridge cases were found a short distance from the cabin. A suspect was eventually located and, although no weapon could be found, several fired cartridge cases were found in the vicinity of his home. These were found to have been fired in the same weapon as those found at the scene. The suspect was charged with the double murder and convicted. However, a review of the case by an independent firearms examiner found that the headstamps on the cartridge cases found at the scene were not in production at the time of the murder. It was also evident that the man convicted of the killings had used the area for hunting small game and that the located cartridge must have been from one of his hunting expeditions. He was released from jail on appeal.

This whole case rested on the fact that fired cartridge cases found at the scene years after the incident were linked to those found in and around the suspect's house. The firearm itself could not be located, as it had been sold on several times. If the ammunition had been carefully examined in the first instance, it would have been obvious that it had not lain in the ground for many years. It would have also been obvious that it was not in manufacture at the time of the incident. These were serious failures, primarily by the firearms examiner but also by the defence for not looking more deeply into the case.

Forensic Ballistics in Court: Interpretation and Presentation of Firearms Evidence, First Edition. Brian J. Heard.
© 2013 John Wiley & Sons, Ltd. Published 2013 by John Wiley & Sons, Ltd.

4.3.2 Basics

The interpretation of these markings alone could fill several volumes and many books have been written on the identification of 'headstamps'.

Basically, the headstamp is a series of marks, letters and/or numbers impressed upon the base of the cartridge by the manufacturer to indicate the calibre and by whom it was manufactured.

Commercial ammunition usually contains little more information in the headstamp other than to show the maker and calibre. The date of manufacture is rarely, if ever, included in commercial ammunition headstamps. Often, the only way in which this information can be obtained is from the packaging material (i.e. the box) in which the ammunition was supplied.

The advertising value of a cartridge headstamp has been recognised for a long time. As a result, many firearms dealers will have ammunition marked with their own name or trademark. Under these circumstances, it is very difficult to ascertain the actual manufacturer.

With large volume users of ammunition, such as police forces, it is possible, at very little extra cost, to have marking included on the headstamp that not only identifies the force, but also the batch number for the ammunition. Such information can be vital for those cases where stolen police ammunition has been used in a crime. It can also greatly assist where there has been an exchange of fire and it is necessary to determine who fired and from where.

Military ammunition is much more informative than commercial ammunition. If one can understand the system of letters and numbers, details such as the calibre, year and month of manufacture, batch number, cartridge case material and bullet type (e.g. tracer, incendiary, armour-piercing, etc.) can be ascertained.

Military ammunition usually has its headstamp applied to a rigid set of rules, with each country rarely deviating from the official pattern. It is thus often possible to identify the source of the ammunition without needing to be able to decipher the headstamp itself. Another identifier of ammunition with a military origin is that, almost without exception, the year of manufacture will be included in the code system.

One anomaly with respect to military ammunition is Japan. Up until 1945, only the Japanese Navy headstamped their ammunition; all the rest were bereft of any markings. When deciphering post-1945 Japanese headstamps, it should be remembered that the Japanese calendar was used for the year markings – thus, the Japanese year 2600 relates to the Western year 1940.

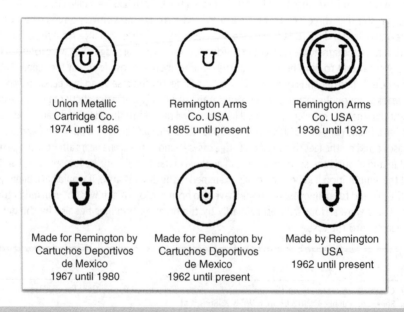

Union Metallic
Cartridge Co.
1974 until 1886

Remington Arms
Co. USA
1885 until present

Remington Arms
Co. USA
1936 until 1937

Made for Remington by
Cartuchos Deportivos
de Mexico
1967 until 1980

Made for Remington by
Cartuchos Deportivos
de Mexico
1962 until present

Made by Remington
USA
1962 until present

Figure 4.3.1   .22″ calibre headstamps.

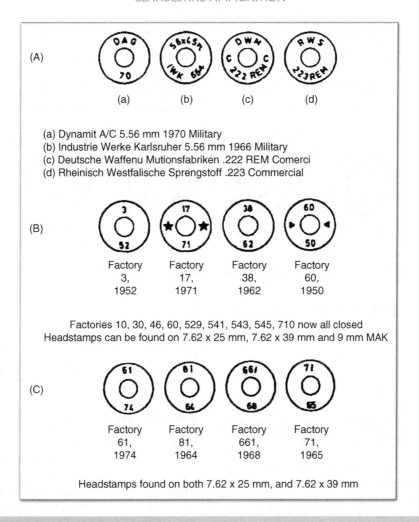

(a) Dynamit A/C 5.56 mm 1970 Military
(b) Industrie Werke Karlsruher 5.56 mm 1966 Military
(c) Deutsche Waffenu Mutionsfabriken .222 REM Comerci
(d) Rheinisch Westfalische Sprengstoff .223 Commercial

| Factory 3, 1952 | Factory 17, 1971 | Factory 38, 1962 | Factory 60, 1950 |

Factories 10, 30, 46, 60, 529, 541, 543, 545, 710 now all closed
Headstamps can be found on 7.62 x 25 mm, 7.62 x 39 mm and 9 mm MAK

| Factory 61, 1974 | Factory 81, 1964 | Factory 661, 1968 | Factory 71, 1965 |

Headstamps found on both 7.62 x 25 mm, and 7.62 x 39 mm

Figure 4.3.2   Examples of headstamps: (A) German (B) USSR (C) China.

Taiwan has its own calendar system based on 1912, the year which signalled the end of dynastic China and the formation of the Republic of China.

Mexico also uses 1912 as the starting point for its headstamps, this being the year of the Mexican Revolution.

4.3.3   Clandestine ammunition

In cases of insurgency or irregular warfare, friendly nations will often attempt to hide their part in the supply of arms and ammunition. Obviously, fired and live ammunition recovered after an incident is a potentially valuable source of information as to the other side's supporters.

Broadly, there are three methods which are used to disguise the origins of the ammunition:

• Complete omission of the headstamp.

• Omit all but the date or code identifying the date.

• The use of a completely false manufacturer's code.

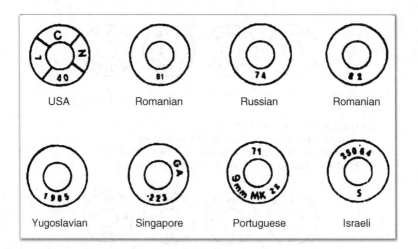

Figure 4.3.3   Some examples of clandestine ammunition and their origins.

Some examples of clandestine ammunition include:

- Ammunition smuggled into Ireland in 1914 for the use of the IRA.

- Ammunition supplied to General Franco during the Spanish Civil War.

- British manufactured ammunition supplied to the Norwegian underground during WWII.

- Ammunition supplied by the USA for use in the Bay of Pigs operation in Cuba.

- Brazil supplying Argentina during the Falklands war.

4.3.4   Colour coding of ammunition

In addition to the headstamp, military ammunition often has some form of colour coding, in the form of bands of coloured lacquer round the bullet, a stripe across the bullet/case joint or around the joint between the primer and cartridge case (primer annulus). Caution should be exercised when attempting to identify the stripe of colour round the bullet/case joint or the primer annulus, as this is often no more than a waterproofing varnish. As a general rule, if there is no coloured varnish on the bullet, then it is a standard ball (military nomenclature for standard bullet) round.

Examples of the coloured lacquer used by various countries and its significance follows.

China

Originally, China used the Russian system of colour coding as their ammunition was originally supplied from this source. In 1967, however, China adopted her own system as follows:

Bullet tip code

Green	Tracer
Black & red	Armour piercing/incendiary – pre-1967
Black	Armour piercing/incendiary – post-1967
Violet & red	Armour piercing/incendiary/ tracer – pre-1967
Violet	Armour piercing/incendiary/ tracer – post-1967
Red	Incendiary
White	Mild steel bullet core – pre-1967

Israel

Bullet tip	Primer annulus	Bullet type
None	Purple	Ball
Red	Green	Tracer
Black	Green	Armour piercing
Black	Red	Armour piercing/ incendiary
Blue	Green	Incendiary

United Kingdom (prior to formation of NATO in 1955)

Primer annulus

Purple	Ball or Practice
Green	Armour Piercing
Red	Tracer
Blue	Incendiary
Yellow	Proof (a special high pressure cartridge)
Black	Observation

Bullet tip

Blue	Incendiary
Black	Observation
Green	Armour Piercing
White	Short Range Tracer
Grey	Dark Ignition Tracer
Red	Long Range Tracer

USA

7.62 × 51 mm ammunition	uses NATO code
.30″ Carbine and .45″ ACP	Red tip for tracer
.50″ Browning machine gun	NATO code plus:

Red tip silver band	Armour piercing /incendiary /tracer
Yellow tip red band	Observation/tracer
Brown tip	Tracer
Light blue tip	Incendiary

NATO countries

All NATO Countries use the same bullet tip colour coding system:

Red	Tracer
Black	Armour piercing
Silver	Armour piercing/incendiary
Blue	Incendiary

Yellow	Observation (a bright flash and smoke on impact)
Yellow/red	Observation/tracer
Orange	Dark ignition tracer

USSR

In the 1930s, the colour coding was very poor, but during and after the 1939–45 war it was regularised and expanded. The following bullet tip colour code system is now standard for all Warsaw Pact countries.

Yellow	Heavy ball
Silver	Light ball
Green	Tracer
Black	Armour piercing
Black/red	Armour piercing/incendiary (now obsolete)
Black/yellow	Armour piercing/incendiary (current)
Purple/red	Armour piercing/incendiary/tracer
Red	Incendiary/tracer
Black/green	Reduced velocity for silenced weapons

Further reading

1 *Military Cartridge Headstamps Collectors' Guide*. Charles Conklin Heritage Books. ISBN-10: 0788441175.

2 White, H.P. & Munhall Burton. D.H.P. (1963). *Cartridge Headstamp Guide*. White Laboratory. ASIN: B003WVQWTM

3 Curtis, L.E.III (1998). *9 mm Parabellum Headstamp and Case Type Guide, Volume I: Headstamps A–F;*First Edition. GiG Concepts, Inc. ASIN: B003D6ALT8.

4 White, H.P. (1963). *Cartridge Headstamp Guide*. White Laboratory. ASIN: B0000EGNUT.

5 Barnes, F.C. (2009) *Cartridges of the World: A Complete and Illustrated Reference for Over 1500 Cartridges;*12th Revised edition. KP Books. ISBN-10: 0896899365.

6 Hogg, I.V. (1982). *The Cartridge Guide*. London/Melbourne, Arms and Armour Press. ISBN 13: 9780853684688.

4.4

Non-toxic and Frangible Bullets

4.4.1 Introduction

Ingestion of lead has been a problem among those involved in firearms training facilities for many years. In indoor ranges, whatever extraction systems are in place, it is particularly serious due to the inherent confines of such a range. Even outdoor ranges, despite their open environment, still present a problem due to the proximity of the trainer to the trainee.

Lead poisoning (also known as plumbism, colica Pictonum, saturnism, Devon colic, or painter's colic) is a medical condition caused by increased levels of the heavy metal lead in the body. Lead interferes with a variety of body processes and is toxic to many organs and tissues, including the heart, bones, intestines and kidneys, as well as the reproductive and nervous systems. Symptoms include abdominal pain, confusion, headache, anaemia, irritability and, in severe cases, seizures, coma, and death.

The main tool for diagnosis is measurement of the blood lead level. When blood lead levels are recorded, the results indicate how much lead is circulating within the blood stream, not the amount being stored in the body. There are two units for reporting blood lead level – either micrograms per decilitre (μg/dl), or micrograms per 100 grams (μg/100 g) of whole blood, which are both numerically equivalent. The Centre for Disease Control has set the standard elevated blood lead level for adults to be 25 (μg/dl) of the whole blood.

Anyone working in a firearms laboratory or range facility who fires weapons on a regular basis will be subjected to increased blood lead levels. This increase is not just though inhaling the micron-sized lead particles, but also through ingestion after becoming contaminated through handling lead-covered clothing and firearms.

There have been a significant number of claims by firearms laboratory personnel, range instructors, range cleaners and others working with or using firearms, and it is conceivable that this will continue.

The (US) National Bureau of Standards claims that 80 per cent of airborne lead on firing ranges comes from the projectile, while the remaining 20 per cent comes from the combustion of the lead styphnate primer mixture.

4.4.2 Elimination of lead in ammunition

In the early 1980s, a determined move was made towards eliminating this health hazard, especially at training facilities and indoor ranges.

The first step in this process was to eliminate the lead in the priming mixture and, as a result, most ammunition manufacturers now retail a line of ammunition with a non-lead-based priming compound. However, the problem of lead being torn off a plain lead bullet as it passed down the bore and lead being volatilised from the base in normally jacketed bullets still existed, with concomitant toxic levels of lead in the air.

Forensic Ballistics in Court: Interpretation and Presentation of Firearms Evidence, First Edition. Brian J. Heard.
© 2013 John Wiley & Sons, Ltd. Published 2013 by John Wiley & Sons, Ltd.

To counter this, manufacturers produced a totally jacketed bullet (TMJ), which had a thick coating of gilding metal electroplated over the lead core. However, as the bullet core was still made from lead, then, on impacting with the butts, it would disintegrate, leading to the release of large quantities of lead dust. As a non-toxic training round, TMJ bullets were not entirely successful.

The obvious answer was to follow the example of non-toxic shotgun ammunition and utilise a frangible and/or totally non-toxic bullet, using materials other than lead in the production of the bullet. As a result, virtually every major ammunition manufacturer now has a line of frangible and/or non-toxic small arms ammunition.

There appears, however, to be some confusion between frangible ammunition and non-toxic ammunition. To delineate between these two rounds, it must be understood that while frangible ammunition may be loaded with non-toxic materials, frangible projectiles completely turn to powder upon impact with any surface that is harder than the bullet itself. However, non-toxic projectiles can ricochet or splash back, akin to a conventional bullet.

4.4.3 Materials used in non-toxic ammunition

Many alternative substances are presently being used in the manufacture of frangible or non toxic ammunition, for example: iron powder; zinc; tungsten; combinations of nylon, zinc, and/or tin coupled with tungsten; bismuth; copper; and bullets containing steel cores.

While copper and steel both have the desired weight factor, these bullets are much harder than lead, causing a serious ricochet factor or bullets which may return back down the line of flight to the firing line.

In soft tissue, a frangible bullet performs in exactly the same way as a full metal jacketed bullet, which clearly makes it a lethal round. Frangible ammunition is, however, an ideal round to use on indoor ranges, due to the elimination of ricochets and splash back.

Frangible bullets have been in production since 1845, in the form of compressed iron or lead dust. These were designed for use in the Flobert indoor

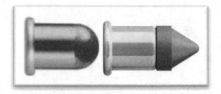

Figure 4.4.1   .22″ calibre BC Cap and BB Cap ammunition.

target ranges and were fired from rimfire weapons known as 'saloon' or 'parlour' pistols and rifles. The rounds were designated CB (conical ball) Cap and BB (bulleted breech) Cap, and they were generally .22″ (6 mm Flobert in Europe) calibre (see Figure 4.4.1).

In 1975, Glazer Co. introduced the Glazer Safety Slug. This was simply a gilding metal jacket filled with No. 12 birdshot (0.05″). The voids between the shot were filled with Teflon, and a flat polymer cap sealed the front end of the casing. To improve ballistic performance, a polymer-tipped ball round was introduced in 1987. The current compressed core form was first sold in 1988. The formation of the polymer was also changed in 1994 to improve fragmentation reliability.

On hitting the target, the jacket broke open, distributing the shot inside the target. It was thus a non-ricocheting round, which completely removed any chance of over-penetration. However, being filled with lead shot, it was hardly non-toxic.

4.4.4 The current situation

As with non-toxic lead shot, frangible and non-toxic bullets are areas of intense research, and the development of new combinations of binding agents and metals is ongoing, with new combinations being released on virtually a weekly basis.

Some examples of the currently available non-toxic and frangible bullets follow.

Blount/Speer ZNT

These rounds are made with lead-free primers and feature a newly designed projectile. This projectile has a fluted copper jacket combined with a cast zinc alloy core, and it is designed to break into small pieces upon impact with steel targets, backstops or other similar objects.

Delta Frangible Ammunition, LLC

Delta Frangible Ammunition (DFA) produces a line of frangible cartridges utilising a nylon composite bullet. The nylon projectile will break apart into small pieces upon impact with hard surfaces, resulting in the reduced penetration of objects which are not intended to be penetrated.

DFA also has a reduced ricochet potential, reduced maximum range capability, and eliminates airborne lead contamination and lead-contaminated environments.

Currently, DFA provides these bullets, which are then loaded and distributed by Winchester for law enforcement use only.

Longbow, Inc

Longbow's frangible bullet is made of a polymer-copper compound. This is claimed to eliminate ricochet and splash back completely, and to be non-toxic.

Remington Arms Co., Inc

Remington manufactures a lead-free frangible called the Disintegrator™. The Disintegrator's lead-free bullet design provides instant and complete break-up upon impact, with no ricochet or lead accumulation. Furthermore, the totally lead-free primer eliminates the hazards of airborne lead residue in enclosed ranges. Point of impact and recoil performance reportedly duplicates that of equivalent standard duty ammunition.

Blount Clean-Fire® Ammunition

While Blount's Clean-Fire ammunition is not totally non-toxic or lead-free, it does eliminate airborne lead

with a totally metal jacketed bullet. It also has a priming mixture that contains no lead, barium, antimony or other toxic metals.

Federal Cartridge Company BallistiClean®

This ammunition uses a copper-jacketed, zinc core bullet, a non toxic copper-coloured primer and is loaded in brass cases headstamped 'NT'. The primer mix is of particular interest as it contains no heavy metals or toxic metals. Instead, the primer mix contains diazodinitrophenol (DDNP) as the primary explosive instead of lead styphnate. Furthermore, the oxidiser is calcium silicate instead of barium and strontium compounds. This round is reportedly the first line of ammunition to be developed that is completely free of toxic metals.

Winchester® Ammunition Super Clean NT

Winchester has introduced a new line of training ammunition called 'Super Clean NT', using tin instead of the zinc that is used in frangible ammunition. The bullets are a jacketed soft point type, non-toxic and lead-free, and they are specifically designed to eliminate pollution from lead dust. Additionally, they are loaded with a primer that is lead-free and does not contain heavy metals.

Winchester has also introduced a new clean centre fire pistol ammunition, primarily designed for indoor ranges, called 'WinClean'. WinClean incorporates Winchester's latest generation primer, which is lead-free and heavy-metal-free. The cartridge features a TMJ bullet.

Remington UMC Leadless

Remington now offers UMC leadless pistol and revolver ammunition. The bullet, of a flat-nose enclosed base (FNEB) design, prevents the hot expanding propellant gases from vaporising lead from the bullet's base.

FrangibleBullets.com

FrangibleBullets.com projectiles are manufactured using a compressed copper/tin powdered metal. The bullets are then heat-treated in a nitrogen furnace and then tumble polished. This results in a non-lead bullet with no jacket or core.

AccuTec USA

This manufacturer produces RRLP Ultra Frangible bullets which are composed of a tungsten polymer mix, and R2X2 Ultra Frangible, which are made from a copper polymer mix.

Sinter Fire Ammunition

A range of copper/tin-based frangible non-toxic bullets containing a 'dry lubricant'. The Cu/Sn sintered powder is compressed, then heated in an inert atmosphere.

Other non-toxic bullets

THV

The French Très Haute Vitesse (THV) was a bullet made from phosphor bronze (see Figure 4.4.2). Intended as an ultra-high-velocity metal penetrating round, it was, however, essentially a non-toxic bullet. The primer was of the normal lead styphnate type.

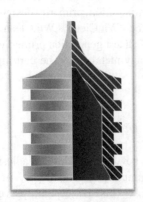

Figure 4.4.2 THV bullet.

Chinese 7.62 × 25 mm pistol round

Up until about 1985, the standard 7.62 × 25 mm round consisted of a very heavily copper-coated steel jacket surrounding a lead core. After that date, the military changed its specification to a sold steel bullet with a copper wash. There was no copper or gilding metal gas check to take up the rifling, merely two raised bands of steel about 1 mm high and 1 mm across. After 50 rounds, the rifling of the Type 54 pistol, which this round was intended to be used in, completely disappears.

While this bullet is 'non-toxic', it was introduced simply to save on manufacturing costs. The primer, however, was definitely not non-toxic and it often contained mercury.

KTW

In the mid-1970s, KTW brought out a range of metal-penetrating rounds, including .357 Magnum, .30 carbine, 9 mm PB and .380 ACP. Originally, the bullets were made from sintered tungsten and were coated in bright green Teflon to enhance the penetration. To prevent barrel wear and to take up the rifling, there was a gas check on the base of the bullet. In the late 1980s, the tungsten was replaced with a hardened phosphor bronze. Once again, the bullet was coated in green Teflon. While this round was intended for metal penetrating, it was, essentially, non-toxic. The primer, however, was not, as it contained lead styphnate.

Further reading

1 *US Military "Green Bullet" Association of Firearm and Tool Mark Examiners Journal* 31 Number 4, Don Mikko.
2 http://www.startribune.com/sports/outdoors/blogs/5169 1207.html
3 *ICC Ammunition Non-Toxic and Frangible Bullets.* www.iccammo.com/frangible.htm
4 *Barnes Non-Toxic Bullets* www.barnesbullets.com
5 Thomas, V.G. *The Policy and Legislative Dimensions of Non-toxic Shot and Bullet Use in North America.* http://www.peregrinefund.org/subsites/conference-lead/PDF/0311 per cent20Thomas.pdf

4.5

Non-toxic Shot

4.5.1 Introduction

In the USA, lead shot has been recognised as posing a threat to waterfowl since 1874. Attempts to phase out lead shot began in the 1970s, but a nationwide ban on lead shot for all waterfowl hunting was not implemented until 1991. Canada and the UK instituted a complete ban on the use of lead shot in 1999, with France following in 2006.

When comparing shot patterns for range of firing estimations, so many different materials and alloys exist that the exact make of cartridge, length of cartridge and loading, in addition to the type of shot and its size, must be used. Any attempt to compare shot patterns with anything other than the exact same cartridge as that used in the crime would be completely useless.

Range of firing can be crucial in determining whether a shooting incident was an accident, self-inflicted or an attempt to snatch the gun away from the holder. However, any attempt at estimating the range of firing (which can be accomplished to quite a high degree of accuracy) without knowing the exact cartridge type and what type of pellet composition it was loaded with is doomed to failure. Even the wads that the cartridge was loaded with can lead to quite dramatic differences in the patterns produced at various ranges.

4.5.2 Materials used in non-toxic shotgun ammunition

Steel shot

The first, and probably still the most common, alternative non-toxic substitute for lead was soft steel shot.

While soft steel shot is relatively cheap to produce, it is only about 70 per cent as dense as lead and, as a result, pellets of the same size differ considerably in the amount of energy they deliver at the target. Another problem is the number of pellets that can be fitted into a cartridge of a given size. This problem is, however, largely offset due to the fact that steel shot is considerably harder than lead, so does not require such thick cushion wads to reduce deformation on firing.

Soft steel shot, despite its name, has a deleterious effect on the bore of the weapon it is fired in. This is especially so at the muzzle end of the barrel, where the shot column is compressed. This appears as peening (dimpling) of the choked area. Many barrels are now provided with a hardened area towards the muzzle end of the barrel and are so marked as being suitable for steel shot.

Lead shot, which is easily deformed upon firing, develops a relatively long, large-diameter shot string. However, as steel shot is three times harder than lead, it deform less on firing and develops a shot string that is 50–60 per cent shorter and 60–70 per cent

Forensic Ballistics in Court: Interpretation and Presentation of Firearms Evidence, First Edition. Brian J. Heard.
© 2013 John Wiley & Sons, Ltd. Published 2013 by John Wiley & Sons, Ltd.

Table 4.5.1 Chart Showing the Number of Pellets per Ounce for Various Sizes of Steel and Lead

Size	Diameter	Pellets per Oz – Lead	Pellets per Oz – Steel
BBB	.190″ (4.83 mm)	No equivalent lead pellet	62
BB	.180″ (4.57 mm)	50	72
1	.160″ (4.06 mm)	81	103
2	.150″ (3.81 mm)	87	125
3	.140″ (3.56 mm)	108	158
4	.130″ (3.30 mm)	135	192
5	.120″ (3.05 mm)	170	243
6	.110″ (2.79 mm)	225	315

Table 4.5.2 Comparisons of the Various Densities for Some of the Non-Toxic Shot Compositions with that of Lead

Steel	7.86 grams/cc
Hevi-Steel®	9.06 grams/cc
Bismuth	9.60 grams/cc
Tungsten/iron	10.30 grams/cc
Tungsten matrix	10.60 grams/cc
Lead	**11.10 grams/cc**
Hevi-Shot®	12.0 grams/cc
Tungsten/iron/bronze (HD Shot®)	12.0 grams/cc

narrower than lead. This can be crucial in determining the range at which the shot was fired from the diameter and density of the pattern.

From the patterns shown in Figure 4.5.1, it can be seen that:

- The steel-pelleted load gives a shot pattern that is 60–70 per cent narrower than the lead pellets.

- The steel-pelleted load gives a shot string that is 50–60 per cent shorter than the lead pellets.

Other alternatives to lead

The list of other materials used or under review is exhaustive, and many more are likely to follow in the future. At present, the following are just some of those either used or currently being considered:

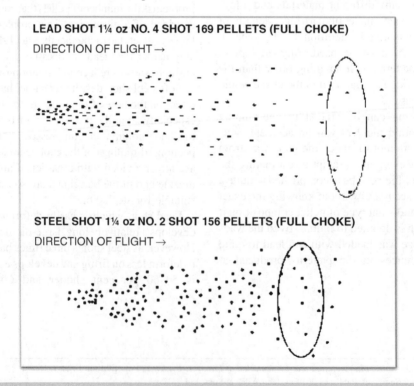

LEAD SHOT 1¼ oz NO. 4 SHOT 169 PELLETS (FULL CHOKE)

DIRECTION OF FLIGHT →

STEEL SHOT 1¼ oz NO. 2 SHOT 156 PELLETS (FULL CHOKE)

DIRECTION OF FLIGHT →

Figure 4.5.1 Comparison of shot strings for lead and steel shot.

1. Soft steel (often copper coated to reduce corrosion)

2. Iron-scrap-tungsten (Hevi-Steel®)

3. Bismuth-tin

4. Bismuth-tin-copper

5. Tungsten-iron

6. Tungsten-iron-bronze (Remington HD Shot®)

7. Tungsten polymer

8. Sintered tungsten-nylon

9. Tungsten matrix

10. Tungsten-bronze

11. Tungsten-nickel-iron

12. Tungsten-tin-bismuth

13. Tungsten-tin-iron-nickel (Hevi-shot®)

14. Nitro-steel (zinc galvanised steel) – Remington

An impression of the relative shot sizes that must be used to generate the same ballistics with various non-toxic alternatives to lead can be appreciated from Table 4.5.3.

Table 4.5.3 Ballistically Equivalent Shot Types and Common Factory Load Parameters

Material	Shot No.	Density (g/cc)	Load (oz.)	Velocity @3ft. (ft/sec)
Steel	BB	7.86	$1\frac{1}{2}$	1,375
Bismuth	2	9.6	$1\frac{5}{8}$	1,250
Tungsten-iron	3	10.3	$1\frac{1}{8}$	1,400
Tungsten-matrix	4	10.8	$1\frac{5}{8}$	1,330
Tungsten-poly	4	10.7	$1\frac{3}{8}$	1,330
Lead	**3**	**11.34**	**$1\frac{5}{8}$**	**1,350**
Hevi-Shot®	5	12.0	$1\frac{1}{2}$	1,375

Table 4.5.4 No. 4 Pellet Performance

Shot Type	Yards	Velocity (fps)	Energy (ft. lbs.)	Penetration (in.) in Ballistic Gel
Hevi-Shot®	20	1,023	8.13	3.63
	40	799	4.95	2.64
	60	647	3.25	1.95
Tungsten matrix	20	986	6.56	3.02
	40	749	3.80	2.12
	60	594	2.39	1.53
Tungsten iron	20	981	6.45	2.97
	40	745	3.72	2.08
	60	590	2.33	1.49
Bismuth	20	962	5.79	2.71
	40	721	3.25	1.86
	60	563	1.99	1.30
Lead	**20**	**1,001**	**7.16**	**3.26**
	40	**770**	**4.25**	**2.33**
	60	**616**	**2.72**	**1.70**
Steel	20	906	4.17	2.04
	40	647	2.13	1.30
	60	485	1.19	.83

For comparison purposes, the velocity has been adjusted to 1,350 fps.

Table 4.5.5 The Much Higher Velocity Attained by Steel Pellets, as Readily Demonstrated by a Comparison of Various Commercial Bismuth, Tungsten and Lead Loads

Manufacturer	Velocity	Number of Pellets
Winchester		
Bismuth BBs $1\frac{5}{8}$ oz.	1267 ft/sec	81
Bismuth No. 2 shot $1\frac{5}{8}$ oz.	1246 ft/sec	138
Federal		
Tungsten BBs $1\frac{1}{8}$ oz.	1358 ft/sec	59
Tungsten No. 2 shot $1\frac{1}{8}$ oz.	1388 ft/sec	106
Federal		
Steel BBs $1\frac{1}{8}$ oz.	1402 ft/sec	81
Steel No. 2 shot $1\frac{1}{8}$ oz.	1428 ft/sec	141
Federal		
Lead BBs 2 oz.	1087 ft/sec	94
Lead No. 2 shot 2 oz.	1123 ft/sec	174

A relative comparison of the energy and penetration in standard ballistics gelatine of the various pellet materials for number 4 size shot can be seen in Table 4.1.4.

As this table is for comparison purposes, it has been left in the Imperial system.

It has been noted that many of the non-toxic alternatives to lead possess pellets with a less than uniform shape, which might be expected to result in extensive 'flyers'. However, this does not appear to be the case, as the patterns are dense, uniform, and often equivalent or better to those produced by lead shot fired from a barrel with a choke size one quarter greater.

It should be noted that lead shot is sometimes copper-coated to increase its hardness. This can be mistaken for copper-coated steel shot. It is, however, readily identified by use of a magnet.

Suggested further reading

1 Guns & Ammo Magazine Hevi Hitter by Ralph Lermayer.
2 Remington Arms Catalogue.
3 Winchester Arms Catalogue.
4 Heavi-Shot Brochure.

4.6

A Brief History of Propellants

4.6.1 Introduction

The subject of propellants is a fairly specialised area, but one that can crop up in a surprising number of investigations.

Black powder is the primary material used in firework manufacture and, due to its ready availability by dismantling such, and its propensity to produce fairly violent explosions, it has been used by terrorists for bomb-making. It is also widely used in bombs used for fishing. Its purchase in powder form is, however, highly restricted, as it is treated as an explosive.

Nitrocellulose propellants have also been used for the production of bombs in terrorist incidents, but their control is less restricted than black powder. They can be purchased fairly freely in bulk for reloading used cartridge cases. They are not explosive under normal conditions, but simply burn extremely quickly, with the burning rate increasing exponentially with pressure. However, nitrocellulose propellants can, under the right conditions, be made to detonate with great violence.

Some of the companies producing these propellants have proposed the tagging of firearms propellants with micro-sized coloured metallic discs. This is done with conventional explosives for the identification of the manufacturer, year and date of manufacture and batch number. If used by terrorists or criminals for bomb-making, these tags can assist in tracing the origin of the explosives. Whether this is currently undertaken with firearms propellants is unknown.

4.6.2 Basics

Gunpowder, whether it is 'black powder', 'nitrocellulose' or a 'double based powder', is a solid substance that, on combustion, is converted into a very large volume of gas within a very short period of time. While nitrocellulose-based powders can be detonated, in small arms ammunition they are merely propellants which, on ignition, produce a very large volume of gaseous materials that propels the missile down the bore.

During combustion, the rate of reaction is exponentially proportional to the pressure. Thus, unconfined gunpowder or a nitrocellulose powder will gently burn at a fairly steady rate. However, if the powder is confined within the chamber of a weapon with a bullet in the bore, the rate of burning will increase dramatically as the pressure builds up. This will continue until the bullet begins to move down the barrel. If the type and quantity of propellant have been correctly chosen for the bore size, bullet weight and barrel length, the rate of burning will proceed at a level where the pressure will be maintained until the bullet leaves the barrel. At the point at which the bullet leaves the barrel, all the propellant should have burned to its gaseous components.

Should the bullet, for some reason, be unable to move down the barrel, the pressure would rise to such an extent that a gaseous explosion would occur. In this instance, the weakest part of the gun would rupture, with catastrophic consequences. This would normally be the cylinder in a revolver, or the chamber in a self-

Forensic Ballistics in Court: Interpretation and Presentation of Firearms Evidence, First Edition. Brian J. Heard.
© 2013 John Wiley & Sons, Ltd. Published 2013 by John Wiley & Sons, Ltd.

loading pistol or rifle. Conditions under which this could occur are many, but the basic causes of such an incidence are a barrel obstruction, a propellant with a burning rate too high for the bullet weight/bore size combination or too great a charge of propellant.

Propellants can be loosely divided into three classes:

- Black powder.

- Black Powder substitutes.

- Nitrocellulose based powders.

Although all three types of propellants are commercially available, the use of black powder and its substitutes tend to be restricted to enthusiasts firing muzzle-loading weapons. Virtually all modern cartridges are loaded with some form of nitrocellulose powder. A brief history follows.

4.6.3   Black powder

Black powder was, undoubtedly, the earliest form of gunpowder or propellant used in firearms. It is, however, impossible to determine to any degree of authority who invented it, although the following will give an indication as to its historical use:

- The use of 'Greek Fire' to capture the city of Delium by the Boetans in 424 BC is well recorded, although it was probably used as no more than an incendiary device.

- The Chinese are known to have fired incendiary and explosive devices from a bow or catapult as early as 1000 AD, and their name for gunpowder (Huo Yao – fire chemical) was standardised by 1040 AD. This Chinese gunpowder probably spread to Europe via the Mongols under Genghis Khan.

- The earliest European reference to gunpowder is found in the writings of Friar Roger Bacon, who lived in England (1214–1294) and prepared his manuscript on the subject around 1250. He was familiar with its explosive properties, but he does not appear to have had any idea as to its use as a propellant. His formula of 7 parts of potassium nitrate, 5 parts of sulphur and 5 parts of charcoal remained standard until improved upon by the French in 1338.

- Another document written by an obscure monk, Marcus Graecus, also deals with gunpowder. The original portion of the document is dated 846 A.D. and is written in Greek. That portion dealing with gunpowder was added to Graecus's document at a later date and in Latin and is dated 1240. Roger Bacon spent some time in Spain and his knowledge is thought to have originated from the Marcus Graecus document.

- Berthold Schwartz, a famous monk of Freiberg, Germany, studied the writings of Bacon and carried out considerable experimentation. It was following his announcement of his researches, in 1320, that gunpowder really started to spread through central Europe.

- Mr Oliver of Boklerberry appears to have been one of the first English dealers in gunpowder, and its manufacture as an industry dates back to Elizabeth I (1533–1603) when gunpowder mills were first established in Kent.

From time to time, various changes have been made to the composition of gunpowder to make it burn faster or slower. In 1781, it was found that by '**Corning**' gunpowder (i.e. wetting the powder, then compressing it and then, after allowing it to dry, grinding it up again into the desired grain size), a much more efficient powder could be produced. It was also found that with each successive 'corning', the powder improved in performance.

Between 1890 and 1900 a type of powder called 'cocoa' or 'brown powder' appeared. This was made by substituting semi-burned charcoal for the regular charcoal. This probably represents the highest development of black powder.

A simple, commonly cited, chemical equation for the combustion of black powder is:

$$2KNO_3 + S + 3C \rightarrow K_2S + N_2 + 3CO_2$$

Black powder is sold according to the size of the grains. Large-bore devices, such as cannon, use coarse granules (up to several millimetres). Small-bore devices, such as shoulder arms, use much finer grain size.

In America, the following sizes are utilised:

- 1F: coarse, for .69″ to .75″ calibre muskets.

- 2F: medium, for .45″ to .58″ calibre rifles and muskets.

- 3F: fine, for .31″ to .45″ calibre rifles and most handguns.

- 4F: extra-fine, only for priming flintlock arms.

In the UK, the sizing is a little different:

- Fg: large bore rifles and shotguns.

- FFg: medium and small bore arms such as muskets.

- FFFg: small bore rifles and pistols.

- FFFFg: short-barrelled pistols, but more commonly for priming flintlocks.

Modern alternatives to black powder

Due to its ability to absorb water from the atmosphere, its high propensity for ignition by static electricity and its low impact ignition tolerances, black powder is difficult to store and keep. Also, due to the aforementioned properties, it is a difficult material to have transported and, in many countries, a special explosives licence is required before it can be purchased.

To overcome the problems associated with the requirement for an explosive licence, a propellant called **Pyrodex** was introduced in the early 1970s by the Hodgdon's Powder Company of America. Pyrodex has the same burning characteristics as black powder and has the same bulk characteristics (i.e. a given volume of Pyrodex will give the same performance as the same volume of black powder). It does not, however, have the same drawbacks as black powder and is much easier to transport, being regarded as a very low grade explosive. Also, its flameless temperature of ignition is 750°F, while that of black powder is only 500°F.

Pyrodex is similar in composition to black powder, consisting primarily of charcoal, sulphur, and potassium nitrate, but it also contains graphite and potassium perchlorate, together with additional ingredients protected by trade secret. Originally available as loose powder in two granularities (RS (rifle/shotgun), equal to FFG black powder, and P (pistol) equal to FFFg black powder), Pyrodex is now becoming available in solid pellet varieties. However, while it offers improved safety and increased efficiency (in terms of shots per pound of powder) over black powder, the level of fouling is similar in that the residues are caustic and corrosive.

Triple Seven, Black Mag3 Goex Clear Shot, Alliant Black Dot and **IMR White Hots** are all black powder substitutes. All are more energetic than black powder and produce higher velocities and pressures, but without the drawbacks.

Western Powders Company introduced **Blackhorn 209** in 2008. Like many other black powder substitutes, it is made to be a volumetric substitute.

Illustrative Case 1

While working in a Hong Kong firearms laboratory, the author required a quantity of black powder propellant for controlled tests in a bomb-making case. None of the airlines flying into Hong Kong would consider carrying a one kilogramme tin of said propellant, due to its explosive nature. However, they suggested that if the powder were decanted into small aluminium tubes, each of which could contain 50 grams, they could be classified as 'un-primed blank cartridges' and they would have no objection to carrying them as freight!

4.6.4 Nitro propellants

The development of smokeless powder was closely associated with the discovery of guncotton and nitroglycerine, both of which are high explosives. Nitrocellulose is, as its name implies, the nitrated form of cellulose, i.e. cotton, wood, paper, etc.

The equation for the nitration of cellulose via nitric acid is as follows:

$$3HNO_3 + C_6H_{10}O_5 \rightarrow C_6H_7(NO_2)_3O_5 + 3H_2O$$

When they were first discovered, attempts were made to use these nitro explosives as propellants. However, detonation occurred with such instantaneous violence that the weapons were blown apart before the bullet even started to move down the barrel. Therefore, some way needed to be found to tame the violent detonation of the explosive into a controlled and progressive burning that would produce large volumes of gas in a predictable manner.

The first form of 'smokeless powder' was probably made by Vieille, a French chemist, in 1884 by dissolving nitrocellulose, or gun cotton as it is also known, in a mixture of ether and alcohol. A gelatinous colloid is formed, which can be rolled into sheets or extruded into rod or tube form. When dried, it forms a hard, stable material which can be handled easily. This type of smokeless propellant is called a **'single base powder'**.

Another form of propellant was developed by Alfred Nobel in 1887. In this form, the nitrocellulose was dissolved in nitroglycerine (nitrated glycerol). Vaseline was added as a lubricant and stabiliser, and the material so formed could then be extruded or rolled and cut into the shape or size required. This type of propellant was called a **'double based powder'**. Probably the most familiar form of a double based powder is the British military propellant **'Cordite'**. Until quite recently, this propellant was used in all British military rifle and pistol ammunition. Cordite contains 37 per cent nitrocellulose, 58 per cent nitroglycerine and 5 per cent Vaseline. It burns with extreme heat and is a very energetic propellant.

Moderation of nitrocellulose-based propellants

When a propellant is ignited within the confines of a cartridge case enclosed in the breech of a weapon, large quantities of gas are produced. The pressure so formed pushes the bullet down the barrel and so discharges it from the weapon. The problem is that, once the bullet starts to move down the barrel, the space occupied by the gases increases and the pressure starts to fall. Some method of modifying the burning rate of the propellant is thus necessary to ensure that the pressure exerted on the base of the bullet is fairly consistent during its progress down the length of the barrel.

Small thin flakes of powder will obviously have a larger surface area than solid lumps, and these are thus preferable for short barrelled, small calibre weapons. The problems come, however, when longer barrels and larger calibres are used. Under these circumstances, other methods to moderate or alter the rate of burning are required. The simplest of these is to perforate the grains of powder. On ignition, both the inside surface of the perforation and the outside surface of the grain burn together. As the grain burns, the outside surface diminishes, as does the production of gases. This is, however, countered by the inside surface becoming larger as it burns. By altering the number of perforations and the ratio of the inside diameter to the outside diameter, the burning rate can be closely controlled.

Other methods of modifying the burning rate include the addition of chemical 'moderators' during manufacture and/or the coating of the grains with graphite and other surfactants to reduce the rate at which the grains ignite.

The range of additives and moderators is enormous (see Table 4.6.1), and many are very tightly controlled trade secrets. The identification of these components can, however, be extremely important in the identification of propellants and their origin.

While moderators do control the rate of burning and, thus, the rate at which the gaseous products are formed, if the bore is obstructed, or the incorrect weight of bullet is used, or there is too much propellant, the rate of burning can rise exponentially. Under these conditions, the pressures produced can give rise to a catastrophic destruction of the weapon. In extreme cases, it can even lead to the propellant detonating, with even more catastrophic results.

Illustrative Case 2

An example of how important the identification of additives and moderators can be involved the use of propellants in a terrorist device which was used to kill a police officer. The device was a very simple pipe bomb using a simple twist of thin wire connected to a battery and switch for ignition. Fragments of un-burnt firearms propellant found at the scene were, at a later date, successfully matched to similar fragments found in the suspect's pockets. The propellant particles were quite unusual in that they were of an American variety not often seen in the UK. As it was a single based propellant, it was necessary to analyse the moderators before a successful identification could be made.

Illustrative Case 3

In the 1970s, a British police force was issued with WWII Webley .380″ revolvers. These weapons were designed to fire .380″ fully jacketed ammunition to conform to the Hague Convention. Unfortunately, this ammunition was no longer available in commercial quantities, so .38″ calibre Smith & Wesson ammunition was used instead. This ammunition has a slightly larger bullet than the .380″ ammunition and, as the supplier was somewhat lax in its quality control, some of the ammunition contained 50 per cent more powder than it was designed for. As a result of the larger bullet and the overcharge of propellant, the revolvers used for training were blowing up at the rate of ten a week. Several serious injuries resulted in the weapons and ammunition being withdrawn from service.

Table 4.6.1   A List of the More Commonly Known Additives and Moderators

Additive	Purpose
Resorcinol	Plasticiser
Triacetin	Plasticiser
Dimethyl sebacetate	Plasticiser
Dimethyl phthalate	Plasticiser
2:dinitro diphenylamine	Plasticiser
Calcium carbonate	Adsorb free nitrogen dioxide for long-term propellant stability
Diphenylamine	Adsorb free nitrogen dioxide for long-term propellant stability
Dinitrotoluene	Gelatiniser to slow the rate of burning
Dibutylphthalate	Gelatiniser to slow rate of burning
Carbamate	Gelatiniser to slow rate of burning
Barium nitrate	To increase rate of burning
Potassium nitrate	To increase rate of burning
Graphite	Surface moderator
Wood meal	A fuel – only found in shotgun ammunition

Other additives include:

- Cresol

- Nitroglycerine

- Carbazole

- N-nitrosodiphenylamine

- Carbanilide

- Trinitrotoluene

- Nitrophenylamine

- NN-dimethylcarbanilide

- Dinitrocresol

- 24-dinitrodiphenylamine

- Triacetin

- Dibutylphthalate

- Nitrotoluene

- Pentaerythritol

- Tetranitrate

- Cyclonite (RDX)

- NN-dibutycarbanilide

- Diethylphthalate

- Methycentralite

Metal fouling

In an attempt to combat metal fouling (from jacket material stripped off the bullet and welded to the bore during firing) in rifles, du Pont, the American powder manufacturer, added powdered metallic tin to the propellant. The patent for this was taken out in 1918 and, to identify those powders containing tin, a '$\frac{1}{2}$' was added to the powder designation (e.g. Powder $17\frac{1}{2}$ contained tin, while Powder 17 did not). These powders originally contained approximately 4 per cent of metallic tin. It was found, however, that while the old Cu/Zn fouling from the bullet jacket was eliminated, metallic tin volatilised by the heat of combustion was condensing inside the bore near the muzzle. The percentage of tin was slowly decreased to one per cent, then was eliminated altogether.

Lesmok ammunition

One peculiar propellant introduced around 1910 was called '**Lesmok**'. Primarily used in .22″ calibre ammunition, it was a mixture of 85 per cent black powder and 15 per cent pure guncotton. Although this was a distinctive improvement over plain black powder, it still left a considerable quantity of corrosive residues in the bore. Consequently, it had a very short life. As far as can be ascertained, the last batch of .22″ calibre Lesmok ammunition was made by Winchester in February 1947.

Nitro propellants versus black powder

The advantages of nitro-based propellants over black powder are many and include:

- A very small quantity of a nitro based propellant is required in comparison to black powder.

- It can be modified with ease to fit almost any circumstance.

- There is a negligible quantity of combustion residues left in the bore.

- The low corrosive nature of the combustion residues.

The flameless temperature of ignition for nitrocellulose propellants is rather low, at approximately 350°C. However, if ammunition is subjected to a fire, it is the primer which will almost invariably ignite first, as the ignition temperature of this is around 250°C. In fires, ammunition never explodes, nor is the bullet propelled with sufficient force to cause any damage. The primer ignites first, setting fire to the propellant, which either pushes the bullet out of the case mouth or splits the side of the case, allowing the gases to escape.

Burning rate for nitro powders

How fast a propellant burns gives an indication as to its intended use. Very fast burning powders are best suited for use with light weight bullets and short barrels, while the slower burning ones are for heavy Magnum calibre weapons with long barrels. Propellants for use in shotgun ammunition also tend to be fast burning, as most of the acceleration imparted to the shot has to occur in the relatively heavy breech end of the barrel. Rifle calibre propellants are slow burning and become progressively more so as the power increases to Magnum calibres.

Powder burn rates can, and do, change from one batch to another, or as manufacturers change product specifications

4.6.5 Dating of ammunition

It is possible, in some instances, to approximately date commercial ammunition by the type of propellant it contains (see Table 4.6.2).

Table 4.6.2 Some Examples of Dating of Commercial Ammunition

Ammunition Type	When Manufactured
Lesmok	1910–1947
Ball Powder	1941 to date
Cordite	1885–1956
Schultzite	1867–1935
Smokeless Diamond	1920–1939

4.6.6 Reduced loads for target shooting

Target shooters tend to use very small quantities of a very fast burning powder (often a shotgun propellant) in their hand-loaded ammunition to ensure accuracy. While this is perfectly safe as long as only small loads of propellant are used, to do the same with a slow burning powder can cause catastrophic consequences.

While the actual mechanism involved is unclear, it would appear that a pressure wave is set up within the cartridge case, which reflects back off the base of the bullet. This is reinforced by the still burning propellant, giving rise to sufficient internal pressure to detonate the remaining powder. Such an instantaneous release of energy is too great for the weapon to handle, and the chamber of the weapon explodes. There have been numerous instances of this effect, including high-power rifles being totally destroyed by a charge of propellant so small that the bullet would normally only just reach the end of a 50 yard range.

Illustrative Case 4

One other instance of propellant detonating has been experienced by the author, but this was for a different reason altogether. This involved a packet of World War I .455″ revolver ammunition which, although very old, appeared to be perfectly good condition. After several rounds were fired, the weapon completely exploded, depositing the barrel, the top strap and the cylinder into the walls and ceiling of the range. On carefully opening some of the rounds, it was discovered that the cordite had started to deteriorate and nitroglycerine was leeching out of the propellant. The amount of free nitroglycerine was sufficient to cause detonation within the rest of the charge, destroying the weapon.

Further reading

1 Kelly, J. (2005). *Gunpowder: Alchemy, Bombards, and Pyrotechnics: The History of the Explosive that Changed the World*. Perseus Books Group, ISBN 0465037224.

2 Davis, T.L. (1943). *The Chemistry of Powder & Explosives*. (Angriff Press [1992] ed.). John Wiley & Sons Inc. ISBN 0-913022-00-4.

3 Matunas, E.A. (1978). *Winchester-Western Ball Powder Loading Data*. Olin Corporation.

4 Heramb, R.M. & McCord, B.R. (2002). AT The Manufacture of Smokeless Powders and their Forensic Analysis. *FBI Forensic Science Communications* 4 (2).

4.7

Priming Compounds

4.7.1 Introduction

Gunshot residues (GSR) are the residues left over when a round of ammunition is fired. They are sometimes also referred to as firearms discharge residues (FDR).

These residues are made up of two major components: organic residues from the modifiers, oxidising agents and stabilisers; and the inorganic components which are mainly from the explosive compounds and the fuels.

The analysis of gunshot residues (GSR) via the scanning electron microscope using an energy dispersive X-ray analyser (EDX) is arguably one of the most important parts of modern forensic firearms examination.

The examination of these residues will be more fully covered in Chapter 14 (Gunshot Residue Examination).

The primer composition used in Western countries is all fairly similar in composition, but in other parts of the world there can be huge differences, not only from country to country, but from one factory to another and even from one batch to another.

An intimate knowledge of primers, their history and development, what chemicals are involved and their function is and essential for presentation of this evidence at court. While the names of some of the chemicals involved can be quite daunting, it is not an insurmountable problem.

Illustrative Case 1

A serious armed robbery occurred in which the robbers were armed with Chinese Type 56 assault rifles (a copy of the Russian AK47) and Chinese Type 54 pistols (copy of Russian Tokarev). Shots were fired at random, killing two and injuring many others. CCTV images showed that all of the robbers were wearing long black nylon coats to hide their weapons. Arrests were eventually made and, during searches of their premises, several long black nylon coats were recovered. In the pocket of one were found several particles of gunshot residue. These were of an extremely unusual type, which had only been encountered once before, and that was in cartridge cases at the aforementioned robbery. While this evidence could not stand alone, it was highly important supportive evidence which assisted in the conviction of the arrested persons for robbery and murder.

Forensic Ballistics in Court: Interpretation and Presentation of Firearms Evidence, First Edition. Brian J. Heard.
© 2013 John Wiley & Sons, Ltd. Published 2013 by John Wiley & Sons, Ltd.

4.7.2　Basics

A **priming compound** is a highly sensitive explosive chemical which, when struck by the firing pin or hammer of a weapon, will explode with great violence, providing the flame to ignite the propellant.

This explosive chemical is often mixed with other chemicals that provide oxygen to assist in the production of the flame, a fuel to increase the length and temperature of the flame, and ground glass as an abrasive to assist in the initial ignition of the explosive.

In the realms of forensic science, the detection of primer discharge residue on the hands can provide crucial evidence as to whether a person has recently fired a weapon.

To fully utilise the evidential value of GSR analysis, a basic understanding of the history, composition and manufacture of primers is essential.

4.7.3　A short history of priming compounds

The earliest priming compound was almost certainly mercury fulminate, as used in the Forsythe Scent Bottle priming system which was introduced around 1806. This compound is highly sensitive and liable to explode spontaneously for no apparent reason. As a result, the Forsythe Scent Bottle, which required a considerable quantity of this compound to be carried in a container on the side of the pistol, did not achieve a great deal of popularity.

In 1807, Forsythe introduced a priming compound with a formula consisting of 70.6 parts potassium chlorate, 17.6 parts sulphur and 11.8 parts of charcoal. While this was somewhat more stable than mercury fulminate, it was terribly corrosive.

The first real percussion cap (a small metal cup containing the priming composition which was placed on a nipple at the rear of the barrel) was introduced by Joshua Shaw in 1814 and contained mercury fulminate. As a result of the unpredictability of plain mercury fulminate, it was superseded in 1818 by a mixture of mercury fulminate, potassium chlorate, sulphur and charcoal. The residues produced by this mixture were, however, still terribly corrosive, requiring the weapon to be cleaned immediately after firing.

In 1828, Dreyse patented the 'Needle Gun', which had a paper cartridge case with the primer cup inside the case with the propellant (see Chapter 1.0). The firing pin on this weapon was a very long, thin needle that penetrated the paper case, striking the primer within. This primer cup contained a mixture of potassium chlorate and antimony sulphide.

It was found that purification of the mercury fulminate would lead to a more stable compound and, in 1873, a mixture of mercury fulminate, potassium chlorate, glass dust and Arabic gum became the standard US military priming compound. However, this mixture suffered from two major drawbacks:

- The brass cartridge cases were made brittle by the mercury in the primer, which led to case failure on firing and dangerous leakage of high-pressure gases from the breech of the weapon.

- The potassium chlorate left terribly corrosive residues in the bore of the weapon after firing.

As a result of these problems, the search began for a non-mercuric, non-corrosive primer composition. Early attempts revolved around the use of potassium chlorate as the main ingredient. Potassium chlorate is, however, a fairly unstable material and is very deliquescent (i.e. it absorbs water from the atmosphere). It also forms potassium chloride on decomposition, which is also deliquescent and is also very corrosive to the weapon's bore.

Just prior to the First World War, it was discovered that thiocyanate/chlorate mixtures were sensitive to impact. These, however, had the same drawbacks as straight chlorate primers, in that they produced corrosive residues on firing.

The German company of RWS was the first to substitute the potassium chlorate with barium nitrate. Lead styphnate was used as the main explosive component, giving the first 'rust free' primer. This was patented in 1928 under the name Sinoxid.

The first true non-corrosive, non-mercuric (NCNM) primers were commercially produced in America sometime between 1935–1938. These, however, did not meet the stringent US government specifications as to storage, misfires, etc., so military ammunition continued to use the old corrosive chlorate mixtures right through World War II.

In the UK, the change to non-corrosive military primers was even slower, and it was not until the early 1960s that all calibres of military and commercial primers used NCNM priming compounds.

Up to early 2000, the most common primer composition encountered was still the lead styphnate, barium nitrate, antimony sulphide and tetrazine type. In this priming compound, the lead styphnate and tetrazine are the sensitive explosive ingredients, the barium nitrate provides additional oxygen to increase the temperature of the flame and the antimony sulphide acts as a fuel to prolong the burning time. Aluminium, and occasionally magnesium, can also be encountered, but mainly in higher-powered Magnum pistol or rifle calibres.

Powdered glass was also often added to the mixture to increase the friction and to assist detonation when the mixture is crushed by the firing pin.

Modern .22″ calibre rimfire ammunition is slightly different in that the composition almost invariably consists of lead styphnate, barium nitrate, tetrazine and powdered glass.

Lead-free and non-toxic primers

It began to become apparent in the early 1970s that, in heavily used training facilities, the range personnel were suffering from the symptoms of lead poisoning. While a large proportion of this lead was being volatilized from the base of the bullets and back-splash of lead dust from the butts, a portion was obviously coming from the lead styphnate primer.

The US National Bureau of Standards claims that when lead-based primers, are used 80 per cent of airborne lead on firing ranges comes from the projectile and 20 per cent comes from the priming composition. These percentages obviously depend on whether the bullet is plain lead or jacketed. In the case of a non-jacketed bullet, the rifling will strip lead from the bullet's surface, thus dramatically increasing the percentage of non-primer-based airborne lead.

The change to a bullet with a Cu/Zn jacket extending over the base was a fairly simple matter of reducing the bullet-sourced airborne lead, but finding a non-mercuric, non-corrosive, non-lead-based primer was another.

The problem was first solved in the early 1980s by Geco, who released a zinc and titanium based primer which they called 'Sintox'. Since then, there have been a number of other lead free primers produced by, for example, CCI Blazer, Speer, Federal and Winchester[1]. The exact composition of the priming compounds used is not available, although SEM/EDX analysis generally shows the presence of strontium in the Speer and Blazer cartridges, potassium in the Winchester cartridges, and calcium and silicon in the Federal cartridges.

Most of the more recent primer formulations contain an initiator explosive compound called 'Dinol', the chemical name of which is diazodinitrophenol.

Other components

Other **initiator explosives** include:

- dinitrodihydroxydiazobenzene salt (diazinate);

- dinitrobenzofuroxan salts;

- potassium dinitrobenzofuroxan;

- various diazo, triazole and tetrazaole compounds;

- perchlorate or nitrate salts of metal complexes of ammonium, amine, or hydrazine, an example of which is 2-(5-cyanotetrazolato) pentaaminecobalt (III) perchlorate (CP).

Oxidisers include:

- zinc oxide;

- potassium nitrate;

- strontium nitrate;

- zinc peroxide.

---

[1]Haag (1995). American Lead Free 9mm-P Cartridges. *AFTE Journal* **27**, 2.

Fuel components include:

- amorphous boron;

- metal powders, such as aluminium, zirconium, titanium, nickel and zinc;

- carbon;

- silicon.

Metal sulphides include:

- antimony sulphide;

- bismuth sulphide;

- iron sulphide;

- zinc sulphide.

Metal silicides include:

- calcium silicide;

- copper silicide.

The **explosive sensitizer** is generally Tetrazine. '**Fast fuels**' may also be included, such as:

- potassium styphnate;

- nitrate esters such as nitrocellulose-based propellants;

- PETN.

Additional ingredients include:

- PVA (polyvinyl acetate);

- karaya;

- tragacanth;

- guar;

- gum arabic;

- powdered glass.

A typical non-toxic, non lead priming composition would be:

- diazodinitrophenol;

- potassium nitrate;

- nitrocellulose;

- boron metal;

- nitro-glycerine;

- tetrazine;

- nickel.

A timeline of primer development (Table 4.7.1)

Table 4.7.1	Timeline of Primer Development	
Date	Primer Type	Primer Composition
1898	US Krag cartridge	Potassium chlorate, antimony sulphide, glass powder
1901	German RWS	Mercury fulminate, barium nitrate, antimony sulphide, picric acid
1910	US Frankford Arsenal	Potassium chlorate, antimony sulphide, sulphur
1910	German RWS	Mercury fulminate, antimony sulphide, barium peroxide, TNT
1911	Swiss Military Primer	Mercury fulminate, barium nitrate, antimony sulphide, barium carbonate
1917	US Winchester Primer	Potassium chlorate, antimony sulphide, lead thiocyanate, TNT
1927	US commercial primers	Mercury fulminate, barium nitrate, lead thiocyanate

Table 4.7.1 (*Continued*)

Date	Primer Type	Primer Composition
1928	German RWS Sinoxid Primer	Lead styphnate, barium nitrate, antimony sulphide, calcium silicide, tetrazine
1930	Herz/Rathburg Non-Mercuric Primer	Nitro-amino-guanyltetrazine, lead styphnate, barium nitrate, antimony sulphide/calcium silicide
1938 (approx)	American commercial primers	Lead styphnate, antimony sulphide, barium nitrate, tetrazine
1940	American P-4 Primer	Red phosphorous, barium nitrate, aluminium hydroxide
1943	British .455 military revolver	Mercury fulminate, sulphur, potassium chlorate, antimony sulphide, mealed black powder
1962	Stabenate Primer	Lead nitroaminotetrazole, lead styphnate, barium nitrate, antimony sulphide, aluminium dust, tetrazine
1983	Geco Sintox Primer	Zinc and titanium-based priming compound containing no lead compounds

4.7.4 Manufacture

The loading of the highly explosive and exceedingly sensitive mixture into the primer cup or cartridge rim of rimfire ammunition is a very delicate and dangerous undertaking. With most commercial primers, this is done with the compound slightly wetted, but in military primers it is carried out as a dry powder to give a more consistent result.

In the 'Eleyprime' process, a mixture of dry, relative safe chemicals, are placed into the primer cup. On the addition of a small quantity of water the chemicals react to form an explosive composition. Basically, the mixture consists of tetrazine, lead monoxide, lead dioxide, antimony sulphide, styphnic acid, barium nitrate and calcium silicide.

Other considerations

The sensitivity of primers is a difficult subject, due to the varying standards not only from country to country, but also between the commercial and military sectors.

In the UK, the commercial standard for 9 mm Parabellum primers states that the primer should discharge when a 57 gram steel ball falls from a height of 330 mm onto a firing pin. The lower limit for this must not be less than 203 mm.

Military standards vary enormously, but the NATO standard for 9 mm Parabellum ammunition is that all primers should fire when a 1.94 oz steel ball is dropped onto a firing pin from a height of 12 inches and none shall fire from a height of 3 inches.

The NATO standard 7.62 × 54 mm rifle ammunition uses a 3.94 oz steel ball, with all firing from 16 inches and none from 3 inches.

It should be noted that the sensitivity for military primers will always be less than that for the equivalent commercial primer. This is to take into account the harsher conditions and treatment accorded to military weapons and ammunition.

4.7.5 Accidental discharge of primers

Following on from the subject of primer sensitivity is the oft-mentioned possibility of cartridge cases exploding in the pocket through coming into contact with keys or loose change, and of cartridges exploding when dropped onto the ground. Experience and an extensive series of tests have shown this to be exceedingly unlikely.

Both rimfire and centre fire cartridges have been repeatedly thrown with great force onto their base without the slightest effect. Cartridges have been dropped down lubricated tubes in excess of 30 feet in length onto small pebbles, and even firing pins, with hardly even a dent on the primer.

Illustrative Case 2

An unusual case of accidental discharge occurred where a cartridge discharged due to a very light impact on its primer. This involved a batch of ammunition which was known to have primers that were slightly softer than would be normally expected. Firing pin impressions were noticed to be particularly deep on fired ammunition and, even when fresh out of the box, small dents were observed on some of the primers. These dents probably resulted from a manufacturing process whereby the finished rounds are tumbled in corn husks, or some other slightly abrasive material, to polish them.

The accidental discharge in this case happened during a range course which was being held in the mid-day sun, with measured temperatures of over 35°C in the shade and over 50°C in the sun.

During the range course, the live ammunition was held base uppermost in boxes at the firer's feet and had, at the time of the incident, been baking for nearly an hour in the direct sun. After one cylinder had been fired, the empty cartridges were tipped on to the ground straight over the unfired cartridges. The rim of one of the fired cartridges struck the extremely hot primer of a live round and it exploded, slightly injuring the firer.

It is known that the sensitivity of the priming compound rises exponentially with temperature and it is assumed that this, together with the softer than normal primer, caused the discharge. While such a discharge should, in theory, be impossible, there was no other logical explanation for this event.

Illustrative Case 3

Another case of accidental discharge occurred when a fully loaded 9 mm Browning HP magazine was dropped into a large tub of live ammunition. The lip on the base plate struck a primer, causing it to discharge. Not being contained, the cartridge case merely split open, causing virtually no damage to the rest of the ammunition.

Ignition of primers in a fire

As far as spontaneous combustion of the priming compound is concerned, the flameless ignition temperature of small arms priming compounds is generally in the region of 190–260°C. This is considerably lower than the ignition temperature for most small arms propellants, which is the region of 350°C. Therefore, it can be assumed that, during a fire, the first thing to ignite spontaneously will be the primer, which will, in turn, ignite the propellant.

Such ignitions are virtually harmless, as the soft brass case of the round and the lightly held bullet in the case mouth do not allow pressures to build up sufficiently for the case to explode. At most, the case wall will rupture, with no more than the odd piece of brass being projected a few feet and the primer being pushed out of its pocket.

Further reading

1 Barnes, F.C. (2003) *Cartridges of the World* (10th edition). Krause Publications. ISBN 0-87349-605-1.
2 Hawks, C. *Primers, the Sparkplug of Centerfire Cartridges.*
3 Hackley, F.W. (1967). *History of Modern U.S. Military Small Arms Ammunition.* Macmillan.
4 Wallace, J.S. (2008). Chemical Analysis of Firearms Ammunition and Gunshot Residue. CRC Press. ISBN 978-1-4200-6966-2.

5.0

An Introduction to Ballistics

5.0.1 Introduction

This is a terribly complicated subject, previously only accessible to ballisticians working with reams and reams of incomprehensible (to the layman at least) tables and charts. Nowadays, however, this subject is easily available via a PC and appropriate software.

It is, however, necessary to have an insight into the factors which control a bullet's flight, both inside and outside of the barrel and in the target. Myths abound as to what affects the bullet's flight through the air, whether the earth's rotation effects it, the effect on right- and left-rifled barrels fired north and south of the equator, maximum ranges of various bullets, the terminal velocity of a bullet at maximum range, whether a revolver bullet will pass through a filled wooden water butt, and so on.

Many of these myths have been perpetrated by the film industry for visual effect but are completely untrue. Unravelling these myths is extremely important if one is to have a clear picture of what happens to a bullet once it is fired, and whether witnesses' accounts can be believed.

5.0.2 Basics

There are basically three types of ballistics: **internal, external and terminal.**

For the purpose of this book, much of the mathematics dealing with **internal ballistics** is purely academic. However, a brief outline of the subject is given here merely for the sake of completion.

External ballistics is likewise of little relevance in normal forensic case work, as the vast majority of shooting incidents occur over a fairly short range. There are, however, those occasions where much longer distances are involved and where a working knowledge of the subject is consequently a distinct advantage.

Terminal ballistics, which deals with the results of a missile striking a body or some other object, is a far more important topic as it has applications to the majority of cases examined.

5.0.3 Background

Internal ballistics is the study of what happens within the barrel of a weapon, from the moment the firing pin hits the primer to the time the bullet exits from the barrel. It is mainly concerned with propellant pressures, acceleration of the missile while it is in the bore, muzzle velocity and recoil.

Esoteric considerations such as primer ignition time, primer pressure/time curves and temperature also come within the general subject matter of interior ballistics. These considerations are, however, far too specialised to be dealt with in this book.

External ballistics deals with the flight of the bullet from the muzzle of the weapon to the target. This is a hugely complicated subject involving parameters such as bullet shape, sectional density,

Forensic Ballistics in Court: Interpretation and Presentation of Firearms Evidence, First Edition. Brian J. Heard.
© 2013 John Wiley & Sons, Ltd. Published 2013 by John Wiley & Sons, Ltd.

atmospheric pressure and even, in larger calibre weapons, the rotation and curve of the earth. With the advent of powerful personal computers, this subject has, however, now come within the realms of the average person. What took hours of complex calculations and much reference to books and charts of flight timetables can now be achieved in a few moments.

Terminal ballistics deals with the behaviour of the missile once it reaches the target. This is not only concerned with simply piercing a paper target, but what the missile does once it encounters a material considerably denser than air. While this will usually be concerned with the missile's performance and wounding capabilities in animal or human tissue, it could also include the missile's performance in water, soil, brick, concrete, wood or bullet-resistant materials.

Further reading

1 US Army (1965). *Interior Ballistics of Guns, Engineering Design Handbook*. Ballistics Series. United States Army Materiel Command, AMCP 706-150.
2 Baer, P.G. & Frankle, J.M. (1962). *The Simulation of Interior Ballistic Performance of Guns by Digital Computer Program*. Aberdeen Proving Ground, MD: Ballistic Research Laboratories, BRL Report No. 1183.
3 Hatcher, J. S. (1962). *Hatcher's Notebook* (3rd edition). Harrisburg, PA: Stackpole Company, ISBN 8117-0614-1.
4 Horst, A.W. (2005). *A Brief Journey Through the History of Gun Propulsion*. Aberdeen Proving Ground, MD: United States Army Research Laboratory, ARL-TR-3671.
5 Rinkler, R.A. (1999). *Understanding Firearms Ballistics*. ISBN-10: 0964559846
6 http://www.ballistics.org/docs/InteriorBallistics.pdf

5.1

Internal Ballistics

5.1.1 Introduction

It could be asked, 'What has the internal ballistics of a firearm got to do with the examination of firearms evidence?' Such esoterica as 'cartridge case capacity vs. pressure curves' has very little to do with it, but **recoil** and **barrel lift** can have a profound effect on the understanding of the ability to control a weapon when fired and the difference between where the weapon is aimed and what and where the bullet actually strikes. So many cases have rested upon the question of where the barrel was pointing at the time the weapon discharged. "The gun was pointing at the ground when I fired and it was the recoil which resulted in him being shot." is one of the most frequently quoted defences for murder.

A simple look at the mathematics of internal ballistics and recoil will show that;

- yes, the barrel does lift on firing;

- but only by a very small amount, and this has been compensated for the factory sight settings;

- however, using a different weight of bullet can have a distinct effect on the point of impact;

- and, yes, the recoil does result in the barrel lifting way above the point of aim;

- but the bullet has long left the barrel by the time that this happens.

These questions can be simply answered by reference to the following facts.

5.1.2 Basics

Internal ballistics is an enormous subject, and one on which many books have been produced. The mathematics involved can be highly complex and, once again, are outside the realms of this book. It is, however, possible to give an insight to the subject by use of a few simplified equations.

When the firing pin strikes the primer, the priming compound explodes with great violence, causing an extremely high-temperature jet of flame to pass through the flash hole and into the propellant charge. This jet of flame, which is about $2,000\,°C$, ignites the propellant, which burns at high speed to form a large volume of gas. This high-pressure gas accelerates the bullet down the barrel and out of the muzzle. At this juncture, it must be made very clear that is *not* an explosive reaction.

Nitrocellulose propellant will, if ignited in an unconfined space, gently burn. If it is in a confined space, the build-up of heat and pressure will accelerate the rate of combustion exponentially. If there is nowhere for the gas to escape (i.e. by pushing the bullet down the barrel), then the pressure and temperature will cause the rate of reaction to rise so rapidly that the weapon will explode with great violence.

Here, the nature of an explosion should be explained.

Forensic Ballistics in Court: Interpretation and Presentation of Firearms Evidence, First Edition. Brian J. Heard.
© 2013 John Wiley & Sons, Ltd. Published 2013 by John Wiley & Sons, Ltd.

An explosion creates a shock wave. If this shock wave is a supersonic detonation, then the source of the blast is called a 'high explosive'. Subsonic shock waves are created by low explosives through the slower burning process known as deflagration. This is not a true chemical explosion – merely extremely high pressure gases rupturing the vessel in which they are confined. It is this sub-sonic deflagration that occurs in weapons that explode.

In a weapon, the propellant is confined within the cartridge case, the mouth of which is closed with a bullet. The round of ammunition is then supported by the chamber walls and the standing breech of the weapon. Under these conditions, the pressure build-up will continue until it is sufficient to overcome the inertia of the bullet and start its acceleration down the bore. Basically, there are two factors which apply here:

- The heavier the bullet, the greater the resistance and the higher the pressure.

- The higher the pressure, the greater the rate of combustion and, consequently, the greater the velocity of the missile.

Cartridge case capacity

Another factor affecting the rate of combustion is the density of the propellant load, i.e. the ratio of case volume to propellant volume. Thus, the larger the unfilled space in the cartridge case, the slower the initial rate of combustion.

Internal pressure

When the propellant burns, most of it turns into gas, comprising mainly of carbon dioxide and water vapour. At first, the gases are contained completely within the cartridge case and the pressure is exerted equally on the base of the cartridge, its walls and the base of the bullet. Once the bullet starts to move, the volume filled by the gases increases and the pressure starts to fall.

In modern propellants, this fall in pressure can be compensated to a certain extent by '**moderating**' the propellant grains (See Chapter 4.7). This involves the addition of various chemicals and the surface coating of the powder grains. In some propellants, the grains are also pierced with holes. Moderation has the effect of increasing the rate of burning as the propellant is consumed. As a result of this, the internal pressure does not drop so drastically once the bullet begins to move.

The moderation of the propellant grains has to be carefully regulated to ensure that they are totally consumed just before the bullet reaches the end of the barrel. Any propellant not consumed before the bullet exits the barrel will not only result in a low efficiency rate for the cartridge, but will also produce a large muzzle flash. This muzzle flash can be extremely disconcerting when firing at night, as it has the effect of destroying the firer's night vision.

Moderation is generally designed for a particular length of barrel, for example a revolver with a four-inch (10 cm) barrel. If that cartridge is then fired in a two-inch (5 cm) barrel, then the combustion of the propellant will not be complete. Not only will there be unburnt propellant exiting from the barrel, but the loading will be less efficient than when fired in the barrel length for which it was designed, and the velocity of the bullet will be lower. If, on the other hand, it is fired in a six-inch (15 cm) barrelled weapon, the propellant would have finished burning before the bullet reaches the end of the barrel, and friction between the bullet and the inside of the barrel will then slow down the bullet.

5.1.3 Recoil

This considers the forces acting on a fired weapon which cause a handgun either to rotate gently in the hand or to bite violently into the palm, or a rifle to push gently against one's shoulder or to produce a bone-bruising kick.

Recoil is probably one of the most misquoted subjects in the field of firearms, and a basic knowledge of the forces involved and how their vectors are calculated is a real asset for anyone dealing with the science of forensic firearms examination. Consequently, it can also be a distinct advantage when dealing with cases where the defence rests upon the weapon having recoiled to an extent that the bullet did no go where the weapon was pointed.

Illustrative Case 1

For the purposes of crime, shotguns virtually always have their barrel shortened to about a third of their normal length. This increases the spread of shot slightly, causes an absolutely huge noise and a flame up to 10 ft (3 metres) in length. This has a number of advantages for the criminal:

- The weapon is easy to carry and conceal.

- It looks very intimidating.

- It produces a noise so loud that most people are shocked senseless.

- The flame is of such severity that it can cause temporary blindness.

- Few people will survive being shot with such a weapon.

During the firing of a weapon, the pressure on the inside of the cartridge case acts not only on the base of the bullet, but also on the standing breech of the weapon. It is this mechanism that causes the pistol rifle or shotgun to recoil. This is Newton's third law of motion, i.e. the mutual forces of action and reaction between two bodies are equal, opposite and co-linear.

Knowing the pressure produced (from the manufacturer's published figures) and the weight of the bullet enables the recoil energy to be calculated.

For example, the pressure in the chamber of a .45″ calibre self-loading pistol is 14,000 pounds per square inch. The base of a .45″ bullet being 0.159 square inches, the total pressure on the base of the bullet is 2,225 pounds, i.e. $14,000 \times 0.159$. This means that when the pistol is fired, there is a pressure of over one ton pushing the bullet forwards and the gun backwards. With a rearwards pressure of over one ton, the only thing that prevents the gun from being impossible to control is that the pressure is only exerted over a fraction of a second. The duration of this pressure is dependent on the period over which the bullet is still in the barrel. Once the bullet leaves the barrel, there is no longer any pressure being exerted on its base and, therefore, there is no pressure on the base of the cartridge case.

Recoil and muzzle lift

As mentioned earlier, the force which acts on the rear of the bullet to propel it forwards is also exerted on the base of the cartridge case to move the gun backwards. It is this force that causes the weapon to recoil. This force not only drives the gun to the rear but, because the barrel is situated above the hand and, therefore, above the rotational axis of the wrist, it also rotates the gun in an upwards direction. As the bullet is travelling down the bore during the period in which the barrel is lifting, it will strike the target above the point at which the barrel was pointed when the trigger was pulled.

As was seen earlier, the actual time the bullet is in the barrel is very short (e.g. with a .45″ calibre self-loading pistol, it is only 0.00102 seconds). During this very short period of time, the muzzle lifts above its point of aim only a fraction of an inch. This does, however, have a pronounced effect on the striking point of the bullet, as only a minute ($\frac{1}{60}$th of a degree) of barrel lift will change the impact point by 1.047″ inches (2.565 cm) at 100 yards (91.5 metres).

To compensate for this, the sights of a weapon are set, or **regulated**, at the factory. The sights are regulated for a certain weight bullet travelling at a certain velocity. If a heavier bullet is used, it will remain in the bore longer. The longer the bullet is in the bore, the more time the recoil has an effect on the hand and the greater the degree of barrel rotation. Thus, *a heavier bullet will strike above the point of aim and a lighter one below.* This is exactly the opposite of what common sense would indicate.

To give an example of the magnitude of barrel lift, when a standard military P14 .303 rifle is fired with standard military ammunition, weapon recoil will cause the barrel to rise by 0.1″ (0.245 cm) between the time the trigger is pulled and the bullet leaves the barrel.

Muzzle lift due to recoil is an oft-quoted excuse in firearms cases. However, as can be seen from the above, this is simply not the case. Basically, the place where the sights are pointing at the instant of firing is where the bullet will (with only slight discrepancies) strike. What usually happens, however, is that the aim is disturbed before the firing pin strikes the primer. There are three main causes for this:

- **Flinching**, which is a subconscious reflex caused by anticipating the recoil from firing.

- **Trigger snatch**, which results from attempting to fire the weapon the instant the sights are aligned with the target.

- **Trigger pull-through**, where there is considerable trigger movement (also called backlash) after the firing pin has been released.

In the case of a right-handed person, these three factors tend to pull the weapon up and to the right, whereas with a left handed person, it will be up and to the left. This obviously causes the bullet to strike the target high and either to the left or the right. The degree of severity depends upon the experience of the shooter and the weapon's design. However, this will never be sufficient to cover the much-quoted excuse that the weapon was pointing at the ground when the shot was fired and flinching/trigger snatch/trigger pull-through and recoil caused the bullet to hit the deceased in the chest!

To reduce these problems, target weapons have a very light trigger pull, which reduces trigger snatch, and a stop to prevent the trigger moving past the point of firing pin release. Flinching is something which has to be mentally controlled, and only experience can overcome this problem.

The **theory of recoil**, **recoil velocity** and **recoil energy** have little relevance in forensic firearms examinations. These subjects are covered in the author's previous book, *A Handbook of Firearms and Ballistics, Examining and Interpreting Forensic Evidence* (2nd edition).

5.1.4   Barrel pressure

Barrel pressure has, once again, little relevance in day to day forensic examinations, although it can occasionally be very important.

Illustrative Case 2

A cash in transit robbery occurred during which the transit guard was shot in the mouth with a revolver and killed. At the post mortem, it became obvious that he was not killed with a revolver bullet, but a revolver loaded with shotgun cartridges. Eventually, a suspect was arrested and in his possession was a WWI Webley .455″ calibre revolver together, with a number of .410″ calibre shotgun cartridges. Normally, these would have been too long to fit into the chamber of a .455″ revolver, but they had been cut down in length. This would normally have left very little room for the shot, but most of the wads had been removed, so that approximately two-thirds of the original load remained. To keep the shot from falling out, molten wax had been poured over the top of the shot.

The first couple of test shots that were fired showed that the modifications to the cartridge worked quite well, with the rifling producing a spiral pattern to the shot. However, the third shot fired completely destroyed the weapon, with only the grip being left in the hand of the firer. A number of cartridges were loaded in an attempt to duplicate those found with the gun, and tests in a pressure barrel found that if the wax was allowed to run down into the shot load, rather than being just a film over the top, the pressures produced would rise to alarming levels. It was obvious that the waxed shot came out of the cartridge as one solid piece rather than individual pellets. When this solid plug of wax-encased shot reached the forcing cone, it became stuck, causing massive pressures.

Table 5.1.1   Some Illustrative Chamber Pressure Figures for Modern Ammunition

Cartridge	Velocity	Bullet Weight	Pressure
0.22″ LR	1,200 ft/sec	40 grain	15,300 psi
	(365 m/s)	(2.56 gram)	(1,071 kg/cm^2)
0.32″ ACP	960 ft/sec	71 grain	21,700 psi
	(292 m/s)	(4.54 gram)	(1,519 kg/cm^2)
0.38″ Special	650 ft/sec	148 grain	21,700 psi
	(198 m/s)	(9.5 gram)	(1,519 kg/cm^2)
9 mm PB	1,200 ft/sec	125 grain	35,500 psi
	(365 m/s)	(8 gram)	(2,485 kg/cm^2)
0.45″ ACP	855 ft/sec	234 grain	14,000 psi
	(260 m/s)	(15 gram)	(98 kg/cm^2)
5.56 mm M16	3,250 ft/sec	56 grain	52,000 psi
	(990 m/s)	(3.6 gram)	(364 kg/cm^2)
12B shotgun	1200 ft/sec	490 grains	10,000 psi
2$\frac{1}{2}$″ cartridge	(365 m/s)	(31.36 gram)	(700 kg/cm^2)

Further reading

1 US Army (1965). *Interior Ballistics of Guns, Engineering Design Handbook*. Ballistics Series. United States Army Materiel Command, AMCP 706-150.

2 Heard, B.J. (2008). *A Handbook of Firearms and Ballistics, Examining and Interpreting Forensic Evidence* (2nd Edition). Wiley-Blackwell, ISBN978-0-470-69460-2.

3 Baer, P.G. & Frankle, J.M. (1962). *The Simulation of Interior Ballistic Performance of Guns by Digital Computer Program*. Aberdeen Proving Ground, MD: Ballistic Research Laboratories, BRL Report No. 1183.

4 Hatcher, J. S. (1962). *Hatcher's Notebook* (3rd edition). Harrisburg, PA: Stackpole Company, ISBN 8117-0614-1.

5 Horst, A.W. (2005). *A Brief Journey Through the History of Gun Propulsion*. Aberdeen Proving Ground, MD: United States Army Research Laboratory, ARL-TR-3671.

6 Rinkler, R.A. (1999). *Understanding Firearms Ballistics*. ISBN-10: 0964559846.

7 http://www.ballistics.org/docs/InteriorBallistics.pdf.

5.2

External Ballistics

5.2.1 Introduction

External ballistics is the study of the missile's flight from when it leaves the muzzle until it strikes the target. Like internal ballistics, this is an extremely complicated subject and, before the advent of powerful desktop computers and ballistic software programs, the calculations were laborious and time-consuming, requiring the use of many mathematical tables and graphs. With modern computers and ballistic programs, it is now possible to calculate the most complex trajectory equations with just a few keystrokes.

While this may seem to have little relevance in normal case investigations, it can, in certain circumstances, be of immense importance.

Illustrative Case 1

A five star hotel was holding a buffet function on the podium level pool area. Some of the guests were commenting on the flavour of the food and the 'crunchy' nature of several dishes. The head chef could not understand this, as there should not have been such a texture in any of the dishes he had produced. Then someone happened to look up at the sky and noticed that it appeared to be snowing, which was a little unusual as this was in the tropics!

A quick look at the 'snow' showed, in fact, that it was crushed glass, and it was this that was giving the food the crunchy texture. A quick search of the rooms above the patio showed that some ten windows on the upper floors had been broken, apparently by bullets. On examination, it was found that the damage was non-penetrating, but it was sufficient to craze the panes of glass and cause the glass dust that was falling into the food below. This was typical of the damage caused by a low-powered air weapon firing steel BB missiles.

The problem, however, was figuring out where the missiles were being fired from, as the nearest building was over 200 metres away. To determine from what direction the missiles had originated, laser sightings were taken from each damaged window to show not which direction the missiles had been fired from, but rather what direction they could not have been fired from (i.e. due to lack of buildings, protrusions such as ledges and framing struts on the hotel structure, trees, etc.). This eventually gave a very accurate direction and pointed to only one building. By carrying out the laser sighting in reverse at the suspected building, it could be narrowed down to a number of flats in a vertical strip.

Forensic Ballistics in Court: Interpretation and Presentation of Firearms Evidence, First Edition. Brian J. Heard.
© 2013 John Wiley & Sons, Ltd. Published 2013 by John Wiley & Sons, Ltd.

The trajectory was easily calculated by entering the assumed velocity of the missile, the range of the building, wind direction and speed into a ballistic program. This gave an exact location for the firing position. When a raid was carried out on the flat, a low-powered, smooth-bored air rifle was located, together with a box of steel BBs. Unfortunately, no missiles were found at the hotel, but the weapon was confiscated and no further shootings were reported.

Illustrative Case 2

Before 1997, China did not, officially, have any political representation in Hong Kong. It did have the New China News Agency (NCNA), but little if any news was ever sent or received from this building. One evening, while one of the 'news reporters' was working late at his desk, a .357 Magnum bullet came crashing through his window. This obviously produced considerable concern, and armed police, together with armed men from inside the building, were in great numbers. A short time later, another bullet penetrated an adjacent window, then two more through windows in adjacent offices.

From the impact sites on the walls and the holes in the windows, it appeared that all the shots had been fired from a low-flying aircraft, as the only building in the sight line had no windows on the side facing the NCNA building. However, by consulting a very sophisticated ballistics program, it was determined that the shots had been fired from a building on the other side of the one facing the NCNA, and the extreme range had caused a trajectory which took the bullet over the top of the building.

Eventually, the building from which the shots were fired was located at a range in excess of 0.75 miles (1.2 km). The search was narrowed down to one flat, inside of which a number of weapons were found. Microscopic comparisons showed these to have fired the shots which hit the NCNA. The owner of these weapons said that they were simply firing at targets on the roof of the building and thought that the bullets would have fallen harmlessly into the harbour!

Illustrative Case 3

During a shoot-out between police and an armed gang, numerous shots were fired. After an extensive search of the surrounding area, all of the fired bullets could be accounted for, apart from one which had been fired from a 7.62×25 mm calibre pistol. Approximately 200 yards (185 m) from the crime scene was a bullet hole in a high wooden fence. Using a ballistics program, it was possible to calculate the trajectory of the bullet after passing through the fence. This led to a hole in a third-storey window some 400 yards (370 m) further on from the fence. Inside the small office behind the damaged window was the owner, with a bullet hole straight though his heart.

From the above three illustrative cases it can be seen how important external ballistics can be in certain cases.

5.2.2 Basics

The two main factors which affect the performance of a bullet on leaving the barrel are air resistance on its nose and the effect of the gravitational pull of the earth. As a result of these forces the bullet will, on leaving the barrel, describe a downward curved path or trajectory.

The exact shape of this trajectory can be predetermined by knowing:

- the gravitational effect;

- the muzzle velocity;

- the angle of elevation of the barrel;

- the velocity;

- the sectional density of the bullet;

- the bullet shape.

The rate of fall can easily be determined by using the formula:

$$h = \frac{1}{2}gt^2$$

Where:

h = drop of missile
g = gravity which is 32.1725 feet per second per second (32.17 ft/sec^2)
t = time in seconds

Thus, a bullet would have dropped one foot below the line of flight in 0.25 seconds of flight (i.e. $h = \frac{1}{2} \times 32.17 \times 0.25 \times 0.25$), four feet in half a second, and sixteen feet in one second.

The drop is, of course, totally independent of the velocity and weight of the bullet. All bullets, no matter whether they are travelling at 200 ft/sec or 4,000 ft/sec, will drop four feet (1.22 metres) in half a second of flight. The only difference is that the 4,000 ft/sec bullet travels much further in half a second than the bullet which is only going at a speed of 200 ft/sec.

It is obvious, however, that the bullet does not continue at the same velocity throughout its flight. Air pressure on the nose of the bullet causes resistance, which gradually reduces its velocity. The amount of resistance caused by the air is dependent upon the shape of the bullet. Thus, a sharp-pointed bullet will have less air resistance than one with a blunt or flat front.

This difference in air resistance is referred to in ballistics as the '**form factor**' and is given the symbol 'i'. The form factor can vary from 0.6 for a sharp-nosed missile to 1.3 for a wadcutter-type profile.

Another important factor is the proportion of the missile's diameter to its weight. The weight is what gives the bullet its 'carrying power', while the cross-sectional area is what causes the air resistance. This is called the **sectional density** of the bullet, and is the weight divided by the retarding area, which is the square of the diameter.

Thus, the sectional density of a bullet is given by:

$$\text{Sectional density of bullet} = \frac{w}{d^2}$$

If we take as an example a .38″ Special 158 grain bullet, which has a diameter of .357″ (see section of ammunition nomenclature), the sectional density is given by the following equation:

$$\text{Sectional density} = \frac{158}{0.357 \times 0.357} = 1239$$

A much lighter, 125 grain, bullet of the same calibre will give a sectional density of:

$$\text{Sectional density} = \frac{125}{0.357 \times 0.357} = 980$$

As can be seen, the sectional density of the lighter bullet is much lower, indicating a lower carrying power.

Ballistic coefficient

The sectional density is not the only factor effecting the retardation (the degree of velocity loss due to the air) of a bullet, as the shape also plays a very large part. If the form factor 'i' is inserted into the formula, the resulting figure is called the '**ballistic coefficient**' of the missile and is the proportion of the bullet's diameter to its weight.

The ballistic coefficient (C) is calculated using the formula:

$$C = \frac{w}{id^2}$$

Where:

C = ballistic coefficient
w = weight of bullet
i = form factor
d = diameter of the bullet

The form factor is basically a measure of how streamlined a bullet is. For example, a wadcutter bullet will have a form factor of about 2.0 and a sleek highly streamlined pointed bullet will have a form factor of 0.55. These figures are published by the various ammunition manufacturers and are available on-line.

Thus the larger the ballistic coefficient, the better the bullet will retain its velocity and the lower the bullet drop for any given distance.

5.2.3 Maximum range of missiles

The instant a missile leaves the barrel of a weapon, gravity starts to act, and the missile will accelerate towards the ground at a speed of 32 ft/sec/sec. The maximum range which a missile will obtain when fired is dependent upon the elevation of the barrel, the bullet shape and the initial velocity.

The computations to accurately determine the external ballistics of a missile are exceedingly complicated and outside the scope of this book. There are, however, a few approximations and rough calculations that will give figures of sufficient accuracy for use in normal crime scene examinations.

Angle of elevation of the barrel

With small arms bullets, it is found that the **maximum range** is attained at an elevation of about 29°. From 29° up to 35°, there is little increase in range. The angle of elevation at which maximum range is obtained is called the **critical angle**.

At elevations in excess of 35°, the maximum range attained begins to decrease. A full study of this can be found in the *British Textbook of Small Arms* (1929).

Formula for calculating maximum range of bullets

There is no simple and accurate way of determining the maximum range of a bullet. The use of ballistics tables or ballistics software based on the Siacci/Mayevski G1[1] drag model, introduced in 1881, is usually considered the most appropriate method for general use. A more modern alternative is probably that presented in 1980 by Prof. Arthur J. Pejsa.[2]

These are, however, far too specialised to delve into within this book.

Other factors affecting maximum range

Bullet shape also has a pronounced effect, with sharply pointed bullets and those with a streamlined base (boat tailed) having a far greater range than a round ball.

As can be reasonably expected, the higher the velocity, the greater the range.

Maximum range for round balls

For calculating the maximum range of shotgun pellets and round balls, it is possible to obtain a very approximate figure using **Journee's Formula**. This states that the maximum range in yards of a spherical ball is 2,200 times the diameter in inches. This is, of course, only applicable to lead pellets.

Thus:

- a 12-gauge ball will have a maximum range of $2,200 \times 0.645'' = 1,420$ yards (1,299 metres);

- a No. 6 pellet will have a maximum range of $2,200 \times 0.1 = 220$ yards (201 metres).

Considering the relatively primitive instrumentation then available, Journee's work was quite remarkable. His omission of the muzzle velocity in his formula for maximum range was not a matter of ignorance of its effect, but recognition that makes no important difference within the practicable levels of shot shell velocities, as can be seen in Table 5.2.2.

Table 5.2.1 includes the maximum ranges for various lead shot sizes, computed by Journee's Formula.

N.B. Tables 5.2.1, 5.2.2, 5.2.3 and 5.2.4 have been left in the Imperial system. To give the metric

---

[1] *'QuickLoad'* computer ballistics program by Siacci/Mayevski.

[2] Pejsa, A.J. *Modern Practical Ballistics.*

Table 5.2.1   The Maximum Ranges of Various Rounds

Cartridge	Bullet Weight Grains (grams)	Muzzle Velocity ft/s (m/s)	Maximum Range Yds (metres)
.22″ LR	40 (2.56)	1,145 (349)	1,500 (1,372)
.22″ HV LR	40 (2.56)	1,335 (407)	1,565 (1,424)
.380″ ACP	95 (6.08)	970 (296)	1,089 (991)
.38″ Spl	148 (9.50)	770 (235)	1,700 (1,547)
.38″ Spl+P	158 (10.1)	890 (271)	2,150 (1,956)
.357″ Magnum	158 (10.1)	1,235 (376)	2,350 (2,138)
9 mm PB	125 (8.0)	1,120 (341)	1,900 (1,729)
.40″ S&W	180 (11.5)	1,000 (305)	1,800 (1,638)
.44″ Magnum	240 (15.36)	1,390 (424)	2,500 (2,275)
.45″ ACP	234 (14.97)	820 (250)	1,640 (1,492)
.223″ Remington	55 boat tailed bullet (3.52)	3,240 (987)	3,875 (3526)
.30″ M1 Carbine	110 (7.04)	1900 (579)	2,200 (2,002)
.30-30	170 (10.88)	2,220 (677)	2,490 (2,266)
.30–06″ Rifle	180 flat base bullet (11.50)	2,700 (823)	4,100 (3,731)
.30–06″ Rifle	180 boat (11.50) tailed bullet	2,700 (823)	5,700 (5,187)
.300″ Win Magnum	200 (12.80)	2,700 (823)	5390 (4,905)
.30–40″ Krag	220 (14.08)	2,000 (609)	4,050 (3,685)
.308″ Win (7.62 NATO)	175 (BT) (11.2)	2,600 (792)	4,800 (4,368)
.375″ H&H	270 (17.28)	2,695 (821)	3,370 (3,066)
.50″ Browning AP	718 (45.95)	2,840 (866)	10,000 (9,150)
12-bore shotgun ball	583 (34.43)	1,200 (366)	1,420 (1,292)
16-bore shotgun ball	437 (27.96)	1200 (366)	1,340 (1,219)
20-bore shotgun ball	350 (22.4)	1,200 (366)	1,200 (1,092)
.410″ shotgun ball	104 (6.65)	1,200 (366)	850 (773)
00 buck	54 (3.45)	1,200 (366)	726 (660)
1 buck	40 (2.56)	1,200 (366)	660 (600)
No. 2 shot	4.86 (0.311)	1,200 (366)	330 (300)
No. 3 shot	4.00 (0.256)	1,200 (366)	308 (280)
No. 4 shot	3.24 (0.207)	1,200 (366)	286 (260)
No. 5 shot	2.58 (0.165)	1,200 (366)	264 (240)
No. 6 shot	1.95 (0.125)	1,200 (366)	242 (220)
No. 7½ shot	1.25 (0.08)	1,200 (366)	209 (190)
No. 8 shot	1.07 (0.068)	1,200 (366)	198 (180)
No. 9 shot	0.75 (0.048)	1,200 (366)	176 (160)

equivalent would result in an almost unreadable table. The conversion factors for the figures can be found at Appendix 7.

A muzzle velocity of 1,200 fps was assumed for all shot sizes to afford a direct comparison with shot of different sizes. As can be seen in Table 5.2.3, the exact muzzle velocity makes little difference to the maximum range.

Table 5.2.2 illustrates that no great error is introduced by neglecting the effect of muzzle velocity on the maximum range of small shot. This results from the poor ballistic shape of spheres, which causes the aerodynamic drag to be very high at supersonic velocities. However, small shot soon drops to the velocity of sound, irrespective of the velocity at which they are launched.

For example, a No. 7½ shot fired at a muzzle velocity of 2,400 fps – twice that of a normal target load – would have its velocity reduced to 1,120 fps (the speed of sound) within about the first 26 yards of

Table 5.2.2   Maximum Ranges for Various Lead Shot Computed by Journee's Formula

Shot Size (Lead Shot)	Diameter (ins)	Maximum Range	Striking Velocity ft/sec
12	.050	110	63
9	.080	176	79
8	.090	198	82
7½	.095	209	85
6	.110	242	89
5	.120	264	94
4	.130	286	96
2	.150	330	99
BB	.180	396	107
4 Buck	.240	528	125
1 Buck	.300	660	135
00 Buck	.330	726	139

Table 5.2.4   Remaining Velocity for Various Lead Shot Fired Vertically

Shot Size	Return Velocity (ft/sec)
12	63
9	79
8	83
7½	85
6	91
5	95
4	98
2	105
BB	115
No.4 buckshot	132
No.1 buckshot	147
No.00 buckshot	154

flight. Doubling the velocity would, therefore, increase the maximum range by only about 26 yards.

Table 5.2.3 Shows the remaining velocity for various sizes of shot at its maximum range achieved at a firing elevation of 22°.

For all shot from No. 12 to 00 buckshot, the maximum range is achieved at firing elevations of about 20–25°. It is important to note, however, that a firing elevation of only 10° produces nearly 90 per cent of maximum range.

Although the striking velocity of about 80 fps for these small shot would not be fatal in itself, a pellet in the eye could cause serious injury, from which death could result. In the case of No. 2 or BB shot, the maximum range exceeds 300 yards and the striking

velocity is about 100 fps. This would produce a much more serious injury.

Many shooters want to know the velocity of shot returning to earth after it has been fired upward at very steep angles. The answer is that the returning velocities are not much different from those shown in Table 5.2.2 for shot fired vertically.

For any body falling through the atmosphere, there is some velocity at which the force of aerodynamic drag equals the weight of the body. When that velocity is reached, the body ceases to accelerate under the influence of gravity and falls at constant velocity, sometimes called the 'terminal velocity of return', regardless of how far the body falls.

It should also be mentioned that other factors not considered in the calculations can affect the maximum range of shot. Since the time of flight is several seconds, a strong wind could materially affect the maximum horizontal range. Deformation of the individual pellets will also generally shorten the maximum range.

It is also possible for several pellets to be fused together if hot propellant gases leak past the obturating wad into the shot charge. This is far less likely now, due to efficient plastic obturating wads, than it was with felt and card wads. However, when it does happen, the clusters of shot can travel considerably farther than individual pellets in the charge.

Table 5.2.3   Maximum Range in Yards of Small Shot at Various Muzzle Velocities

Shot Size	MV = 1,200 ft/sec	MV = 1,500 ft/sec	MV = 2,400 ft/sec
7½	210	219	236
2	303	317	343
00 buck	561	591	650

Table 5.2.5   Terminal Figures for No. 6 Shot Fired at Various Elevations

Firing elevation (Degrees)	Distance to Impact (Feet)	Angle of Fall (Degrees)	Time of Flight (Seconds)	Impact Velocity (ft/sec)
0	0	0	0	1200
1	119	2.6	0.75	224
5	187	18.8	2.28	100
10	212	37.8	3.53	83
15	231	51.1	4.48	82
20	236	59.5	5.23	80
25	236	64.8	5.82	92
30	231	69.0	5.73	95
35	222	71.2	6.63	97
40	209	73.0	6.78	97
45	193	74.0	6.84	96

All figures are for No. 6 shot fired at a velocity of 1,200 ft/sec.

Illustrative Case 4

The sports master at a prestigious private school thought that he would inject some incentive into his cross-country runs by taking pot shots at the children with a 9 mm shotgun. At the ranges he was firing from, there was little, if any, chance of the pellets even reaching the children, let alone injuring them – in theory. Unfortunately, the shot in one of the rounds 'balled', which resulted in a single 9 mm projectile with a muzzle velocity of 1,200 fps (366 mps). This struck one of the children in the chest, coming to rest in his heart, where the 'balled' shot broke up and was pumped round his body. The boy did survive, but only after having each and every one of the pellets removed via extensive surgery.

With other missiles, the figures in Table 5.2.6 give an approximate range when fired at an elevation of approximately 30°.

An elevation of between 29° and 35° will give the greatest range.

Table 5.2.6   List of Maximum Range for Various Missiles Fired at an Elevation of 30°

Cartridge	Bullet Weight	Muzzle Velocity	Maximum Range
0.22″ LR	40 grn (2.56 gram)	1,145 f/s (350 m/s)	1,500 yds (1,372 m)
0.30″ M1 carbine	110 grn (7.04 gram)	1,900 f/s (363 m/s)	2,200 yds (2,013 m)
0.30″ M1 rifle	180 grn (11.52 gram) flat base bullet	2,700 f/s (823 m/s)	4,100 yds (3,751 m)
0.30″ M1 rifle	180 grn (11.52 gram) boat-tail bullet	2,700 f/s (823 m/s)	5,700 yds (5,215 m)

(continued)

Table 5.2.6   (*Continued*)

Cartridge	Bullet Weight	Muzzle Velocity	Maximum Range
0.38″ Spl	148 grn (9.42 gram)	770 f/s (234 m/s)	1,700 yds (1,555 m)
0.38″ Spl+P	158 grn (10.12 gram)	890 f/s (271 m/s)	2,150 yds (1,967 m)
9 mm PB	125 grn (8.0 gram)	1,120 f/s (341 m/s)	1,900 yds (1,738 m)
0.357″ Magnum	158 grn (10.12 gram)	1,235 f/s (376 m/s)	2,350 yds (2,150 m)
0.45″ ACP	230 grn (14.72 gram)	855 f/s (260 m/s)	1,460 yds (1,336 m)
0.44″ Magnum	240 grn (15.36 gram)	1,390 f/s (424 m/s)	2,500 yds (2,287 m)

5.2.4 Maximum altitude that a bullet will attain

As with many other subjects that one comes across in forensic firearms examinations, this has little real relevance in everyday case examinations. There are occasions, however, when it can be extremely important especially in cases involving terrorism.

In 1909, Major Hardcastle fired a number of rounds vertically into the air, and shortly after World War I Julian S. Hatcher carried out a similar set of experiments using the 30–06 rifle round.

A very simple rule of thumb was found to be that the maximum altitude that a bullet will reach will be approximately two-thirds the maximum horizontal range.

The results of some actual test firings are shown in Table 5.2.7.

Table 5.2.7   Maximum Height Attained for Various Missiles Fired Vertically

Calibre	Bullet Weight (grns.)	Velocity (fps)	Maximum Height (ft)
.22 LR	40	1257	3,868
.25 ACP	50	751	2,287
.44 Magnum	240	1,280	4,518
5.56 mm SS109	50	3,200	2,650
7.62 NATO	150	2,756	7,874
30–06 M2	150	2,851	9,331
.303	175	2,785	9,420
30–06	180	2,400	10,105
12B	No.2 shot (US)	1,312	330
12B	No.4 (US)	1,312	286
12B	No.6 (US)	1,312	242
12B	No.7½ (US)	1,312	209
12B	N.8 (US)	1,312	198

Illustrative Case 5

On landing at Heathrow Airport, a commercial airliner which had been flying in the air space above Northern Ireland was found to have a 7.62mm calibre hole in one side of the tailfin. Unfortunately, the airline concerned was unwilling to have the tailfin taken apart, due to the costs involved, so it was not possible to determine the exact calibre of the weapon used.

The question was, therefore, what type of weapon could have fired a bullet with sufficient velocity to reach an altitude of 9,000 feet (2,743 m) at which the airliner was flying?

From the limited data in Table 5.2.7 it can be seen that only the 30-06 or .303" rounds have sufficient velocity to reach an airliner flying at 9,000 feet. There are, however, a vast number of hunting cartridges that would be equally capable of reaching such an altitude.

5.2.5   Terminal velocity

The terminal velocity of a missile is obviously much more relevant to the investigator, as any bullet fired vertically into the air will come down with potential wounding capability. The ability to calculate the actual terminal velocity of a missile could, therefore, be critical to the investigation.

When any object falls through the atmosphere, eventually the retarding force of drag will balance with gravity, and the object's terminal velocity will be reached. It is easy to calculate this terminal velocity if the drag coefficient is known.

When the forces are balanced:

$$Mm_2 v^2 = Mg$$

Where:
  M = mass of object
  m_2 = ballistic coefficient
  g = gravity
  v = velocity

Illustrative Cases 6

- December 31, 1994: A tourist from Boston was killed by a falling bullet from celebratory firing while walking on the Moonwalk in the French Quarter of New Orleans, Louisiana.

- July 22, 2003: More than 20 people were reported killed in Iraq from celebratory gunfire following the deaths of Saddam Hussein's sons Uday and Qusay in 2003.

- January 1, 2005: A stray bullet hit a young girl during New Year celebrations in the central square of downtown Skopje, Macedonia. She died two days later.

- February 25, 2007: Five people were killed by stray bullets fired at a kite festival in Lahore, Pakistan, including a six year old schoolboy who was struck in the head near his home in the city's Mazang area.

- July 29, 2007: At least four people were reported killed and 17 others wounded by celebratory gunfire in the capital city of Baghdad, Iraq, following the victory of the national football team in the AFC Asian Cup.

- January 1, 2012: A 15 year old girl, Karla Michelle Negrón Vélez, was wounded in the head by celebratory gunfire ten minutes after midnight in Puerto Rico.

- January 1, 2012: 12 year old Diego Duran was wounded in the head by celebratory gunfire while watching fireworks around 1 AM in Ruskin, Florida.

Table 5.2.8 Some Examples of the Terminal Velocities of Everyday Items

Object	Speed (mph)	Speed (fps)	Speed (mps)
Raindrop	15	22	6.7
Table tennis ball	20	29	8.8
Golf ball	90	131	40
Baseball	95	139	42

The mass of the bullet (M) drops out of the equation, which at first may seem strange, since mass clearly should have an effect on terminal velocity. Actually, the ballistic coefficient itself depends on mass (e.g. bullet shape, air density, and cross-sectional area, among several other things), so M dropping out of the above equation is merely illusionary.

Because air resistance depends largely on surface area, while weight depends on volume, larger bullets will drop faster than smaller bullets.

Table 5.2.9 Some Examples of the Terminal Velocities of Bullets

Calibre	Bullet Weight	Initial Velocity	Terminal Velocity
.22″ LR	40 grn	1,257 ft/sec	197 ft/sec
.44″ Magnum	240 grn	1,280 ft/sec	250 ft/sec
30-06	150 grn	2,756 ft/sec	325 ft/sec
.50″ Browning	750 grn	2,900 ft/sec	500 ft/sec

Small bullets will start to tumble and they will come down relatively slowly, whereas larger bullets can maintain their stabilising rotation and will come down much faster.

These figures are well within the penetration limit for skin, showing that a falling bullet does have the potential to wound.

5.2.6 Use of sight to compensate for bullet drop

To compensate for the bullet drop due to gravity, the sights are raised to give the barrel sufficient elevation so that the bullet will strike the target at a set distance. For handguns, this is generally ten yards, for a .22″ rifle it is 25 yards and for full bore rifles it is generally 200 yards.

With the rear sight so elevated, the sight line would be parallel to the ground and the sight line along the barrel axis considerably elevated above the target. Thus, the bullet leaves the barrel below the sight line but along the barrel axis. At some point from the barrel, it passes through the sight axis line and describes a trajectory between the barrel axis and sight line, eventually striking the target at the point of aim.

5.2.7 Other influencing factors

In addition to air resistance and gravity, there are other forces that influence the flight of the bullet. For example, **wind** will cause the bullet to drift

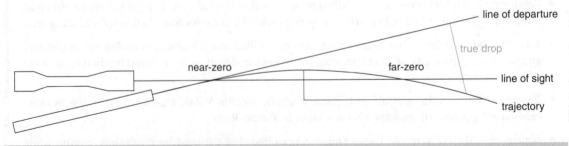

Figure 5.2.1 Line of sight vs. bullet drop.

Illustrative Case 7

While at the top of a ladder, painting his house, a man suddenly fell off and, upon examination, was found to be quite dead. The post mortem examination revealed an extremely small hole in the neck by the right shoulder blade and a bullet lodged in his heart. This was obviously the cause of his death, but the question was, 'from where was the bullet fired?'

From the direction the bullet took, it appeared that the bullet had been fired from a plane, but this was hardly likely. On close examination, bullet it was found to have, in addition to the clear rifling marks, a series of deep spiral scratches from the bullets nose to its base. Obviously, the bullet had struck something else before hitting the deceased. Back-calculating the angle of entry showed that the bullet had been falling almost straight down. Estimating its final velocity showed that the bullet was obviously falling under gravity alone and, by consulting a ballistics computer program, it was determined that the shot was fired from nearly two miles (3.2 km) away.

The only range within that distance from the deceased was a military small arms training facility. On consulting the firing logs, it was found that one group of soldiers had been practising with a general purpose machine gun (GPMG). During a demonstration by the officer in charge of the correct firing technique, the weapon had escaped his grasp and the bullets had started to strike the top of the retaining bank at the end of the range. It was a simple matter of collecting test fired bullets from the weapon concerned and comparing them against the bullet recovered from the deceased to show that the bullet had been fired from that weapon.

---

with it in proportion to the wind's direction and velocity.

Thus, a wind blowing from the right of the bullet will cause it to drift to the left. Rear winds will have an increasing effect on the velocity, and nose winds a decreasing effect. The amount of wind drift, when striking the bullet at 90°, can be calculated by the following:

$$D = \left(T - \frac{R}{V} \right) W$$

Where:

D = deflection of bullet by wind
R = range
V = muzzle velocity
T = time of flight
W = cross wind speed.

Drift is caused by the rifling of the bullet and is as a result of the gyrostatic properties of the rifling-induced spin. This effect gives bullets with a right-hand spin a drift to the right and left-hand spinning bullets a drift to the left. It is hardly of any significance in rifles, and virtually none at all in handguns.

With a .303″ rifle, the drift will be approximately 13 inches to the right at a range of 1,000 yards.

Yaw is something that only has real relevance to rifle ammunition. It is due to a slight destabilisation of the bullet as it leaves the barrel and is probably a consequence of excessive spin on the bullet. This results in the bullet describing an air spiral while, at the same time, having a spin around its own tail axis. At close ranges, this results in a larger target group than would be expected. As the range becomes greater, the effect disappears and the target groups return to their expected dimensions. The effect is very similar to that of a spinning top which wobbles slightly before settling down into a stable spinning condition.

It is this yaw in rifle bullets which produces far greater wounds at close range than would normally be expected. With the bullet rotating around its axis, it is easily destabilised when entering tissue or some medium denser than air. This destabilisation causes the bullet to start tumbling, giving up its energy very quickly. So violent can this tumbling be that many

---

Illustrative Case 8

During filming for a documentary, it was decided to fire various rounds at modelling clay to illustrate the various wounding capabilities of the weapons under test. Modelling clay is not the ideal medium for this purpose, but for the filming it was acceptable. Various pistol rounds were fired, with predicable effects, but when it came to a .303 rifle, the director wanted the shooter and the block of clay to be in frame together. It was suggested that this would not give an accurate representation, due to the yaw of the bullet at close range. When the first shot was fired at a range of 25 metres, the table-sized block of modelling clay exploded into small fragments. Not one piece of the bullet itself could be found. When the shot was fired at a range of 200 metres, the bullet made a small entry and a small exit hole, with a tunnel connecting the two which was only slightly larger than the bullet.

Illustrative Case 9

A range accident occurred involving a military 7.62 × 51 mm round fired from a FNL rifle. It was assumed that the rifle was empty when the soldier left the firing point but, on pulling the trigger, it was discovered that there was still a round in the chamber. Another soldier in the target practice detail was shot in the abdomen at a range of no more than ten metres. On entering the body, the bullet destabilised and started to break up, causing an absolutely massive wound right through the body and out the back. The rifle was test fired at tissue simulants at ranges from 5–200 metres, and it was found that up to about 150 metres, the bullet would destabilise and break up. At ranges in excess of 150 metres, the bullet was stable and would pass through the tissue simulant, causing no more than a very small 'through and through' hole.

---

bullets will completely break up, causing even more massive wounds. Once the spin slows down, the bullet will stabilise, giving rise to far more typical bullet wounds.

5.2.8 Muzzle energy

Muzzle energy is probably the most important property when dealing with ballistics. This figure gives an indication of the overall power of the bullet as it leaves the barrel and, as a result, an indication of its wounding potential. It is also extremely important when determining whether a low-powered gas- or air-powered weapon fits within certain firearms regulations.

Naturally, many other factors have to be taken into consideration when dealing with wound ballistics, but these will be dealt with at a later stage.

Muzzle energy is the potential work energy possessed by the missile as it exits the muzzle. It is quoted in terms of kinetic energy, which is the ability to do work. The formula for calculating the muzzle energy of a missile is:

$$KE = \frac{1}{2}MV^2$$

Where:
  $KE =$ kinetic energy
  $M =$ mass of the projectile
  $V =$ velocity of the projectile

When using imperial measurements, it is usually quoted in foot pounds (ft/lbs), with the weight of the projectile being measured in grains (7,000 grains = 1 pound) and the velocity in feet per second.

When the appropriate figure for gravity (32.174) is placed into the formula, it becomes:

$$KE \text{ (ft lbs)} = \frac{MV^2}{2 \times 32.174 \times 7000}$$

When working in the SI system, the kinetic energy is quoted in **Joules** (J), with the mass of the bullet in kilograms and the velocity in metres per second. The equation then becomes:

$$KE \,(\text{Joules}) = \frac{MV^2}{2}$$

The elimination of g in the SI system occurs simply because the two systems have different sized relationships between their physical units.

The conversion factor for ft/lbs to Joules is to multiply by 1.3558

5.2.9   Momentum

The most important property of momentum, as far as ballistics is concerned, is that it is conserved in collisions. That is, if two or more objects collide, the total of their momenta is the same after collision as it was before. The importance of this will be seen in the next section (5.3, Terminal Ballistics).

Momentum is the quantity of motion of a moving body and is calculated by the formula:

$$\text{Momentum} = M \times V$$

Where:
  M = Mass of projectile
  V = Velocity

In the Imperial system, momentum expressed in pounds feet per second (lb ft/sec). In the SI system, it is quoted in kilogram metres per second (kg m/s)

Further reading

1 Whelen, T. (1945). *Small Arms Design and Ballistics*. Small Arms Technical Publishing Co, Georgetown, SC. ASIN: B001NZQ8U2.
2 Rinker, R.A. (1999). *Understanding Firearm Ballistics*. Mulberry House Pub Co; ISBN-10: 0964559846.
3 The War Office (1929; New edition 2003). *Textbook for Small Arms 1929*. Naval and Military Press. ISBN-10: 1843428083.
4 Hicks, J.W. (1919). *The Theory of the Rifle and Rifle Shooting*. London, C. Griffin & Company, Limited.

5.3

Terminal Ballistics

5.3.1 Introduction

Terminal ballistics is the study of missiles' penetration in solids and liquids. It can be subdivided into **penetration potential**, which is the capability of a missile to penetrate various materials, and **wound ballistics**, which is the effect the missile has on living tissue.

The misinformation surrounding these two subjects is staggering. It is therefore extremely important to have an overview of the main concepts surrounding these topics, as well as a basic understanding of the mechanisms involved.

Lawyers need a good grasp of wound ballistics to promote rules limiting the use of force and prohibiting certain types of bullets, and forensic firearms examiners require such an understanding to present evidence in court about cause of death.

It was mentioned earlier that the basic definition of a firearm is a 'lethal barrelled weapon' – but what criteria must be satisfied for a gun to be classified as 'lethal'? The UK Firearms Act defines a firearm as 'a weapon capable of firing a projectile with sufficient force to inflict more than a trivial injury, i.e. with sufficient force to puncture skin'. The Home Office considers the lowest level of muzzle energy capable of inflicting a penetrating wound is one foot pound (1.35 Joules). Hence, guns producing less than 1 ft/lb. are not covered by the Act and therefore not classified as air weapons or subject to any restrictions.

To place this into perspective, a pellet fired from a low velocity .177" (4.5 mm) calibre air gun, for example producing 1 ft/lb. (1.35 J) of KE, may only cause a trivial injury to a fit young person; however, if an elderly person is shot in the eye, the trauma could conceivably lead to their death. On the other hand, a low velocity air weapon designed to fire steel BBs may be incapable of penetrating skin, but a dart fired through the same weapon could pierce an artery close to the surface of the skin, which could cause death through excessive blood loss.

A weapon's 'lethality' could be therefore be age-related or missile-related. This chapter will attempt to clarify such points and to clear up some of the misconceptions which surround this subject.

5.3.2 Basics

Penetration potential

The penetration of various materials can be of great assistance in the investigation of shooting incidents. It is also of considerable general interest to show how often movie makers and novel writers make appalling blunders.

Forensic Ballistics in Court: Interpretation and Presentation of Firearms Evidence, First Edition. Brian J. Heard.
© 2013 John Wiley & Sons, Ltd. Published 2013 by John Wiley & Sons, Ltd.

Illustrative Case 1

In virtually all Western movies, there is a shoot-out with one or both sides hiding behind tables or water butts. The weapons used are normally Colt Single Action Army Model 1873 revolvers in .45″ Colt calibre and the Winchester Model 1873 under-lever rifles in 44–40″ calibre. The bullets from both the .45″ Colt and .44–40″ cartridges would pass straight through a normal 2″ (50 mm) thick tabletop or an empty water barrel. A water barrel full of water would appreciably slow down the .45″ Colt bullet, but it would still come out of the other side with considerable velocity. The 44–40″ bullet, on the other hand will still have most of its energy left after penetrating such a water-filled water barrel.

One of the very many ways in which movie and TV producers get it completely wrong is with sawn-off shotguns. The firing of such a weapon is generally shown with a shower of sparks emanating from the barrel, and with virtually no recoil whatsoever. In reality, there will be a huge gout of flame, along with a vicious recoil which most people would have the greatest difficulty in controlling. In test firings with sawn-off shotguns (unpublished work by author), there have been broken fingers, split skin on the palms of the hands, dislocated thumbs, severe bruising and weapons which have recoiled out of the hands of the firer.

Bullet penetration

In the past, one of the standard tests performed to assess bullet and cartridge performance was the penetration of 7/8″ (2.14 mm) thick pine boards. This, as with any other type of penetration test, is plagued with inaccuracies. Many factors, including the moisture content, knot content, tree age and even the separation of the boards, can give rise to highly variable results. Other than for general interest this type of test is of little use in the scientific examination of firearms related situations. For the sake of historical documentation some of the published results for this test follow.

The following are some indicators of the penetrative powers of various types of ammunition:

- A .22″ lead air gun pellet requires a minimum of 250 ft/sec (72 m/s) velocity to penetrate fresh human skin.

- A .177″ lead air gun pellet requires a minimum of 300 ft/sec (91.5 m/s) velocity to penetrate fresh human skin.

- A .22″ lead air gun pellet at 450 ft/sec (137 m/s) will make a hole in, but not penetrate, $\frac{1}{4}$″ (0.63 cm) plate glass.

- A .22″ lead air gun pellet at 600 ft/sec (183 m/s) will penetrate $\frac{1}{4}$″ (0.63 cm) plate glass.

- A steel BB (.170″ ball bearing) at 200 ft/sec (61 m/s) will make a hole in, but not penetrate, $\frac{1}{4}$″ (0.63 cm) plate glass.

- A steel BB or .177″ (4.5 mm) lead pellet at 200 ft/sec (61 m/s) will detach part of the coloured portion (iris) of a human eye, leaving what appears to be a second pupil.

- A steel BB or .177″ (4.5 mm) lead pellet at 450 ft/sec (137 m/s) will burst a human eye.

Table 5.3.1 Penetration of 7/8″ (2.14 mm) pine boards for various pistol calibres

.22″ LR	5 boards
.32″ ACP	5 boards
.38″ S&W revolver	5 boards
.38″ Special	7 boards
9 mm PB pistol	9 boards
.45″ ACP	7 boards
30–06 rifle	72 boards
45–70 govt. rifle	15 boards

- A.177″ (4.5 mm) steel air gun dart will penetrate to shank in skin at 120 ft/sec (36.5 m/s).

- A 158 grain (10.1 gram) .38″ Special plain lead bullet will generally not penetrate the outside skin of a car body.

- A 158 grain (10.1 gram) .357″ Magnum semi-jacketed bullet will penetrate the outside skin of car door and sometimes just penetrate the inside skin.

- A 125 grain (8 gram) 9 mm PB fully jacketed bullet will generally penetrate both skins of a car door.

- A 158 grain (10.1 gram) .38″ Special plain lead bullet will only penetrate one side of a human skull.

- A 158 grain (10.1 gram) .38″ Special plain lead bullet will generally not exit from a human body.

- 158 grain (10.1 gram) .38″ Special + P and .357″ Magnum semi jacketed bullets will penetrate both sides of a human skull.

- A.38″ Special + P, 158 grain (10.1 gram) non-expanding bullet will, unless it strikes bone, pass straight through a human body.

- Virtually all calibres (excepting air weapons) will penetrate the tread or side wall of a motor vehicle tyre.

The above figures are the results of unpublished work by the author.

The following are illustrative penetration capabilities of a 30–06 full-jacketed rifle bullet at a velocity of 2,700 ft/sec (823 m/s) and at a range of 200 yards (182 m):

- ¼″ (0.6 cm) of armour plate

- 7″ (17 cm) of gravel

- 4.5″ (11 cm) of brick

- 4.0″ (10 cm) concrete

- 32″ (78.5 cm) of oak wood

- 6.5″ (16 cm) of dry sand

- 7″ (17.1 cm) of moist sand

- 26″ (64 cm) of loam

- 24″ (59 cm) of clay

- 19″ (46.5 cm) of loose earth

- 60″ (147 cm) of 1″ (2.45 cm) pine boards

The above figures are taken from the *Textbook for Small Arms 1929*. Naval and Military Press. ISBN-10: 1843428083.

5.3.3 General wound ballistic concepts

There are three concepts generally held by most people as to the effect of a bullet striking a human being:

1. The first is that the bullet 'drills' its way through, leaving a small entry and an equally small exit wound.

2. The second is that the bullet leaves a small entry and an enormous exit wound.

3. The third is that when someone is shot by anything other than an air rifle, the impact is enough to lift the person off their feet and flying through the air.

Basically all three concepts are incorrect in one way or another. Let us look at these misconceptions in more detail.

Misconception 1

As a bullet passes through human tissue, it imparts some or all of its kinetic energy to the surrounding tissue. The energy so supplied throws the tissue away from the bullet's path in a radial manner, leaving a temporary wound cavity much larger than the diameter of the bullet. The temporary nature of this cavity results from the natural elasticity of animal tissue, which allows it to regain its original structure after the bullet has passed.

There is also a permanent cavity which results from the destruction of tissue caused by the bullet itself. This permanent cavity is dependent on the cross-sectional area of the bullet and any secondary missiles which may be produced from the break-up of the bullet during its passage. The temporary cavity has a very short life span and is followed by a number of after-shocks decreasing in severity. The final, permanent, cavity may be many times greater than the diameter of the missile, but it is also many times smaller than the temporary cavity.

Unlike the temporary cavity, where the tissue is merely being thrown away from the wound track and no permanent damage is being caused to the tissue, the permanent cavity is caused by the actual destruction of the tissue by the passage of the bullet. The dimensions of this cavity are dependent upon the shape, weight, size and velocity of the missile and the elasticity of the surrounding structures.

With extremely high velocity missiles, in excess of 3,000 ft/sec (914 m/s), there is an explosive movement of the tissue away from the wound track. This results in enormous temporary cavities, as well as extensive fracturing to bones and damage to veins and arteries in the immediate vicinity. In addition, there is often a back splash of tissue out of the entry hole, giving the impression of an exit wound. This explosive movement of the tissue away from the bullet track is sometimes referred to as 'tissue quake'. This is not the best of terms to use.

An example of the relationship between the permanent and temporary cavity can be seen in Figure 5.3.1. which has been caused by a 12-bore shotgun cartridge loaded with AAA pellets that are 0.2″ (5.2 mm) in diameter.

Misconception 2

The second misconception is that the entry hole is always small and the exit hole large. This can be a major problem when interpretation of close range or suicide wounds is called for.

When dealing with high-power handgun ammunition firing hollow point ammunition, it is often the case that the entry hole is smaller than the exit hole.

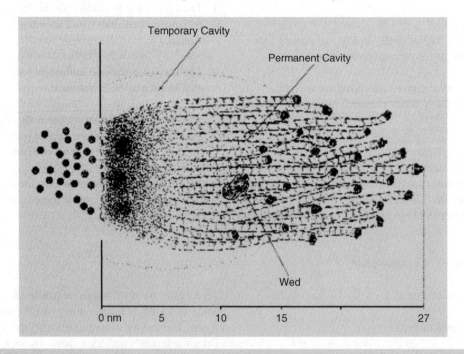

Figure 5.3.1 Permanent and temporary cavities caused by a 12-bore shotgun cartridge loaded with AAA shot.

Tissue entering the hollow point cavity causes the bullet to expand, increasing the permanent wound cavity and hence the exit wound size. In some cases, this can increase the surface contact area of the bullet by up to 200 per cent. Not only does this increased surface area enable the missile to transmit more of its energy to the target, but it also increases the possibility of the bullet damaging a vital organ or blood vessel due to the much larger permanent cavity of the wound track. If the bullet does exit from the body, this expansion of the hollow point bullet within the tissue will give rise to an exit hole considerably larger than the entry hole.

Expansion of a hollow point bullet in soft tissue does not appear to be dependent upon its calibre. It does, however, generally require a velocity in excess of 900 ft/sec (274 m/s) for it to happen. At velocities below this, the bullet will not expand at all unless it hits bone.

Another factor influencing the expansion of hollow point bullets is bullet yaw. A yawing bullet will not strike the target at 90° and, as a result of this, bullet expansion will not occur (Knudsen & Sørensen, 1994).

There is, however, some controversy over the necessity for a hollow point bullet to strike at 90° for expansion to take place. Poole *et al.* (1994) are of the opinion that, at striking angles of up to 45°, this is not the case.

Plugging of the hollow point by fabric from the bullet's passage through clothing or any other intermediate material will also inhibit the expansion of hollow point bullets. If, on the other hand, even a moderately powered handgun is held with the

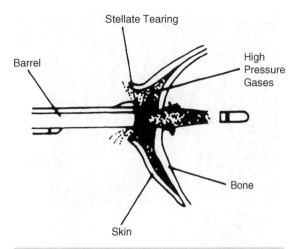

Stellate Tearing

Barrel

High Pressure Gases

Bone

Skin

Figure 5.3.2 Diagram showing contact wound to the head.

muzzle in tight contact with the skin, the entry hole can be massive. In this case, the high pressure gases which follow the bullet out of the barrel have nowhere to go other than into the wound behind the bullet. These gases expand at a rate grater than the speed at which the bullet is passing through the tissue and, as they have nowhere else to go, they burst back out through the bullet entry hole. The resultant hole can be enormous and, to the inexperienced eye, this can give every indication of an exit wound. The presence of partially burnt propellant in the wound, and blood and tissue in and on the barrel of the weapon, will correctly identify the wound as an entry rather than an exit wound. Another identifier is the deep cruciform tearing around the wound, called **'stellate tearing'**.

Illustrative Case 2

A married police officer was having an affair with an unmarried female. She became pregnant and was pressing him to leave his wife and children and live with him. He decided that he didn't want to lose his wife, so he ended the affair during a very heavy drinking session in an hotel room. When he awoke the next morning, there beside him was the girlfriend, who had been dead for several hours, with a through-and-through wound to the head. On the right side of her head was a very large torn hole, and on the left a small hole. The wounds were typical of those produced by the muzzle of the weapon being held in tight contact with the right temple, causing massive stellate tearing. One question being asked was 'Why wasn't the officer awakened by the sound of a short-barrelled revolver being fired in close proximity to him?' The answer to this is quite simple, in that the woman's head was acting as a large silencer, allowing the gases to expand and thus slow down to below the speed of sound.

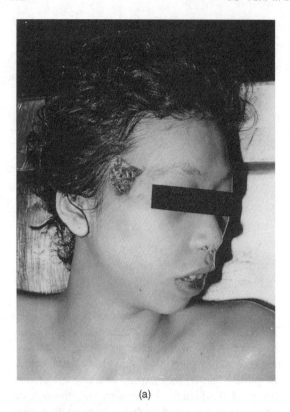

(a)

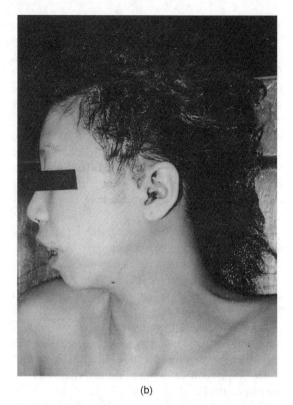

(b)

Figure 5.3.3(a)   An example of contact entry wound exhibiting stellate tearing.

Figure 5.3.3(b)   Exit wound from Figure 5.3.3(a).

Other indicators of a contact wound can be the flare from the side of a revolver's cylinder and, sometimes, the presence of a mark made by the front sight of the weapon. In double-barrelled shotguns, the second, unfired barrel can often leave a large impact-type mark (Figure 5.3.4). This mark results from the high-pressure gases which, before bursting back out, balloon out the tissues, crushing the skin into the other muzzle.

Misconception 3

The third concept, that when someone is shot by anything other than an air rifle, the impact is enough to lift the person off their feet and flying through the air, is completely untrue. This once again enters the realms of mathematical ballistics, but it is a very important concept to be aware of, especially when dealing with multiple-shot suicides (Poole *et al.*, 1994; Stone, 1987).

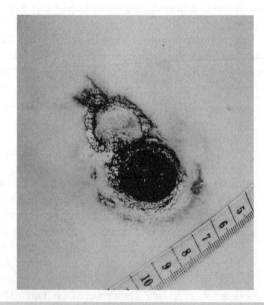

Figure 5.3.4   Wound from O/U shotgun, clearly showing the imprint from the second barrel and the winged foresight.

Illustrative Case 3

A police officer was found dead inside a locked room with five bullet holes from a .38″ Smith and Wesson revolver in his chest. The defence was that the first shot would have thrown the revolver so violently away from his body that he could not have fired a second, let alone a third and a fourth shot. This was a nonsensical argument, as the .38″ S&W revolver is a very low-powered round, with a consequentially low recoil. However, even if it had of been a .357″ Magnum round, the revolver would have done little other than rotate in the shooter's hand.

In this type of case (see Illustrative Case 3), the common misconception is that after the first shot, the body will be thrown away with such force that a second shot would not be possible. This is, of course, completely false, as a brief examination of the mathematics will show.

There are two factors to consider when dealing with the effect of a bullet on the human body, one is **momentum** and the other **kinetic energy**.

Momentum (plural 'momenta') is Mass × Velocity, and possibly its most important property is that it is conserved during collisions. That is, if two or more objects collide, the total of their momenta is the same after collision as it was before. This is Newton's Third Law of Motion.

Consider a rifle bullet of 0.02 lbs (140 grains) being fired at 3,000 ft/sec (914 m/s) into a 200 lbs (90.6 kg) stationary piece of wood (the following calculations are being left in the Imperial System to prevent the equations becoming confused with masses of figures in brackets).

The momentum of the bullet, $M1$, before collision is thus:

$$M1 = 0.02 \times 3000 = 60 \, \text{lb ft/sec (pounds feet per second)}$$

If $M2$ is the momentum of the log plus bullet after being struck by the bullet, then: $M1 = M2$. The log will, after being struck, have a mass of $200 + 0.02 = 200.02$. Thus, $200.02 \times$ velocity of the log must equal the momentum of the bullet before striking the log, i.e. 60 lb ft/sec. By rearranging the equation and substituting the known figures, we have:

Velocity of log after being struck = 60/200.02

$$= 0.2999 \, \text{ft/sec}$$

With such a minimal velocity, it can be easily appreciated that if the log were a person, then the body would not fly very fast or far through the air.

The next question is how far would the body be lifted off the ground by such an impact? If the mass is 200.02 and the velocity 0.2999 ft/sec, then:

$$KE = \frac{1}{2}MV^2$$

Where:

KE = Kinetic Energy

M = Mass of the projectile

V = Velocity of the projectile

$$KE \, (\text{ft lbs}) = \frac{200.02 \times 0.299^2}{2 \times 32.174} = 0.27 \, \text{ft lbs} \, (0.36 \, \text{Joules})$$

A kinetic energy of 0.27 ft lbs is enough to lift 1 lb by 0.27 feet or 200 lbs by 0.00135 feet or 0.016 inches. A distance of 0.016 inches is hardly on a par with the commonly perceived notion of a body being lifted off the floor and flung against a wall or through a window.

The following table comparing the velocity, momentum and kinetic energy for various common objects will place these figures into perspective:

It is an interesting comparison that the most powerful elephant rifle ever commercially produced would have little or no stopping effect on a charging elephant running at 20 mph.

When talking about the wounding capabilities of a bullet, many people wrongly refer to kinetic energy as 'power'. Power is the rate of doing work and is generally measured in 'Horse Power' (SI = kg metres/sec). If the power of a bullet is required, one has to know how long the bullet takes to stop in inches. The kinetic energy of the bullet is then divided by this distance, and then the result is divided

Table 5.3.2   Velocity, Momentum and Kinetic Energy for Some Common Objects

Object	Mass (lb)	Velocity (ft/sec)	Momentum (lb ft/sec)	KE (ft lbs)
.22″ LR (40 grn)	0.0057	1,200	6.85	120
.38″ Special (158 grn)	0.0226	850	19.2	235
Cricket ball (60 mph)	0.328	88	30	40
.303″ rifle	0.025	2,440	61	2,313
12-bore shotgun	0.078	1,300	101	2,051
600 Nitro Express rifle (900 grn)	0.129	1,950	251	7,600
150 lb runner (15 mph)	150	22	3,300	1,128
Elephant (5 ton, 20 mph)	11,200	29.33	328,500	149,700

It should be remembered, when using this table for comparison purposes, that momentum is the ability to move the target or to stop it moving in the opposite direction and the KE is the ability to lift a weight off the floor.

again by 550 to convert the answer into horsepower (horsepower to kg metres/sec: multiply by 75). Thus, the power of the bullet is dependent upon the material into which it is fired. As a result, this is a fairly meaningless figure.

Generally speaking, the only way a body is likely to leave the floor after being shot is via an involuntary muscle spasm caused by a shot to the brain.

5.3.4   Other factors influencing the wounding capabilities of a missile

This is quite a technical subject, but it can explain some phenomena associated with terminal or wounding ballistics which are not well understood.

Immediately after leaving the barrel, the bullet is in a slightly unstable condition. This is a result of three factors: 'yaw', 'precession' and 'nutation'.

Yaw can be described as the deviation of a bullet in its longitudinal axis from the straight line of flight (see Figure 5.3.5). It exists before the bullet achieves full gyroscopic stability.

Angles of yaw have only received detailed examination in military weapons. For example, the measured angle of yaw for a .303″ rifle is 1.5°, and for a 5.56 mm M16 rifle bullet it is 6°.

This yaw does have a pronounced effect on the wounding capabilities of the missile. The greater the degree of yaw, the greater the wounding effect of the bullet. This yaw effect also explains the commonly observed effect of a rifle bullet having greater penetrative powers at 200 yards than at the muzzle.

Precession is the rotational effect of the bullet about its mid-axis (see Figure 5.3.6).

Nutation is the progressive corkscrew motion of the bullet until it attains stability (see Figure 5.3.7). This action is very similar to the wobble observed immediately after a top or gyroscope is initially set spinning, and it is a function of the spin rate being too great.

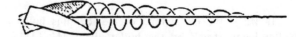

Figure 5.3.6   Precession of bullet.

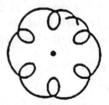

Figure 5.3.7   Nutation of a bullet.

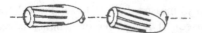

Figure 5.3.5   Bullet yaw.

As with a top, these factors eventually settle down to a stable flight pattern which, in rifles, can be anything up to 200 yards (183 m). It is this initial instability that often accounts for the far greater wounding effects of hard-jacketed bullets at close ranges when compared to those at greater distances.

There is a fourth condition which imparts a sideways drift to the bullets path called either 'spin drift' or 'gyroscopic drift'. This is to the right for a right-handed rifling and left for left-handed rifling. It is caused by air pressure under the slightly nose-up attitude of the bullet as it descends its trajectory. This effect is really only noticeable on extreme range rifle bullets or artillery shells.

Rate of spin imparted by the rifling

The rate of spin imparted to a bullet by the barrel's rifling is calculated to ensure that the bullet is stable in air. Once it enters a denser medium, however, the spin is insufficient to stabilise the bullet and it begins to wobble. As this exposes a greater cross-sectional area of the bullet to the tissue, the wobble becomes greater until, eventually, the bullet begins to tumble end over end. As the tumbling bullet exposes a much greater area of the bullet, the wound track and the kinetic energy loss will be tremendously increased. In lightly jacketed bullets, this tumbling can also cause the bullet to break up, causing a massive increase in the kinetic energy loss and a consequential increase in the temporary and permanent wound cavities. This effect is much greater in short projectiles (e.g. the .223″ (5.56 mm) M16 bullet) than with longer bullets (e.g. the .303″ British military round). Some bullets, such as the Japanese 6.5 mm Arisaka, were specifically designed to be only marginally stable in air, thus causing tremendous wounding when the bullet hits denser materials such as muscle.

The wounding effect of a missile is also dependent on the shape of the bullet nose. A round-nosed bullet will be retarded more than a sharp-pointed bullet. An expanding hollow point bullet will be retarded even more.

The amount a bullet will deform during passage through soft tissue will depend very much on the construction of the bullet. A fully jacketed bullet will hardly deform at all, while a soft lead hollow point bullet will deform very easily.

For a hollow point soft-nosed bullet to expand, a velocity of at least 900 ft/sec (275 m/s) is required. A round-nosed plain lead bullet will enquire at least 1,200 ft/sec (366 m/s).

Numerous reports exist to the effect that the 5.56 mm (.223″) M16 bullet 'blows up' on striking soft tissue. This is nonsense. What does happen, however, is that the thinly jacketed bullet, which is only just stable in air, becomes very unstable in tissue and starts to tumble. This tumbling action presents a much larger surface area of the bullet to the retarding tissue. This causes tremendous strain on the bullet's structure, which results in the jacket rupturing and the lead core fragmenting. With an initial bullet velocity of over 3,000 ft/sec (914 m/s), the kinetic energy loss is already tremendous, but as the bullet breaks up it becomes even greater. Massive permanent cavities, huge temporary cavities and tremendous damage to organs, blood vessels and bone remote from the wound track give rise to an appearance which many associate with the result of the bullet exploding. Some bullets are now provided with a scoped nose to induce this tumbling action and thus increase its wounding capabilities.

5.3.5 Bullet performance and 'wounding capabilities'

This is another subject which is surrounded by a great deal of myth and misinformation. In many ways, this is understandable as the number of factors influencing how a bullet reacts on entering a human body are so diverse as to make a scientific study of the subject nigh on impossible.

If the body were made uniformly from a material of constant density, it would be extremely simple to simulate the effects of a bullet. The body is, however, full of voids and has a hard bone skeleton and associated cartilaginous materials. The effects of a bullet hitting the thigh bone and muscle will be completely different to one striking the chest area, which has little muscle or hard bony material.

In an attempt to obtain some meaningful results for the wounding capabilities for handgun ammunition, the United States War Department constituted a board, in 1904, comprising Col. T. Thompson (the inventor of the Thompson sub-machine gun) and Col. Louis A. La Garde. This board was to conduct a series of tests to determine the stopping power and shock effect necessary for a service pistol. The results of the board's experiments were fully described in Col. La Garde's book, *Gunshot Injuries* (www.ebooksread.com/ . . . la-garde/gunshot-injuries). This is one of the most important investigations undertaken into the wounding effects of handgun bullets, as it consisted of controlled shots into human cadavers.

Many of the calibres used in the tests are no longer popular, but the basic findings (i.e. it is the bullet's cross-sectional area and nose shape, rather than the speed, which are the all-important considerations in the wounding capabilities of a bullet) still hold today.

In its tests, the cadavers were suspended by the neck while being shot. The quantity of shock to the cadaver by being struck by the bullet was estimated by the disturbance to the body. The bodies were also dissected to determine the degree of tissue damage.

The ammunition used during these tests was as follows:

- 7.65 mm Parabellum, full jacket

- 9 mm Parabellum, full jacket

- .38″ Long Colt revolver, plain lead

- .38″ Super ACP, full jacket and soft point

- .45″ Long Colt revolver, plain lead and hollow point

- .455″ revolver, 'man stopper' (a flat-nosed bullet with a very large cup-shaped hollow point)

- .476″ revolver, plain lead

The results were quite interesting, in that the higher velocity small calibre bullets, even when they had a soft or hollow point, caused almost no shocking power at all. The shocking power was, in fact, found to be proportional to the cross-sectional area of the bullet, with velocity being only of secondary importance.

These tests were, of course, on cadavers, which could not give any indication of the propensity for a round to incapacitate the subject. To investigate this aspect, a series of rapid firing tests were carried out on live steers in an abattoir. Series of up to ten shots were fired into the lung or intestinal area of the animal, after which it was humanely dispatched. Once again, the smaller calibre bullets had virtually no effect on the animals at all. The .38″ calibre bullets had little effect until the sixth or seventh shot had been fired. Only the .45″ and above calibre bullets were found to have any appreciable effect on the first shot.

This type of testing is the only way in which meaningful results can be obtained as to the actual wounding effect of bullets can be obtained. Firing into human cadavers and live animals are both extremely sensitive subjects and open to much adverse comment.

In an attempt to set some standard by which a bullet's performance may be measured without shooting cadavers or live animals, many different materials have been used to simulate body tissue. Among these are wet telephone books, bars of industrial soap, Plasticine, dukseal, water and 'ballistic gelatine'. While most of these can be used for strictly comparative purposes, they do not give a realistic picture as to how the missile will perform in human tissue.

The only medium which gives a close approximation as to the effects of a bullet on human tissue is **'ballistic gelatine'**.

Water also gives some approximation as to the expansion capabilities of various bullet constructions, but it does not, of course give any indication as to the temporary and permanent cavity produced.

Ballistic gelatine is made by dissolving type 250 ordinance gelatine in water to make a ten per cent solution. During the preparation, the temperature of the gelatine solution should never be allowed to rise above 40 °C, as higher temperatures result in hardening of the gelatine. The solution should be set in a refrigerator at 4 °C for at least 36 hours, and the blocks should be used within 30 minutes of removal.

After use, the blocks may be re-constituted by re-melting at a temperature not exceeding 40 °C, then set in a refrigerator as before.

Theoretically, the wounding effect of a bullet would depend upon its striking energy, i.e. kinetic energy. Here, however, theory and practice decidedly part company. Other factors have a very profound effect on the bullet's effect in animal tissue or other stimulant' including the bullet shape, cross-sectional density, weight, velocity and bullet construction.

5.3.6   Relative stopping power (RSP)

It may appear that the relative stopping power (RSP), the relative incapacitation index (RII) or the average incapacitation time (AIT) might seem to have little interest to the criminal lawyer. However, in cases where there is some controversy over whether adequate ammunition is being issued to law enforcement agencies, or whether the ammunition being used by the criminals has lethal potential, it can be crucial.

Major Julian Hatcher was of the first to seriously attempt to assign a numerical figure to the wounding capabilities of a particular bullet/cartridge combination (Hatcher, 1935). He called the numerical value the '**relative stopping power**' (RSP).

The original formula he used to calculate the RSP was as follows:

$$RSP = \text{bullet cross sectional area} \times \text{muzzle energy} \times \text{shape factor}$$

Hatcher did realise, however, that this formula was flawed, because the factor which permits the transfer of velocity to the surrounding tissue is not the muzzle energy of the bullet, but rather its momentum.

He therefore modified his formula for RSP using momentum, as follows:

$$RSP = \text{bullet cross sectional area} \times \text{momentum} \times \text{shape factor}$$

The shape factor was an empirical figure assigned by Hatcher. The factors he gave for various bullets are as follows:

Round nosed jacketed bullet:	900
Round nosed but with a flat top:	1,000
Round nosed plain lead:	1,000
Plain lead with blunt nose:	1,050
Plain lead with a large flat on nose:	1,100
Wadcutter bullet:	1,250

Table 5.3.3 The RSP for Various Cartridge Types Using Hatcher's Method

Cartridge	Momentum	Cross-Sectional Area	Shape Factor	RSP
.22″ LR	0.097	0.039	1,000	3.8
.25″ ACP	0.083	0.049	900	3.7
7.65 mm PB	0.246	0.075	900	16.6
.32″ ACP	0.147	0.076	900	10.0
.38″ Super Auto	0.347	0.102	900	31.8
9 mm PB	0.288	0.102	1,000	29.4
.38″ Special	0.302	0.102	1,000	30.8
.44″ Special	0.416	0.146	1,000	60.6
.45″ ACP	0.420	0.159	900	60.0

The momentum is measured in pounds feet per second and the cross-sectional area in square inches (these figures have not been converted into SI as the results would not relate to Hatcher's RSPs).

A major contribution of this formula was the recognition that the bullet's cross-sectional area has a very significant effect on its effectiveness in animal tissue. This gave a useful set of figures for direct comparison purposes between various bullet configurations, but it was not in total agreement with actual case incidents.

In 1973, The American National Institute of Law Enforcement and Criminal Justice sponsored research into determining the effectiveness of handgun cartridges as definitively as technology at that time would permit. The effectiveness of a bullet configuration was given a numerical value called the '**relative incapacitation index**'. This was calculated on the basis of three factors: target vulnerability, hit distribution and bullet terminal ballistics.

Target vulnerability was calculated by determining the relative sensitivity of the various areas of the body. This was done by dividing an anatomical model of the human body into one inch thick slices. Each of these horizontal slices was then divided into rectangular solids by vertically imposing a 0.2″ square grid onto the slice. Doctors then assigned a numerical value to each of these rectangular solids, representing the vulnerability of that solid. This formed the basis of the 'computer man' which was used as a vulnerability model for the study.

Hit distribution was obtained by live firing using soldiers firing .45″ Colt self-loading pistols at 'pop-up' targets. The hit distribution data was weighted against the penetration data in the anatomical model with respect to incapacitation potential.

The terminal ballistics data was obtained by an examination of the bullets' behaviour in 20 per cent gelatine (this is counter to the normal use of ten per cent gelatine), a standard set by the US Army Surgeon General. The factor used in determining the potential wounding capability of the bullet was to measure, via high-speed motion picture, the temporary cavity formed in the gelatine.

It is interesting that a dramatic 'ballooning' effect was noted in the temporary cavity when the projectile's velocity exceeded 1,100 ft/sec (335 m/s), which is approximately the speed of sound in air.

In calculating the RII figures, the analysis was run using the centre of vulnerability of the computer man, which is located in the chest area at armpit level.

Table 5.3.4 represents an abbreviated table as there were 142 different cartridges evaluated in the original paper. It does, however, give some

interesting data. For example, the .45″ACP, which has always been considered to be a very effective round, is rated only marginally better than the .38″ Spl LRN, which has long been recognised as being totally inadequate in a combat situation.

Using these figures, it was considered that any round with a RII below a factor of 9.0 was not suitable for a military or police round.

In 1991, a privately funded group was formed to study the physiological effects of bullet impact on medium-sized animals. These are now known as the **Strasbourg tests**. These tests were politically very sensitive in nature, as the animals were shot while in a conscious condition.

The animals selected were French Alpine goats, as their weight and the dimensions of their lung capacity and thoracic cage were very similar to those of human beings. To measure the effects of their being shot, transducers were implanted in the carotid artery and electroencephalograph needles were inserted into the scalp.

The animals were shot in the lung area, as this was considered the most likely place a human being would be struck by a bullet. In all, a total of 611 goats were shot during these tests.

The results for these tests are in the form of **'average incapacitation time'** (AIT), which is deemed to be the average time (usually over tests on five individual goats) which it took the animal to collapse and be unable to rise again.

Table 5.3.4 The RII for Various Cartridges Using the 'Computer Man' Method

Calibre	Weight (grns)	Bullet Type	Velocity (ft/sec)	RII
0.44″ Magnum	200	JHP	1277	54.9
.38″ Spl + P	125	JHP	1108	25.5
.45″ ACP	185	JHP	895	21.1
.357″ Magnum	158	JHP	1030	17.5
.357″ Magnum	158	WC	821	14.7
.357″ Magnum	158	JHP	982	11.1
9 mm PB	125	JSP	1058	9.9
.38″ Special	125	JHP	911	7.0
.45″ ACP	230	FJ	740	6.5
.38″ Special	158	LRN	795	5.0
.22″ LR	37	LHP	872	2.3

JSP = jacketed soft point, FJ = full jacket, JHP = jacketed hollow point, WC = Wadcutter, LRN = lead round nose, LHP = lead hollow point, + P = a very high pressure cartridge available only to law enforcement agencies.

These figures have not been converted to the SI system, as the RII results would not then relate to the original research.

Table 5.3.5 The RII for Various Cartridges From the Strasbourg Tests

Calibre	Weight (grns)	Bullet Type	Velocity (ft/sec)	AIT
9 mm PB	115	JHP	1,175	9.3
9 mm PB	115	FJ	1,165	14.4
9 mm PB	147	JHP	962	9.68
.45″ ACP	185	JHP	939	10.66
.45″ ACP	230	FMJ	839	13.84
.45″ ACP + P	185	JHP	1,124	7.98
.38″ Spl	158	RNL	708	33.68
.38″ Spl	125	JHP	986	14.28
.38″ Spl + P	125	JHP	998	10.92
.38″ Spl + P	158	LHP	924	10.86

Table 5.3.6 'One Shot Stop' Results for Various Cartridges Using the Marshall Method

Calibre	Weight (grn)	Bullet Type	Velocity (ft/sec)	Total Shootings	One Shot Stops	Percentage
.38″ Special	158	RNL	704	306	160	52.28
.38″ Spl + P	158	LHP	926	114	79	69.29
.38″ Spl + P	158	JHP	991	183	126	68.85
.38″ Spl + P	110	JHP	1126	16	11	68.75
9 mm PB	115	FMJ	1149	159	99	62.26
9 mm PB	115	JHP	1126	32	20	62.50
9 mm PB	147	JHP	985	25	19	76.00
9 mm PB +P+	115	JHP	1304	76	68	89.47
.357″ Magnum	158	JHP	1233	23	22	81.48
.357″ Magnum	125	JHP	1391	83	73	87.95
.357″ Magnum	125	JHP	1453	426	418	96.96

Evan Marshall, an ex-patrol officer with the Detroit police force, spent 15 years collecting data on actual shooting incidents. Any incident where one shot was sufficient to incapacitate the assailant so that he was incapable of further fight was classified as a '**one shot stop**'. Table 5.3.6 shows some of his figures.

Of all the various tests and simulations dealing with handgun ammunition effectiveness, probably the most important is the Marshal list of 'one shot stops'. From all the above it is clear, however, that even La Garde in 1904 had it correct in that it is not the velocity which really matters – it is the necessity of getting a large calibre missile deep into the body. Back in 1904 this was done with large calibre (.455″ and .476″), slow-moving missiles which punched their way through the tissue.

Today, the move is towards smaller missiles, but with a hollow point which, when travelling in excess of 900 ft/sec, will expand to give the effect of a large calibre missile.

5.3.7 Bullet resistant vests (BRV)

Introduction

One of the tasks that the forensic firearms examiner is often called upon to perform is the testing and evaluation of bullet resistant vests and jackets, generally called '**soft body armour**'.

As this aspect comes within the realms of terminal ballistics, it would be a good point to review the subject, especially in the light of the occasional death or injury that occurs to an officer when wearing one of these vests. One problem with such vests is that the wearer takes on a 'Superman' persona, where he/she feels invincible. This, however, is never the case, because no vest, no matter how many layers thick and what hard armour is used, can ever be considered truly 'bullet-proof'. A vest can never cover more than a small part of the body, there will always be joins through which a bullet can slip, many materials lose their stopping power when wet and there will always be a harder, faster and more penetrating bullet that will defeat the vest.

Where a lawyer will become involved with BRVs is in the determination as to whether the BRV on issue is suitable for the threat level posed by the weapons generally in use by the criminal. If, for instance, the issue vest is designed to stop .38″ Special ammunition with a round nose bullet, but the weapon used by the criminals is known to be a .357″ Magnum firing jacketed ammunition, then the BRV is clearly inadequate.

History

Body armour, in the form of metal plates, was widely used during the time of hand-to-hand combat with swords, knives and various bludgeoning instruments.

Illustrative Case 4

The BRV issued to a force was an NIJ (National Institute of Justice) Type II vest designed to defeat 9 mm PB full metal jacketed bullets and .357" Magnum jacketed soft-point bullets. The criminals were, however, using Chinese military issue 7.62 × 25 mm pistol rounds loaded with a solid steel bullet. During an exchange of fire with an armed gang, a BRV was compromised, which resulted in a serious injury to the police officer. When tests were carried out with this solid steel ammunition, it was found that the bullet would pass through the front and back of two issue BRVs. The compensation claim made by the officer was more than considerable.

As a footnote, it was found that the only way to reliably defeat this solid steel bullet was by inserting a titanium alloy steel plate in a pocket in the front of the BRV.

With the advent of the crossbow and firearms, however, plain steel suits were found to be inadequate to defeat the missiles, and they rapidly became obsolete.

During World War II, **ballistic nylon** (a co-polymer of the basic polyamide) was used against shrapnel from munitions. This was, however, of little use against bullets other than low-velocity soft lead projectiles.

The major advance in soft body armour came with a generation of what are loosely referred to as 'super fibres', which were introduced by Du pont. The best known of these was a para-aramid fibre called **Kevlar**, which was originally used in fabric-braced radial tires. It did not take long, however, for it to be realised that Kevlar could be woven into a fabric which was so strong that it could be used in bullet-resistant soft body armour.

The Kevlar fibres were simply woven into sheets, with varying thicknesses of yarn and density of weave (called **denier**), to provide the particular properties required. The sheets were then assembled into 'ballistics panels', which were permanently sewn into a carrier in the form of a vest.

It is undeniable that Kevlar does produce a very effective, lightweight and flexible jacket, which can be tailored to stop virtually any handgun missile. It does, however, suffer from a number of problems. First, it is not stable to UV light and has to be kept inside a light-proof pouch. It is also very susceptible to attack by many household chemicals. Also, if wet, it loses most of its ability to stop bullets.

A recent development in the field of soft body armour is the use of an ultra-high molecular weight polyethylene fibre called **Spectra**, which is produced by Allied Signal Inc. This consists of exceedingly fine spun fibres of polyethylene which are laid, in dense mats at 90° to each other, then covered top and bottom with a thin sheet of polyethylene. This is then heat treated to semi-melt the fibres together, or bonded with a plastic resin to form a sheet. As thousands of bonded fibres must be pulled from the matrix to allow the passage of a bullet, the sheets are even more efficient than Kevlar. This material is not affected by water (in fact, it floats), nor is it affected by UV light or any chemical, and it is considerably lighter than Kevlar. If it has a disadvantage, it is that its melting point is much lower than that of Kevlar.

One of the most recent innovations in bullet-resistant materials concerns the use of materials that exist as a semi-solid under normal circumstances, but solidify when subjected to a shock such as a bullet strike. These are called **shear thickening materials** (or **dilatant** materials), and they are composed of hard particles suspended in a liquid. The liquid is generally polyethylene glycol and the particles are nano-sized pieces of silica. The shear thickening liquid is soaked into the layers of a normal Kevlar vest and can reduce the weight of the vest by up to a third. BAE Systems in Bristol, UK, recently carried out tests in which a large gas gun fired metal projectiles at over 300 m/sec into both 31 layers of untreated Kevlar and ten layers of Kevlar combined with the liquid. The tests determined that the liquid-treated armour was as effective as the much thicker untreated one.

Mechanism of bullet-resistant materials

To effectively stop a bullet, the material must first deform the missile. If the surface area of the bullet is large enough and the material has sufficient resistance to the passage of the bullet, then energy transfer to surrounding fibres can occur. A non-deformed bullet will merely push apart the weave and penetrate.

If the bullet is sufficiently soft (e.g. plain lead, semi-jacketed or a thinly jacketed), then the material alone will often be sufficient to cause the deformation. If, however, the bullet is heavily jacketed or of the metal-penetrating type, then some intermediate, much more rigid material will be required to deform the bullet. This generally takes the form of a hard plate which fits in front of the soft body armour.

Ballistic inserts

This is the name generally given to rigid plates that are placed in front of the soft body armour. Their purpose is to break up high-velocity, hard-jacketed and metal-penetrating missiles. Once the bullet's velocity has been reduced and its shape deformed, it will be stopped easily by the underlying Kevlar or spectra material. These inserts are generally made from either a fused ceramic material, heat-treated aluminium, hardened steel or titanium. They can be either solid plates or small overlapping tiles. More modern materials, such as hot-pressed boron carbide and silicon carbide, are being introduced, and these considerably reduce the weight of the insert. One problem with such ceramic and boron carbide plates is that they shatter when struck by a bullet, thus losing much of their stopping potential for a second round.

Soft body armour is not infallible, as the examples in Illustrative Cases 5 and 6 demonstrate.

Standards for BRV threat levels

Body armour standards are regional. Ammunition used in criminal activities varies around the world, and as a result, the armour testing must reflect the threats found locally. Law enforcement statistics show that many shootings where officers are injured or killed involve the officer's own weapon. As a result, each law enforcement agency or paramilitary organisation will have their own standard for armour performance, if only to ensure that their armour protects them from their own weapons.

While many standards exist, a few standards are widely used as models. The US National Institute of

---

Illustrative Case 5

This case involved a police officer wearing a very substantial bullet-resistant vest capable of defeating .357″ Magnum and 9 mm PB calibre bullets. He was shot at close range with a .45–70″ rifle which had a large, soft bullet weighing 400 grains, at a velocity of 1,500 ft/sec (457 m/s). While the jacket was successful at defeating the bullet, it was driven into the officer's chest, killing him.

Illustrative Case 6

Another case involved a live demonstration of a ballistic insert plate made of metal. The plate was designed to defeat an armour-piercing round, but the demonstration was merely to show how effective it was against a full magazine from a sub-machine gun. The soldier wearing the jacket was not killed, but fragments generated by the bullet breaking up on the plate neatly severed the lower part of his jaw.

Table 5.3.7 NIJ Threat Levels for BRVs

Armour Level	Protection
Type I (.22″ LR;.380 ACP)	.22 long rifle lead round nose (LR LRN) bullets at a velocity of 329 m/s (1,080 ft/s ± 30 ft/s) and 6.2 g (95 grn) .380 ACP full metal jacketed round nose (FMJ RN) bullets at a velocity of 322 m/s (1055 ft/s ± 30 ft/s). It is no longer part of the standard.
Type IIA (9 mm;.40″ S&W;. 45″ ACP)	9 × 19 mm parabellum full metal jacketed round nose (FMJ RN) bullets at a velocity of 373 m/s (1225 ft/s); 11.7 g (180 grn) .40 S&W full metal jacketed (FMJ) bullets at a velocity of 352 m/s (1155 ft/s) .45 ACP full metal jacketed (FMJ) bullets at a velocity of 275 m/s (900 ft/s).
Type II (9 mm;.357″ Magnum)	9 mm FMJ RN bullets at a velocity of 398 m/s (1305 ft/s) .357 Magnum jacketed soft point bullets at a velocity of 436 m/s (1,430 ft/s).
Type IIIA (.357″ SIG; .44″ Magnum)	.357 SIG FMJ flat nose (FN) bullets at a velocity of 448 m/s (1,470 ft/s) .44 Magnum semi jacketed hollow point bullets at a velocity of 436 m/s (1,430 ft/s).
Type III (rifles)	7.62 × 51 mm NATO M80 ball bullets at a velocity of 847 m/s (2780 ft/s). It also provides protection against the threats mentioned in Types I, IIA, II, and IIIA.
Type IV (armour-piercing rifle)	.30–06 Springfield M2 armour-piercing (AP) bullets at a velocity of 878 m/s (2880 ft/s). It also provides at least single hit protection against the threats mentioned in Types I, IIA, II, IIIA, and III.

Justice BRV levels are examples of broadly accepted standards. In addition to the NIJ, the UK Home Office Scientific Development Branch (HOSDB – formerly the Police Scientific Development Branch (PSDB)) standards are used by a number of other countries and organisations. These 'model' standards are usually adapted by other counties by incorporation of the basic test methodologies with modification of the bullets that are required for test.

Further reading

1 French, G.R. *Wound Ballistics*. US Government Printing Office.

2 Knudsen, P.J. & Sørensen, O.H. (1994). The initial yaw of some commonly encountered military rifle bullets. *International Journal of Legal Medicine* 107 (3), 141–146.

3 Poole, R.A., Cooper, R.E., Emanuel, L.G., Fletcher, L.A. & Stone, I.C. (1994). Angle: Effect on Hollow Point Bullets Fired into Gelatin. *AFTE Journal* 26 (3), 193–198.

4 Eisele, J.W., Reay, D.T. & Cook, A. (1981) Sites of Suicidal Gunshot Wounds. *Journal of Forensic Sciences* 26 (3), 480–485.

5 Stone, I.C., Jr. (1987). Observations and Statistics Relating to Suicide Weapons. *Journal of Forensic Sciences* 32 (3), 711–716.

6 Gelatine Manufacturers Institute of America Inc. *Gelatine*.

7 Hatcher, J.S. (1935). *Textbook of Pistols and Revolvers*. Small Arms Technical Publishing Company.

8 The War Office (1929; New edition 2003). *Textbook for Small Arms 1929*. Naval and Military Press. ISBN-10: 1843428083.

9 Federal Bureau of Investigation (1989). *Handgun Wounding Factors and Effectiveness*. U.S. Department of Justice.

10 Fackler, M.L. (1997). Book Review, Street Stoppers: The Latest Handgun Stopping Power Street Results. *Wound Ballistics Review* 3 (1), 26–31.

11 Dodson, S. (2001). Reality of the Street? A Practical Analysis of Offender Gunshot Wound Reaction for Law Enforcement. *Tactical Briefs* 4 (2).

12 Shear thickening materials: http://www.gizmag.com/go/5995/

6.0

A Brief History of Forensic Firearms Identification

6.0.1 Introduction

While this subject is often referred to as forensic ballistics, this is not the best of terms to use. As can be seen from previous chapters, ballistics is concerned with the way a bullet behaves inside of the barrel, during its flight path to the target and upon striking the target. Although these matters are often part of the forensic examination of crime incidents, most of the examination will be concerned with the gun, fired ammunition and, where appropriate, the clothing of the injured or deceased. Having said that, it is a title familiar to many, and most are more comfortable with that than forensic firearms examination.

As with any evolving science, the exact origins of forensic firearms identification are shrouded in obscurity. It will never be known exactly when it was first noticed that fired bullets from a given weapon possessed a certain number of equally spaced impressed grooves, all inclined in the same direction and at the same angle, and which were the same on every other bullet fired through that weapon. Likewise, it will never be known when the next logical step was taken, to compare the width, number and degree of inclination of the grooves with those from weapons of a different make. The next step, however, required a quantum leap in lateral thinking, to show that all bullets fired through the same weapon bore microscopic stria (parallel impressed lines) that were unique to the weapon in which they were fired.

While this may seem to be a subject matter that has little bearing on current court cases, if one is not aware of how, where and when the basics of the subject matter originated, then effectively presenting such evidence will be made that much more difficult.

It will also make one aware of the possible miscarriages of justice that have occurred in the past through a basic lack of information of the core subject matter. One of the more infamous cases of such is documented in Illustrative Case 1 below.

Illustrative Case 1

In 1920, two factory workers, Frederick Parmenter and Alessandro Berardelli, carrying the factory payroll, were shot and killed in Dedham, Massachusetts (USA). The trial of the two accused murders, Nicola Sacco and Bartolomeo Vanzetti, started in summer of 1921. The case received worldwide publicity due to the political activities of the accused. At the trial, four 'experts' presented firearms related evidence – two for the prosecution and two for the defence. The firearms identification experts for both prosecution and defence were at odds with each

---

Forensic Ballistics in Court: Interpretation and Presentation of Firearms Evidence, First Edition. Brian J. Heard.
© 2013 John Wiley & Sons, Ltd. Published 2013 by John Wiley & Sons, Ltd.

other throughout the trial. Two examiners provided testimony linking the firearms evidence to the suspect's firearms, while the defence experts stated that the bullets and cartridge casings were not fired by the suspect's firearms. Based on the testimony of the firearms examiners, and other testimony presented to the court, the two suspects were convicted of murder. Many individuals objected to both the trial and the execution, as they felt that Sacco and Vanzetti had been framed because of their political views, and that the firearms evidence was unreliable.

In 1925, Celestino Madeiros, a Portuguese immigrant, confessed to being a member of the gang that killed Frederick Parmenter and Alessandro Berardelli. He also named the four other men, including the Morelli brothers, who had taken part in the robbery. The Morelli brothers were well-known criminals who had carried out similar robberies in area of Massachusetts. However, the authorities refused to investigate the confession made by Madeiros. On 23rd August, 1927, the two convicted men were executed.

Up to the present, most writers have focused their attention on the legal, social, and cultural dimensions of the Sacco-Vanzetti case. The legal dimension, in particular, has been rather exhaustively considered, and its two major issues – the fairness of the trial and the innocence or guilt of the two men – still dominates most of the literature about the case.

Earlier opinion almost unanimously felt that the two men were innocent and had been unjustly executed, but later revisionist points of view emerged – some totally (if implausibly) defending the verdict as correct, while others more plausibly argued that, based on new ballistics tests, Sacco was guilty and Vanzetti innocent. No single account, nor any ballistics test, has been able to put all doubts about innocence or guilt completely to rest, but on 23rd August, 1977, Michael Dukakis, the Governor of Massachusetts, issued a proclamation that effectively absolved the two men of the crime.

Surprisingly, although the Sacco-Vanzetti case is considered the political case par excellence, few accounts have taken the politics of the two men and their anarchism very seriously, and fewer still are knowledgeable about it. However, this is one of the defining forensic firearms cases, and each and every firearms examiner, as well as prosecuting and defence counsels, should be aware of the circumstances surrounding the case and its repercussions for modern forensic firearms examinations.

6.0.2   Early cases involving bullet identification

In June, 1900, an article appeared in the *Buffalo Medical Journal*, by Dr. A.L. Hall, to the effect that bullets fired through different makes and types of weapon, of the same calibre, were impressed with rifling marks of varying type. Unfortunately, Dr. Hall never expanded on his original article.

In 1907, as a result of riots in Brownsville, Texas, where members of the US Infantry opened fire, staff at the Frankfort Arsenal were tasked with identifying which of the weapons had been fired. As a method of identification, magnified photographs of the firing pin impressions on the cartridge cases were used. By this means, they were able to identify positively that, of the 39 cartridge cases

examined, 11 were from one weapon, eight from a second, eleven from another and three from a fourth. The six remaining cartridge cases were not identified. As to the recovered bullets, the examiners concluded that the bullets bore no distinctive markings as to the particular weapon from which they were fired. The only conclusions reached were that they had, by the rifling characteristics, been fired from either a Krag or a Springfield rifle.

6.0.3   Use of photomicrographs

The epochal work by the staff at Frankfort Arsenal was not recognised for a number of years, and it was not until 1912 that Balthazard made the next profound advancement to this science. Balthazard took photomicrographs of bullet lands and grooves in an attempt to identify the weapon from which a bullet was fired. From these examinations, he came to the conclusion that the cutter used in rifling a barrel never leaves exactly the same markings in its successive excursions through a barrel. These markings, which by inference must be unique to that barrel, are then imprinted as a series of striations on any bullet passing through the barrel. He thus reasoned that it is possible to identify beyond reasonable doubt that a fired bullet originated from the barrel of a certain weapon and none other. The significance of Balthazard's work cannot be overestimated, for it is upon this premise that the whole of modern science of bullet identification rests.

Balthazard's work, however, extended beyond that of matching striations on bullets, and included the markings imprinted on fired cartridge cases in self-loading pistols. The markings he identified as being those bearing identifiable stria and markings unique to a certain weapon were those caused by the firing pin, breech face, cartridge extractor and ejector. He reasoned that the final pass made by a cutting or finishing tool in, for example, the cartridge extractor, left a series of striations which were unique to that extractor. Likewise, the finishing strokes made by a hand-held file, for example in rounding off the firing pin tip, once again left marks that were unique to that piece of work.

Balthazard's work was, however, exceedingly labour-intensive and required the production of numerous photomicrographs under exactly the same lighting and magnification. These photomicrographs then had to be painstakingly enlarged, under identical conditions, to produce the photographs which could then be compared with the unaided eye.

In 1923, a paper was published in the *Annales de Medicine Legale* by De Rechter and Mage, which discussed the merits of using firing pin impressions for the identification of the weapon used. While some reference was made in this paper to the work carried out by Balthazard, it did not fully credit him for his work with self-loading pistols.

At about the same time, Pierre Medlinger also mentioned the reproduction of minute irregularities in the breech face on the soft brass of American primers. The matter was, however, taken no further

than that, with no mention of the possibility of identification of the weapon in which it was fired.

6.0.4 Identification of weapon from breech face markings

While it was accepted at this time that it was possible to match a fired bullet and cartridge case with a given weapon, there was no information available to indicate, from fired bullet or cartridge case alone, the make and model of weapon it was fired in. In 1932, Heess, Mezger and Hasslacher rectified this via the publication of an immense amount of data in Volume 89 of the *Archiv fur Kriminologie*, entitled 'Determination of the Type of Pistol Employed, from an Examination of Fired Bullets and Shells'. This article was translated and reprinted in the 1932 edition of the *American Journal of Police Science*. Appended to the paper was an 'atlas' containing photographs of 232 different self-loading pistols, each containing an illustration of the breech face and the markings produced on fired cartridge cases. Measurements of width, number, direction and angle of rifling twist were also included. This atlas was produced commercially as a series of cards, which was added to on a regular basis. Unfortunately, it has been unavailable for several decades, with copies being very sought-after as collectors' items.

6.0.5 Early use of comparison microscope

It was not until 1925 that mention was first made of a comparison microscope that could enable the simultaneous viewing of magnified images of two bullets or cartridge cases for forensic comparison purposes. Calvin Goddard, in a paper published in the 1936 edition of the *Chicago Police Journal*, attributes the development of the comparison microscope to a Philip Gravelle in 1925. This, he states, was a development of the comparison microscope used by Albert Osborn for document examination. The microscope so formed consisted of a Zeiss optical bridge, Spencer microscope bodies, Leitz eyepieces, Bausch and Lomb objectives and bullet mounts constructed by Remington Arms Company.

The optical bridge referred to is a 'Y' shaped tube, the two arms of which fit over the vertical tubes of two microscopes. By means of a series of prisms inside the 'Y' tube, the images are directed into a single eyepiece. The resultant image is a circular field of view, composed of the image from the left microscope in the left side of the field, and that from the right in the right side of the field. The images are separated by a fine line in the centre of the field.

Emile Chamot of Cornell University also described the use of a comparison microscope, using an optical bridge designed by Bausch and Lomb, for examining small arms primers in 1922. The optical bridge, however, dates back to a Russian mineralogist, A.V. Inostrszeff, who, in 1885, designed an optical bridge for the comparing the colour of minerals.

However, it does not matter who actually invented the comparison microscope, for it was Gravelle who first realised its use in the forensic comparison of stria on bullets and cartridge cases.

Shortly after the 1925 publication of the paper in the *Army Ordnance Journal*, the Spencer Lens Company manufactured the first commercial comparison microscope. This was very soon followed by Bausch and Lomb and Leitz.

In 1927, Mr Robert Churchill, the famous English gun maker, became interested in the comparison microscope. After seeing illustrations of a comparison microscope in an American periodical, he had a similar instrument manufactured for himself.

There is some dispute as to when Churchill first used his comparison microscope, with Mathews[1] indicating it was in solving the famous Constable Gutteridge murder case. Major Burrard[2] is convinced, however, that the Gutteridge case was solved by the War Office experts using a simple monocular microscope and photomicrographs.

The brief facts concerning the murder of Constable Gutteridge are as follows: in a motor car used by the murderers of Constable Gutteridge was found a fired revolver cartridge case. After many months of work, the police were convinced that two men,

Brown and Kennedy, were the murderers. Two revolvers were found in the possession of Brown and the whole case hinged on whether one of these was the murder weapon. Eventually it was established that one of the revolvers did, in fact, fire the cartridge case. After trial, Brown and Kennedy were hanged for the murder.

Although the fact that a microscopic comparison had been made was not particularly significant, this was the first time that such evidence had been presented to a court of law in the United Kingdom.

These early commercial comparison microscopes still consisted of the bottom half of two normal microscopes joined by an optical bridge. In the 1930s, the first real purpose-built microscope appeared, in which the objective lenses were attached directly to the optical bridge. This made for a very compact instrument, which could be mounted on a single base stand.

6.0.6 Introduction of the binocular comparison microscope

The next major improvement was the introduction of binocular eyepieces. It should be noted here that this did not give stereoscopic (i.e. 3D) images, as each stage still only had a single objective lens. It merely made operational use of the instrument much more comfortable.

It is often claimed that two-dimensional photographic reproduction of striation comparisons do not represent the three-dimensional views obtained on the microscope. While there is some truth in the statement that photographic representation of striation matches are of little evidential use, this is not due to photographs being only two-dimensional. In fact, the view obtained through the eyepieces is two-dimensional, as the single objective lens system used in comparison microscopes is not capable of representing three dimensions.

Some so-called 'expert witnesses' have used the excuse that a two-dimensional photograph cannot display the three-dimensional image seen using the comparison microscope as an reason for not supplying such photographic images to the courts. This should be strongly refuted, as it simply not true.

---

[1] Mathews, J. (1962). *Firearms Identification*, Vol. 1. The University of Wisconsin Press.
[2] Burrard, G. (1934). *The Identification of Firearms and Forensic Ballistics*. Herbert Jenkins Ltd.

6.0.7   Improvements in illumination

Apart from considerable improvements in optical quality, the only other real improvement in comparison microscope design has been the introduction of optical fibre and co-axial illumination.

Obtaining the correct lighting balance to enhance the micro stria under observation is one of the most difficult aspects of comparison microscopy. To achieve this using a conventional focused tungsten bulb system for each stage, so that the light intensity, colour temperature and angle of illumination are identical for both stages, is exceedingly difficult. To rectify this problem, modern instruments are now supplied with a single source halogen bulb serving two focused fibre optical arms. Each stage is thus supplied with a light source of exactly the same intensity and exactly the same colour temperature. Being highly manoeuvrable, the fibre optic light sources can be positioned with an accuracy previously unobtainable.

More modern instruments use a form of lighting once called the 'Ultrapak' or co-axial lighting system. Originally, this lighting system was used on Leitz microscopes, which were specifically designed for the examination of paint flakes and fibres. In this type of examination, which is usually concerned with colour determination, a shadowless but incident lighting of the object was required. Shadowless lighting required that the light source be vertically over the object being examined, which presents some problems where a microscope is concerned. The problem was solved by introducing the light into the lens barrel around the outside of the lens system. The light was directed down the lens barrel and focused on the object being examined via a lens surrounding the objective lens. As the light source was now coming from around the objective lens, it gave a 360° shadowless illumination of the object.

The system has now been updated and appears on modern Leitz comparison microscopes, giving a brilliantly clear, shadowless lighting. The stria appear not as peaks and furrows, as with normal incident lighting, but more as a series of 'bar codes'. Its real use, however, is in the examination of deeply indented firing pin impressions and deeply drilled holes, where normal incident lighting would be almost impossible due to the shadows produced. This considerably simplifies the examination and reduces the eyestrain of the examiner.

6.0.8   Photography of stria

Although most comparison microscopes have some form of photographic system for recording the striation matches, this is only of any real use in toolmark examination. In toolmark examination, the stria are generally on a flat surface and are easily photographed.

The stria on bullets are, however, on the circumference of a curved surface, and only a small portion of this can be adequately represented in focus on a single photograph. Modern instruments can now be fitted with a CCTV and monitor connected to a video recording device. With this, is it possible to record the striation match around the whole of the circumference of a bullet.

In general, the use of comparison photomicrographs in a court of law to illustrate stria comparisons should be discouraged. At best, they are illustrative of a stria match, and at worse they can be totally misleading to a layman jury. A video recording of the whole circumference of a bullet comparison, or the various parts of a match on a cartridge case could, however, be far more informative and remove some of the perceived 'mysticism' behind striation comparisons.

Where problems still occur, the court can either be taken to the forensic laboratory to witness the match at first hand, or the comparison microscope itself can be taken into court. The author has used both methods to display a striation match on a number of occasions, to great effect.

6.0.9   Modern technology for stria comparison (Figure 6.0.1)

In 1989, drug-related crime in Washington DC, USA, reached a stage where the law enforcement agencies were forced to implement a 'war on drugs' campaign. As a result, the forensic laboratories became overwhelmed with the quantity of fired ammunition submitted. In an attempt to assist the

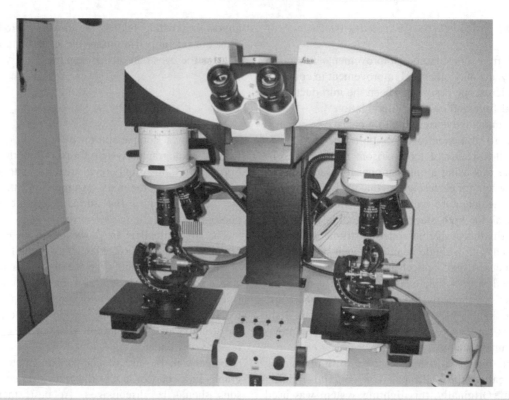

Figure 6.0.1   Modern Leica comparison microscope.

forensic laboratories as much as possible, 'target' cases were selected by the FBI for special attention.

Comparing each bullet and cartridge case in this list with those from a submitted case was, however, still, very manpower-intensive. To simplify matters, large photographs of the bullets and cartridge cases from the targeted cases were pinned onto the wall behind the comparison microscopes. The examiner could use these photographs as a rough screen to determine whether there were any similarities between the exhibits on the comparison microscope and those on the wall. If there were, then the relevant exhibit would be taken from the Outstanding Crime Index (OCI) and compared directly on the microscope.

Realising that this could be carried out more effectively with the use of modern technology, the FBI sponsored research into digitalising the photographs. These were displayed on a high-resolution computer screen in a tiled pattern surrounding the exhibit under examination. The system was called 'Drugfire'.

Drugfire went through a series of developments, until eventually it utilised computer-based comparison algorithms for the matching of stria on digitised images of the fired cartridge cases and bullets. In its eventual form, it was a highly effective system.

Around the same time as the FBI contract was issued, the Bureau of Alcohol, Tobacco and Firearms (ATF) established its own automated ballistics identification system. However, instead of developing a custom-made system like the FBI, the ATF opted to build their network on an existing platform which had already been developed by Forensic Technology Inc. (FTI) for general industrial comparison purposes.

From the very start, the FTI system utilised computer-based comparison algorithms and did not have to go through the same developmental process as Drugfire.

Initially the system was only capable of comparing bullets, and was called 'Bulletproof'. Later, it was upgraded to handle cartridge cases and was then renamed the Integrated Ballistic Identification System (IBIS).

As a result, from 1993 to 1998, the United States had two incompatible automated ballistics identification systems in place: Drugfire, under the FBI; and IBIS, under the ATF. Although there were attempts to interconnect the two systems under the National Integrated Ballistic Identification Network (NIBIN), it was not successful.

In 1999, the FBI and ATF finally decided to phase out Drugfire and standardise NIBIN on the IBIS platform. This decision was arrived at after a thorough joint FBI-ATF evaluation revealed the superiority of IBIS over the other system. The adoption of IBIS as the NIBIN standard made FTI the world's biggest manufacturer of automated ballistic identification systems.

In 2005, FTI released their 'Bullet TRAX' system, and in 2006 the 'Brass TRAX' systems which enabled both 2D and '3D' imaging of bullet and cartridge case stria. This not only enabled users to take qualitative measurements of the surface topography of a bullet and cartridge case, but also considerably enhanced the capability of the IBIS system.

It should be noted that this cannot be true 3D imaging as it is viewed on a 2D monitor. However, the large depth of field, as in an SEM, gives the appearance of 3D images.

Examples of FTI 3D imaging can be seen in Figures 6.0.2 and 6.0.3.

A number of other ballistic identification systems are also in the market, including:

- ARSENAL, by Papillon Systems of Russia.

- CONDOR, by SBC Co. Ltd.

- EVOFINDER, by SCANBII Technology.

- CIBLE, a French system.

- TAIS, another Russian system.

- BALİSTİKA, from Turkey.

- FIREBALL, from Australia.

There are also a large number of issued patents covering this technology, so more systems can be expected in the future.

It should be strongly emphasised that these systems cannot, at present, replace the comparison microscopist. All they do is generate a list of 10–20 top candidates as possible matches. The firearms examiner uses this list to select the actual bullets/cartridge cases from the Outstanding Crime Index for visual examination on a comparison microscope.

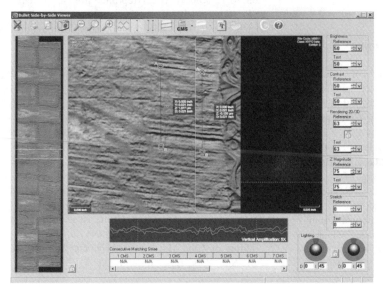

Figure 6.0.2 3D imaging of rifling stria.

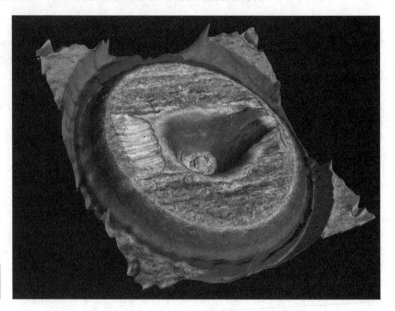

Figure 6.0.3   3D imaging of firing pin indentation on a primer.

It is the examiner who makes the final decision as to whether there is a match, and it is he or she that testifies to this in court. At this juncture, it should be noted that it is standard practice in most laboratories for a senior examiner to re-examine the match and countersign the laboratory report to this effect. All laboratory accreditation systems demand this as a prerequisite.

Suggested further reading

1 Mathews, J. (1962). *Firearms Identification*, Vol. 1. The University of Wisconsin Press.
2 AFTE Glossary. AFTE (Association of Firearm and Toolmark Examiners): 1st Edition published 1980, 2nd Edition published 1985, 3rd Edition published 1994, 4th Edition published (in CD format) 2001.
3 AFTE Training Manual. AFTE (Association of Firearm and Toolmark Examiners): 1st Edition published 1982, 2nd Edition online at www.afte.org.
4 AFTE (1998). Theory of Identification as it Relates to Toolmarks. *AFTE Journal* 30 (1), 86–88.
5 Anonymous (1886). Inostranzeff's Comparison Chamber for the Microscopical Study of Opaque Minerals and other Objects. *Journal of the Royal Microscopical Society.*
6 Anonymous (1943). Criteria of Firearms Identification. *The Technician* 1 (5).
7 Arther, R. (1970). *The Scientific Investigator.* Springfield, IL, Charles C. Thomas.
8 Balthazard, V. (1911). Du l'identification par les empreintes digitales. *Compté. Rend.* 152.
9 Balthazard, V. (1913). Identification des douilles de pistolets automatiques. *Archives d'Anthropologie Criminelle* 28.
10 Goddard, C. (1989). A History of Firearms Identification. *AFTE Journal* 21 (2) (reprinted from the *Chicago Police Journal*, 1936).
11 Hatcher, J. (1933). The Identification of Firearms. *Army Ordnance* 14.
12 Hatcher, J. (1935). *Textbook of Firearms Investigation, Identification and Evidence.* Small Arms Technical Publishing Company.
13 Hatcher, J. (1947). *Hatcher's Notebook.* Harrisburg, PA, Military Service Publishing Company.
14 Hatcher, J., Jury, F. & Weller, J. (1957). *Firearms Investigation, Identification and Evidence*, 2nd Edition, Harrisburg, PA, The Stackpole Company.
15 Smith, S. (1928). The Identification of Firearms and Projectiles. *The Police Journal (London)* 1.
16 Teale, E. (1932). Secrets of Crime Read on Bullets. *Popular Science Monthly.*
17 Editors of *Look* Magazine (1947). *The Story of the FBI.* New York, E.F. Dutton & Co.

7.0

Basic Concepts of Striation Matching

7.0.1 Introduction

"The automatic pistol leaves plenty of evidence of its presence in the form of empty fired cases which the guilty party rarely tarries to recover, his main idea being to get away from there, and these can tell a very revealing story if properly assayed."

> *Calvin Goddard, Address to Southern Police Institute, University of Louisville (May 1953)*

When investigators find a bullet at a crime scene, it can tell an examiner the calibre of the gun that fired it, the type of bullet and, possibly, the manufacturer and model of the firearm. If police find expended cartridge cases, these also indicate the calibre of the weapon used, its type (rifle/shotgun/revolver/semiautomatic pistol) and, possibly, the firearm's manufacturer. If police also recover a gun from a suspect, an expert can usually, if it is the weapon used in the crime, match the bullet and cartridge case to that specific firearm. Experts can do this by looking at the marks the firearm makes on the cartridge and those made on the bullet as it is fired.

When a cartridge is fired, the firing pin strikes the primer. This impresses the firing pin's mark into the soft metal of the primer. When the gun is fired, the pressures produced by the burning of the propellant create pressure on the base of the cartridge, the walls of the cartridge case, and on the bullet. As the bullet is the only part of the cartridge not constrained by the weapons chamber, it is forced out of the barrel,

leaving the cartridge case behind in revolvers or to be ejected if the weapon is a self-loading type.

As the bullet passes through the barrel, it engages the lands and grooves, forcing the bullet to rotate. As the bullet moves down the bore of the weapon, the land and groove impressions and other microscopic details are etched onto the bearing surfaces of the bullet. These fine microscopic details are called **striations** or **stria**. In the case of self-loading or pump-action weapons, a cartridge case will also receive striated marks from the weapon's firing pin, the standing breech, the extractor, ejector, chamber walls, feed ramp and magazine lips in firearms that have these features.

The gross marks will be the same for any bullet fired from any firearm of the same make and model of weapon. These are called **class characteristics**. Reference works list the class characteristics for each manufacturer, which would enable an examiner to determine what type of firearm was used to fire the recovered bullet or cartridge case. This determination has, as mentioned in earlier chapters, little relevance in the investigation of armed crime cases, but it is request often made by police in the investigation of an armed crime incident.

Firearm identification assumes that there are **individual characteristics** that are unique and consistent to one specific firearm. Theory dictates that it is not possible to make two machined surfaces that are microscopically identical. Even rifled barrels manufactured consecutively can be distinguished from one

---

Forensic Ballistics in Court: Interpretation and Presentation of Firearms Evidence, First Edition. Brian J. Heard.
© 2013 John Wiley & Sons, Ltd. Published 2013 by John Wiley & Sons, Ltd.

another because the cutting and grinding tools are blunted and worn each time they are used, leaving minute variations. Similarly, firing pins and the breech also leave unique markings.

Normal wear and maintenance, corrosion, rust, dirt and debris will change markings over time, creating both permanent individual characteristics and **temporary accidental characteristics**. These changes enable the differentiation of one firearm from others made by the same manufacturer. On the other hand, the non-permanence of markings, even from one test firing to the next, makes firearms identification via a striation match much more difficult than either a DNA or fingerprint comparison.

According to the Association of Firearms and Toolmark Examiners (AFTE) Criteria for Identification Committee, an identification means that 'the likelihood another tool could have made the mark is so remote as to be considered a practical impossibility'.

When examining evidence, the examiner can come to four conclusions:

1. *Identification*, defined in the AFTE Glossary as 'agreement of a combination of individual characteristics and all discernible class characteristics where the extent of agreement exceeds that which can occur in the comparison of toolmarks made by different tools and is consistent with the agreement demonstrated by toolmarks known to have been produced by the same tool'.

2. *Elimination*, defined as 'significant disagreement of discernible class characteristics and/or individual characteristics'.

3. *Inconclusive*, defined as either 'some agreement of individual characteristics and all discernible class characteristics, but insufficient for an identification' or 'agreement of all discernible class characteristics without agreement or disagreement of individual characteristics due to an absence, insufficiency, or lack of reproducibility' or 'agreement of all discernible class characteristics and disagreement of individual characteristics, but insufficient for an elimination'.

4. *Unsuitable* for microscopic comparison.

Note that the examiner's conclusion is 'all or nothing'. The recovered evidence can be matched to one, and only one, firearm under this definition. The AFTE definitions are not binding, but most examiners will not offer testimony about statistical probabilities. In reaching this conclusion, the examiner is looking for a certain quality and quantity of agreement which, in turn, is mentally compared to the closest known non-match that the examiner can recall seeing. Some differences always exist between a recovered bullet and a test bullet, even if they come from the same weapon. Similarly, one would expect some differences between cartridges that come from the same weapon.

In 1997, an article by Joseph J. Masson proposed looking for **consecutive matching stria** (CMS). CMS analyses the pattern of striated marks to determine how many consecutive matching stria are needed to minimise the likelihood that another firearm was the source of the markings on the recovered evidence. This is covered more fully in a later chapter.

There is presently a dispute between experts who prefer the CMS method and those who prefer the more subjective approach. They have raised questions about the CMS methodology and about whether CMS should be used to determine whether a match exists, or can be used after the examiner has concluded that a match exists to validate that conclusion.

7.0.2 Basics

Class characteristics

As explained in Chapter 6.1, the rifling of each weapon will possess a series of family resemblances that will be present in all weapons of the same make and model. Correctly called 'class characteristics', these relate to the number of lands and grooves, their direction of twist, inclination of twist, width and profile. While these dimensions can be extremely useful in identifying the calibre, make and model of weapon which fired a particular bullet, they cannot be used to individualise the weapon.

Individual characteristics

Although all weapons of the same make and model will have the same class characteristics, statistically and empirically it can be shown that no two weapons will have exactly the same individual rifling characteristics. These individual characteristics are caused by small defects in the rifling that are produced during the manufacturing process. They are totally random and, as such, are as individual to a particular weapon as fingerprints are to a person. These marks are called 'individual characteristics'.

It is thought by many that the individual characteristics in a weapon's rifling result from the actual cutter which makes the rifling. However, while the actual cutter does wear very slightly with each pass it makes, and factors such as inclusions in the metal of the barrel and swarf build-up do produce individual characteristics, this is not the primary source of the marks used when individualising a weapon.

The marks inside a barrel that characterise that weapon are not longitudinal, as produced by rifling cutters, but are rotational or spiral. These rotational marks are produced during the initial drilling and reaming of the weapon's bore and, as such, they are totally random. They result from wear of the drilling tool, build-up of swarf on the cutting edge and hard inclusions in the metal's crystalline structure. Being rotational, they leave far more characteristic marks on a bullet passing over them than do longitudinal striations.

Despite any actions subsequent to the rifling (e.g. lead lapping and ball burnishing – see Chapter 6.1), it is exceedingly difficult to eradicate totally these rotational marks.

It is the rotational or spiral marks on the barrel's lands which translate into longitudinal striations on the grooves of a bullet as it passes down the bore. Also, it is these striations which enable a fired bullet to be connected, beyond reasonable doubt, to a particular weapon.

While the majority of these individual characteristics will remain with the weapon for its working life, the bore of a weapon will also acquire additional individual characteristics as it ages. These additional marks can include, for example, small corrosion pits, damage caused by improper use of a cleaning rod and accidental damage to the muzzle.

Overzealous cleaning with abrasives and steel wire brushes to remove metal fouling can also damage or alter the appearance of a weapon's individual characteristics. In some instances, the excessive use of force can actually erase some of the individual characteristics. It can thus be seen that the individual characteristics in the bore of a weapon are constantly evolving.

Purposeful eradication of individual characteristics

It is often assumed that the last part of the rifling to touch the bullet before it leaves the barrel produces the only stria of any significance. In part, this is true, as the last part of the bore does have the ability to erase any stria that came earlier. It is also true that if the marks made from closer to the breech were deeper than those at the muzzle, then they will not be erased.

Illustrative Case 1

In one case, a felon used a saw to remove the last two inches of a barrel between his first and second bank robberies. In between subsequent armed robbery cases, he placed the barrel in a lathe and removed the top two-thousandths of an inch of the rifling lands. By the time of his last robbery, no rifling was visible in the bore at all. Matching the bullets from the first and second robberies was straightforward, as the individual characteristics had only been slightly altered. Matching the rest was somewhat problematical, as the tops of the lands had changed so much between subsequent cases that they could no longer be used. It was possible, however, to find an area of accidental damage to one of the grooves, probably caused by a steel cleaning rod, which enabled all the bullets to be matched.

Illustrative Case 2

During his training, the author took a new Webley .380″ calibre revolver and collected the first and second bullets fired, the 500th and 501st, 1,000th and 1,001st, 1,500th and 1,501st, and finally the 2,000th and 2,001th. The bullets were Cu/Zn jacketed and therefore harder than plain lead, but it was still possible to match the first and last bullet fired through the weapon.

There have been many instances where the last few inches of a barrel have been sawn off in an attempt to prevent a weapon from being linked with previous cases.

Life expectancy of individual stria

If a weapon's bore is well maintained, kept clear of metal fouling, regularly cleaned and kept free of rust, it is probable that the individual striations in the bore will not change significantly during a weapon's life. Practically speaking, though, the constant evolution of its individual characteristics will, over time, cause a significant change in these marks.

This evolution of individual characteristics can be so significant that while it is possible to match bullets fired one after the other, bullets fired months apart, or even numbers of rounds apart, may not be matchable.

In this respect, rusting of the bore is the method by which the individual characteristics are most likely to be permanently altered. Such pitting and corrosion of the bore can be so serious that it becomes impossible to match the micro stria from consecutively fired bullets.

7.0.3   Identification of weapon type

When a revolver is fired, the fired cartridge cases remain in the weapon until the weapon is manually opened and the cartridge cases ejected. Unless all the rounds have been fired and the weapon has been reloaded, it is unusual to find fired cartridge cases from a revolver at the scene of a shooting incident.

With fully automatic weapons and self-loading pistols, rifles and shotguns, the empty cartridge case is automatically ejected from the weapon after firing. Unless there is a mechanical fault, a fired cartridge case will always be found at a crime scene where one of these weapons has been fired.

In pump-action, bolt-action and other repeating weapons, it is also possible that after firing, the action will be manually cycled to load a fresh

---

Illustrative Case 3

An example illustrating how easy it can be to make a wrong identification involved the case of a very wealthy woman who was shot five times in the back with a .22″ Magnum calibre weapon. Matching the cartridge cases and bullets proved an extremely difficult task, due to the very fine stria present. Eventually it was concluded that, as the cartridge cases and bullets could be grouped into one batch containing three and the other two, then two self-loading .22″ Magnum calibre self-loading pistols had been used.

Several months after the shooting, a man surrendered to the police and confessed to the murder. It turned out that he had been the woman's butler and had been terribly badly treated by her. Finally he had snapped and had shot her in the back with a .22″ Magnum calibre double barrelled derringer. He had reloaded twice during the shooting, ejecting the fired cartridge cases and leaving one live unfired round, which he took away with him.

cartridge into the chamber. During this process, the fired cartridge case will be ejected from the weapon. As a result, a fired cartridge case will often be recovered from a crime scene where a repeating weapon has been used. The absence of a cartridge cannot, however, rule out the use of a repeating weapon.

As in the case of fired bullets, fired cartridge cases will also possess class and individual characteristics. The class characteristics will include the position and shape of the extractor claw and ejector pin, marks made by the lips of the magazine and feed ramp into the barrel, cut-outs on the standing breech face, marks made by the edge of the ejector port on the slide and, in certain weapons, the actual shape of the tip of the firing pin.

These will, once again, enable the calibre, type, make and model of the weapon to be ascertained with a high degree of accuracy.

7.0.4 Individual characteristics on cartridge cases

The parts of a weapon which imprint class characteristics on the fired cartridge case have, of course, been individually manufactured. The manufacturing process involves cutting, drilling, grinding, hand filing and, very occasionally, hand polishing. Each of these processes will leave individual characteristics, in much the same way as the boring process which is the initial step in making a barrel.

An example which conveniently illustrates the production of individual characteristics would be the final step in the production of a firing pin. After the automated manufacturing processes have produced the rough pin, the final step would be the rounding off of the tip with a smooth file. Each pass of the file across the firing pin tip will involve removal of metal, some of which will be deposited on the cutting edges of the file. This deposited metal will alter the cutting characteristics of part of the file, which will continue to be altered further as the metal build-up continues.

During this whole process, the surface of the file is constantly changing, giving an endless variety of striation marks on the tip of the firing pin. Other variables that will also radically affect the stria left on the pin's surface include:

- the force applied;

- the gradual wearing and blunting of the tool's cutting surface;

- the part of the file being used;

- the direction in which the file is drawn;

- the angle at which the file is used.

Such are the variables involved that the chance of two firing pins having exactly the same manufacturing stria is so low as to be negligible. It is the

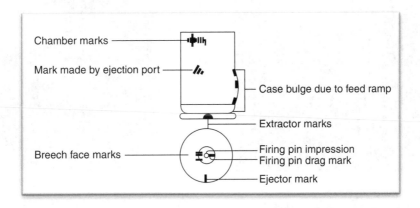

Chamber marks

Mark made by ejection port

Case bulge due to feed ramp

Extractor marks

Breech face marks

Firing pin impression
Firing pin drag mark

Ejector mark

Figure 7.0.1   Diagram showing extractor, ejector, breech face and other marks on a fired cartridge case.

combination of these randomly produced patterns of individual stria which enable a weapon to be matched to fired ammunition with a degree of certainty beyond reasonable doubt.

7.0.5 Formation of stria

During the firing of a weapon, the individual stria are transferred from the hard surface of the weapon's barrel onto the softer surface of the bullet or cartridge case.

As the tremendous pressures build up during the first few moments of firing, the base of the bullet swells to fill, and so obturate, the weapon's bore. As it passes down the barrel, minute irregularities in the bore form longitudinal scores or striations down the length of the bullet. Some of these are obviously rubbed off or modified by subsequent barrel imperfections, while others remain during the bullets flight through the weapon's bore.

Likewise, the tremendous pressures on the base of the bullet are also exerted in an equal and opposite direction on the cartridge case. The case is thus slammed into the standing breech face, replicating, in reverse, the toolmarks thereon. As the cartridge is extracted from the chamber, the extractor claw imparts its own class and individual toolmarks onto the rim of the cartridge. The ejector striking the base of the cartridge to tip it away from the gun will also leave its own class and individual characteristics.

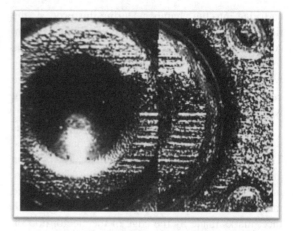

Figure 7.0.3   Example of a striation match on a cartridge case.

Other marks, such as the lips from the magazine, the ramp which directs the round of ammunition into the chamber (feed ramp) and the indicator pin, which shows whether the chamber is loaded, will also leave individual characteristics.

A good example of class and individual characteristics can be found on many of the 7.62×25 mm calibre Type 54 Chinese military pistols. In these, the end milling striations from the standing breech are clearly visible on the fired cartridge case. They are often mistaken for individual characteristics, and it is

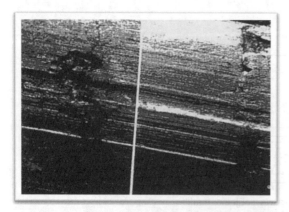

Figure 7.0.2   Example of a striation match on a bullet.

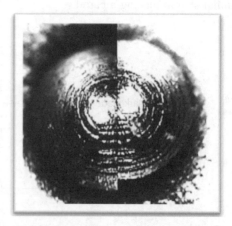

Figure 7.0.4   Striation match of circular marks on the tip of a firing pin.

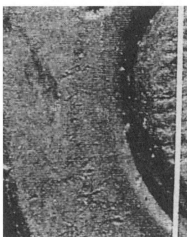
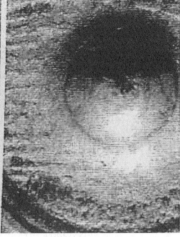

very easy to make an incorrect identification on this basis. If the cartridge is turned through 90°, however, the individual characteristics reveal themselves. This is illustrated by the photomicrographs shown in Figures 7.0.5 and 7.0.6.

7.0.6 Problematical areas

Damaged bullets, bullets fired through rusty barrels, bullet fragments and barrels with little or no rifling all produce their own problems. Polygonal rifling,

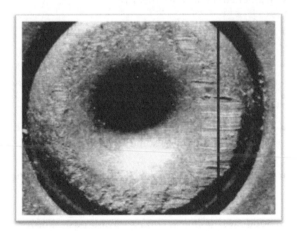

Figure 7.0.6 True match of individual characteristics from a Chinese 7.62 × 25 mm pistol.

however, produces problems of a completely different type.

The main difficulties in trying to match two bullets from a polygonal rifled are:

- as there are no sharp edged rifling grooves, it is extremely difficult to locate land and groove marks;

- as the barrel is hammered onto a mandrill, there will be no reaming marks to replicate themselves on the bullet;

- a mandrill will often be used to make hundreds of barrels so, as there will be little or no wear on the mandrill, each barrel will be virtually identical;

- to improve manufacturing efficiency, the barrel blank is of sufficient length that three or even four barrels can be made with one pass of the mandrill.

Generally speaking, it is possible, although extremely difficult, to match bullets from polygonal rifled barrels. The individual characteristics which are, generally, of most use are not from the rifling but from other barrel finishing processes. These include the production of the 'leade' (also spelt leed and lead) from the chamber or from the 'crowning' of the muzzle.

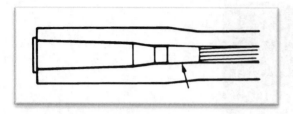

Figure 7.0.7   Chamber throat or leade.

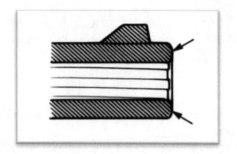

Figure 7.0.8   Muzzle crown.

The leade is the area forward of the chamber where the rifling is slightly cut back. This is to allow the bullet to engage the rifling gradually. Also called 'chamber throat', it is generally cut with a reaming tool. The marks left by the reaming tool will leave individual marks on the bullet.

In crowning, the rifling at the muzzle end of the barrel is very slightly counter-bored (cut back) to reduce the chance of accidental damage to this vulnerable area of the rifling. Whatever process is used, the cutting implement will leave its own individual characteristics, which will be reproduced on the bullet as it leaves the muzzle.

Problems with striation visualisation and matching of non-lead and non-toxic bullets

Most of the non-lead and non-toxic bullet types pose little problem with respect to the visualisation of stria and the subsequent matching on a comparison microscope. Some, however, do have to be treated somewhat differently in order to visualise what stria might be present. The various bullet types available are numerous, and new ones are being added virtually by the day. Some of the currently available ones are listed here:

- Winchester Lubalox, introduced 1991. Some confusion exists over this coating, with Winchester calling it an 'oxide coating similar to blueing' (could be a form of Parkerising) and others referring to it as a molybdenum disulphide coating.

- Federal Nyclad – a bullet coated with a shiny black nylon-type material.

- Molybdenum disulphide and nylon 11 (possibly Nyclad).

- Totally metal jacketed (TMJ).

- Nickel plated copper jacket – sometimes with a copper disc over the exposed area of lead at the base of the bullet.

- Copper plated steel jacket – sometimes with a copper disc over the exposed area of lead at the base of the bullet.

- Solid brass THV.

- Sintered tungsten – early KTW.

- Hardened solid brass – KTW.

- Sintered iron.

- Sintered zinc.

- Nylon/zinc composite.

- Combinations of zinc, tin, tungsten, bismuth and copper with nylon or some type of polymer.

- Steel jacket – copper coated (Chinese 7.62 × 25 mm pre-1985; also current 7.62 × 39 mm).

- Solid steel (Chinese 7.62 × 25 mm post-1985).

As most of the above composites have some softer, usually organic, material blended in with the sintered metal, they pose little or no problem in respect of barrel wear, nor to the transfer of stria from the barrel to the bullet and the subsequent examination on a comparison microscope.

The following information (Table 7.0.1) should, however, be noted:

Methodology for magnesium smoking

Magnesium smoking can be used to:

- render translucent and highly reflective materials such as PVC and nylon opaque so that

Table 7.0.1 Some Problems and Their Solutions

Bullet type	Problem	Solution
Nyclad	A black shiny coating completely covering the bullet. Stria are not visible under normal lighting due to the reflection of light.	Lightly smoking the bullet with burning magnesium will eliminate light reflection and visualise any stria present.
Sintered iron	This is quite a hard material and stria are not easily transferred. Care should be taken not to fire too many rounds, as the bullet can remove the finer stria.	No solution. Limit the number of rounds fired.
Sintered tungsten	Early KTW ammunition was provided with a gas check to take up the rifling. This does tend to fall off on hitting the target.	Ensure that the gas check is not overlooked as the bullet itself does not contact the rifling.
Solid steel	This type of ammunition simply tears out the bore of a weapon. Each round produces a huge ball of sparks as a result of the rifling being removed from the barrel!	Rounds 1–3 will probably be matchable, but 1 and 4 probably not. After 50 rounds, the bore will be all but bereft of rifling.
Steel jacket	Once again, extremely hard on the barrel's rifling.	Not as bad as solid steel, but care must still be taken with the number of rounds fired.
TMJ	Lead core completely covered by an very thick electroplated copper/zinc (Cu/Zn) jacket	Coating tends to be very much harder than a normal Cu/Zn jacket. Problems have been noted with certain weapons which have fairly shallow rifling (older Colt revolvers). It has been found that the rifling is too shallow to gain sufficient purchase on the bullet, and slippage occurs. Not only are the rounds very difficult to match but, as a result of insufficient spin stabilisation, the weapons become very inaccurate.
Saboted bullets	The Sabot is lost once the bullet leaves the muzzle, leaving a completely unmarked bullet. Also, the sabot is manufactured from a somewhat reflective and translucent polyethylene or plastic-type material. This renders a normal microscopic comparison virtually impossible.	As with Nyclad bullets, lightly smoking the sabot with burning magnesium strip will eliminate light reflection and visualise any stria present.
Plastic shotgun wads	Once again, these are manufactured from a shiny, translucent polyethylene-type material which renders a normal microscopic comparison virtually impossible.	Stria from the front sight bead staking, adjustable chokes, etc. can be transferred to the plastic wad. These can likewise be visualised by smoking with burning magnesium.

they can be examined under a comparison microscope;

- for the examination bullets fired through lightly rusted barrels; in this instance, the smoking eliminates the very fine stria that result from the corrosion, leaving the stria due to the weapon's individual signature clearly visible;

- eliminate differences in colour of the areas under examination.

The smoking itself is quite an art[1]. It is, however, non-permanent and non-destructive and, if the layer of deposited magnesium oxide is too thick, it can simply be blown off or brushed clean with a very soft-bristled brush. If the cov-

ering is insufficient, it can be thickened up by re-smoking.

Care must be taken, however, when dealing with low melting point materials such as polyethylene, PVC or nylon, as the heat from the burning magnesium can melt the material under examination.

To carry out the smoking, a short length of magnesium ribbon, about four inches long, is held in a pair of pliers and ignited. The material being smoked is then wafted in the plume of smoke until an even deposit over the entire surface is achieved. Metallic materials are best held at a distance of about three inches above the burning magnesium, and low melting point materials at a greater distance.

A light coating over transparent or translucent materials will enable any stria present to be seen easily under the comparison microscope.

Illustrative Case 4

This case involved a murder committed with a heavily used .22″ RF target rifle. A bore scope examination of the suspect weapon showed the rifling to be heavily fouled and to contain significant quantities of deposited lead. As was normal practice at that time, a clean, tight patch of 4″ × 2″ cotton was pushed through the bore to determine whether the fouling was fresh or otherwise. Subsequent to this, two rounds were fired and the bullets recovered. These bullets were compared as a reference prior to carrying out a comparison with the bullet recovered from the victim. The two found bullets matched perfectly, but there was virtually no similarity between these and the bullet recovered from the body.

There was no question as to whether any other weapon was involved, as it was known for certain that the case exhibit rifle was the murder weapon.

In an attempt to determine why the bullet from the body could not be matched with the controls from the suspect weapon, 20 heavily used .22″ RF target weapons of the same make and model were taken, and the first and second bullet from each was collected. In each case, these two bullets matched perfectly. Fifty more bullets were then fired from each rifle and the next two were collected from each gun. Once again, the 53rd and 54th bullets from each rifle matched each other perfectly. As expected, these two also matched the first and second bullets fired from each gun.

A tight 4″ × 2″ patch was pushed through the barrel of each rifle bore, and then two more bullets were fired through each.

Of the 20 rifles, the bullets fired from 11 (which were the ones that started out with the heaviest fouling) could not be matched with the bullets fired prior to the cleaning. Of the rest, four were marginal matches and the rest were satisfactorily matched[2].

It was obvious that the bullets from the 11 rifles were unmatchable due to the removal of the lead from the rifling by the patch of 4″ × 2″. Once this lead had been removed, the fine stria underneath were exposed. Bullets fired through this clean barrel took up the fine stria, while those fired through the barrel before it was cleaned had no fine stria

---

[1] Burd, D.Q. (1965). Smoking Bullets. A Technique Useful in Some Bullet Comparisons. *The Journal of Criminal Law, Criminology, and Police Science* **56**(4), 523–527.

[2] Unpublished paper by B.J. Heard.

present. The only stria present on the bullets before the barrel was cleaned were the gross stria on the leading and trailing edges of the rifling.

The absence of fine stria on the bullets fired prior to cleaning the barrel rendered a match with bullets fired after cleaning a far from positive undertaking.

In an attempt to reproduce the effect that the heavy barrel leading had on bullets fired through it, the bullets fired after cleaning were smoked with burning magnesium. This effectively covered up the fine stria, leading to matchable bullets in every case. It was noted that the bullets fired through the barrel before cleaning also required a light smoking to ensure that there was no colour difference between the two bullets being compared.

The bullet recovered from the deceased, and the bullets fired from case rifle after the barrel had been cleaned, were smoked in exactly the same way and a positive match was found.

As a result of the findings detailed in Illustrative Case 4, it is strongly suggested that if it is deemed necessary to examine the barrel of .22″ RF weapons for signs of fouling from firing, it be done with great caution – and then only using a very loosely fitting patch.

Problems with manufacturing marks

With the number of processes that a round of ammunition has to go through, it is not surprising that spurious marks are sometimes left on the ammunition. On fired ammunition, these marks can be – and have been – mistaken for individual characteristics, leading to misidentifications. Examiners should be acutely aware of this possibility; although it is preferable to fire exactly the same ammunition as that used in a crime, it is preferable if ammunition from another source can also be fired. Examples of stria produced during manufacture are shown in Figures 7.0.9 and 7.0.10, and a match between manufacturing marks on two unfired cartridges is shown in Figure 7.0.11.

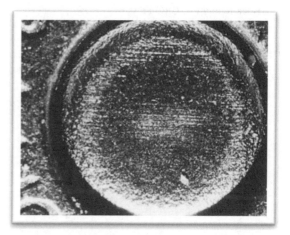

Figure 7.0.10 Manufacturing marks on unfired primer.

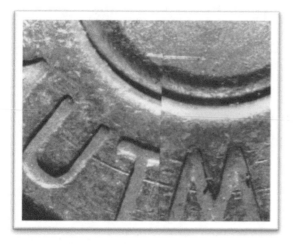

Figure 7.0.9 Manufacturing marks.

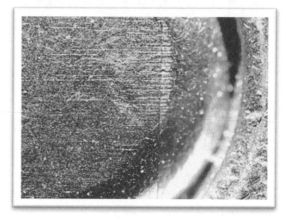

Figure 7.0.11 Striation match of manufacturing marks.

Further reading

1 Biasotti, A. & Murdock, J. (1984). Criteria for Identification or 'State of the Art' of Firearm and Toolmark Identification. *AFTE Journal* 16 (4).

2 Biasotti, A. & Murdock, J. (1997, revised 2002). Chapter 23, Section, 23–2.0, *Modern Scientific Evidence: The Law and Science of Expert Testimony*.

3 Burrard, G. (1962). *The Identification of Firearms and Forensic Ballistics* (1st Am Ed). New York, A. S. Barnes and Co.

4 Butcher, S. & Pugh, D. (1975). A Study of Marks Made by Bolt Cutters. *Journal of Forensic Science Society* 15 (2).

5 Churchill, R. (1929). The Forensic Examination of Firearms and Projectiles. *The Police Journal (London)* 2.

6 Di Maio, D. & Di Maio, V. (1993). *Forensic Pathology*. Boca Raton, FL, CRC Press.

7 Goddard, C. (1993) A History of Firearms Identification to 1930. *AFTE Journal* 25 (3).

8 Goddard, C. (1989). A History of Firearms Identification. *AFTE Journal* 21 (2) (reprinted from the *Chicago Police Journal*, 1936).

9 Hamby, J. (1974). Identification of Projectiles. *AFTE Journal* 6 (5/6).

10 Hamby, J. & Thorpe, J. (1999). The History of Firearm and Toolmark Identification. *AFTE Journal* 31 (3).

11 Hatcher, J. (1935). *Textbook of Firearms Investigation, Identification and Evidence*. Small Arms Technical Publishing Company.

12 Hatcher, J. (1947). *Hatcher's Notebook*. Harrisburg, PA, Military Service Publishing Company.

13 Nichols, R. *Critical Review of 'A Systemic Challenge to the Reliability and Admissibility of Firearms and Toolmark Identification'*. PowerPoint summary on the AFTE website (www.afte.org) to the article by Adina Schwartz that appeared in the Columbia Science and Technology Law Review.

14 Smith, E. (2004). Cartridge Case and Bullet Validation Study with Firearms Submitted in Casework. *AFTE Journal* 36 (4).

15 Thomas, F. (1967). Comments on the Discovery of Striation Matching and on Early Contributions to Forensic Firearms Identification. *Journal of Forensic Sciences* 12 (1).

16 http://www.firearmsid.com/Feature%20Articles/GreenBullets/GreenBullets.htm

7.1

Basic Concepts in Comparison Microscopy

7.1.1 Introduction

Comparison microscopy is, arguably, the most important part of forensic firearms examiners' evidence. Much like DNA and fingerprint evidence, however, it is the one area that can often make or break a case. It is also an area of forensic science which is probably less understood than any other.

In the UK, as in many parts of the world, there is a general acceptability of the scientific basis upon which striation matches are based. Likewise, there is an aura of infallibility accorded to expert witnesses in this field. 'Believe me, I am the expert' is an oft quoted phrase.

In the USA, however, the situation is somewhat different, in that the US Congress has passed Federal Rules of Evidence which control the admissibility of expert witness testimony via a 'generally acceptability standard'.

In 1993, this was built upon as a result of the Daubert vs. Merrell Dow Pharmaceuticals (1993, 509 US 579, 589) case. In Daubert, the Supreme Court held that the judges are the gatekeepers of scientific evidence. Under the Daubert Standard, the trial judge must evaluate proffered expert witnesses to determine whether their testimony is both relevant and reliable.

This has evolved into the Daubert Trilogy for the standard of review, in which the following pertain:

Relevancy

The relevancy of the testimony refers to whether or not the expert's evidence fits the facts of the case. For example, you may invite an astronomer to tell the jury if there had been a full moon on the night of the crime. However, the astronomer would not be allowed to testify if the fact that the moon was full was not relevant to the issue at hand in the trial.

Reliability

The Supreme Court explained that, in order for expert testimony to be considered reliable, the expert must have derived his or her conclusions from the scientific method. The Court offered 'general observations' of whether proffered evidence was based on the scientific method, although the list was not intended to be used as an exacting checklist.

Empirical testing

- The theory or technique must be falsifiable, refutable and testable.

- It must be subjected to publication and peer review.

Forensic Ballistics in Court: Interpretation and Presentation of Firearms Evidence, First Edition. Brian J. Heard.
© 2013 John Wiley & Sons, Ltd. Published 2013 by John Wiley & Sons, Ltd.

- There must be a known or potential error rate and standards concerning its operation must be maintained.

- The theory and technique must be generally accepted by a relevant scientific community.

To paraphrase the above, **the judge is the gate-keeper**: the task of 'gatekeeping', or assuring that scientific expert testimony truly proceeds from 'scientific knowledge', rests on the trial judge.

Relevance and reliability

This requires the trial judge to ensure that the expert's testimony is 'relevant to the task at hand'. Concerns about expert testimony cannot simply be referred to the jury as a question of weight. Furthermore, the judge must find it more likely than not that the expert's methods are reliable and reliably applied to the facts at hand.

Scientific knowledge/methodology

A conclusion will qualify as scientific knowledge if the proponent can demonstrate that it is the product of sound 'scientific methodology' derived from the scientific method.

Relevant factors

The Court defined 'scientific methodology' as the process of formulating hypotheses and then conducting experiments to prove or falsify the hypothesis, and provided a non-dispositive, non-exclusive, 'flexible' test for establishing its 'validity', based on the empirical factors listed above.

Although trial judges have always had the authority to exclude inappropriate testimony, trial courts often preferred to let juries hear evidence proffered by both sides. Once certain evidence has been excluded by a Daubert motion because it fails to meet the relevancy and the reliability standard, it is likely to be challenged when introduced again in another trial. Even though a Daubert motion is not

binding to other courts of law, if something has been found not trustworthy, other judges may choose to follow that precedent. Of course, a decision by the Court of Appeals that a piece of evidence is inadmissible under Daubert would be binding on district courts within that court's jurisdiction.

To summarise, the five cardinal points of Daubert asks from every new technique to be admissible in court are:

- Has the technique been tested in actual field conditions and not just in the laboratory? For example, fingerprinting has been extensively tested and verified not only in laboratory conditions, but also in actual criminal cases, so it is admissible. Polygraphy, on the other hand, has been well tested in laboratories but not so well tested in the field.

- Has the technique been subject to peer review and publication?

- What is the known or potential rate of error? Is it zero or low enough to be close to zero?

- Do standards exist for the control of the techniques operation?

- Has the technique been generally accepted within the relevant scientific community?

While these points are not law in the UK or under other jurisdictions, they can provide a useful pointer for establishing the viability of an expert witness and his/her testimony.

7.1.2   Basic methodology and background to stria comparisons

It has been quoted[1] that up to 25 per cent of the stria in a non-match, and in excess of 75 per cent of the stria in a match, will show concordance. Such a degree of accidentally matching lines is exceedingly high and has not been supported by personal

---

[1] Walls, H.J. (1974). *Forensics Science*. Sweet & Maxwell. ISBN: 0091099609.

experience. There is no dispute, however, that out of the thousands of lines present in any one comparison, a number must, by pure chance alone, show agreement.

Experts should be tasked as to their interpretation of this quoted degree of accidental concordance and should give some idea to the court as to what they consider an acceptable percentage of accidental matching stria before it becomes a true match. They should also be tasked with identifying the number of stria necessary for concordance, especially when considering the limited area available on such areas as a firing pin tip, an extractor claw or the stria produced on a cartridge case by the magazine lips.

When carrying out a microscopic comparison, the accidental agreement in a non-match must be recognised by the examiner and mentally discounted as being non-relevant. It is this ability to reject non-matching stria, while accepting those of relevance, that is the identifying feature of an experienced comparison microscopist.

The actual process of assessing which stria is of relevance is quite simple. First, each of the available fired ammunition components (for this example, fired bullets) is compared with all the other test-fired bullets until one is found that is considered to be representative of a 'match'. This is then used as a reference for comparison with the fired bullets in the actual case. This does not, however, mean that all the other test-fired bullets are discarded, as one of these might eventually be discovered as being a better match with the suspect bullet than the 'representative bullet'.

During this search for a representative 'match', one is attempting to find a pattern of easily recognisable stria that can be mentally retained and used in subsequent comparisons with the case bullets. This identification of a stria pattern can only be obtained through extensive experience in the matching of stria, and it is not a skill that can be taught in a book.

Should there be a suspected match with the case bullet, then each of the other test bullets must also be compared with the case exhibit to determine whether the agreement was accidental or if a match exists that is beyond reasonable doubt. Once a 'match' has been observed, it is normal practice for the match to be confirmed by a senior examiner, and for a note to be made to this effect on the witness statement. While this is not laid down in any legislation, it is a prerequisite for every laboratory accreditation system.

7.1.3 Lighting used for comparison microscopy

This is probably one of the most important aspects of forensic stria comparison, but is probably the least well understood. Even with binocular eyepieces, a comparison microscope is only able to display a

---

Illustrative Case 1

An examiner had made what he considered to be a match between a control cartridge case fired from a seized firearm and one found at the scene of a murder. The firing pin was virtually featureless, as were the breech face and ejector marks. The concordance was found on just part of the extractor mark, under the rim of the cartridge case, and consisted of no more than seven lines. Other stria were present which did not match.

Using the concept of 'consecutively matching stria' (see Chapter [7.2]), concordance is accepted when 'in a two-dimensional toolmark, at least two groups of at least five consecutive matching stria appear in the same relative position, or one group of eight consecutively matching stria are in agreement in an evidence toolmark.'

Under this concept, which the author is not entirely happy with, the match between six lines was non-viable. Possibly this could be stated as a confirmation of the viability of CMS.

Despite another examiner refusing to countersign the match as being positive, the examiner went ahead with confirming his finding in writing via his report. It was possible that the cartridge case had been fired in the seized weapon, but the case should never have been reported as such. The arrested person was convicted, but was successful on appeal largely based on the striation match.

two-dimensional image, as there is only one objective lens. However, by using low-angle lighting to illuminate the stria, the impression of a three-dimensional image of the stria can be obtained. This low-level lighting illuminates the side of the stria closest to the light source and places the side away in shadow. The lower the lighting angle, the greater this effect. Care must, however, be taken to ensure that the two light sources – one for the right stage and one for the left – are at the same angle, otherwise mistakes can be made in the identification. Care must also be taken to ensure that the intensity of light is also the same, for similar reasons.

There are a number of different light sources that can be used with a comparison microscope, each of which has its own advantages and disadvantages. Some of the more common follow.

Simple tungsten bulb or LED light source

This is probably the most commonly used, and it is attached to the table on which the bullet/cartridge case is mounted. It has a full range of movements, allowing the incident light to illuminate the bullet or cartridge case from the right or left, and at different incident angles. When viewing firing impressions, the light must be at a much higher angle than that used for linear striation marks.

The disadvantage with this type of illumination is that the colour temperature of the light is very difficult to adjust in order to ensure that both light sources are the same.

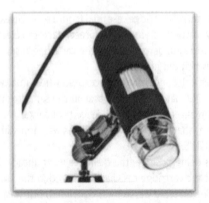

Figure 7.1.1   Single bulb light source.

Single source LED or tungsten light with twin fibre optical cables

Here there is a single light source connected to two fibre optical cables, one for each stage, so the light intensity and temperature is the same for both stages. This is a great deal better than the normal twin light source, but it does have the disadvantage that the light cannot be focused as in a conventional light source. The flexible fibre cables offer a great deal of manoeuvrability but, as with all light sources, the angle of lighting for both stages must be as similar as possible.

Fluorescent or tungsten strip lights

These are less popular than bulb sources, as they have a much smaller range over which the bulbs can be manipulated. Also, as they produce a more diffuse light source, they tend to be less effective than a conventional bulb (which is essentially a spot source light) at producing the illuminated peaks and troughs.

Ring light source

This is very useful for illuminating firing pin impressions and for producing a bar code type of stria image. It does provide a useful and totally reproducible light source, which is required for computerised

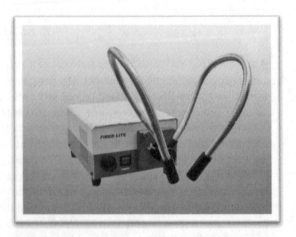

Figure 7.1.2   Single light source with fibre optic cables.

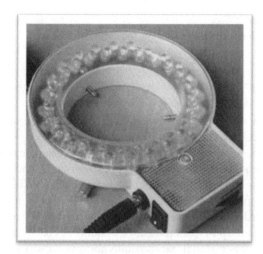

Figure 7.1.3 LED ring light.

stria comparison equipment such as FTI's IBIS (Integrated Ballistics Identification System). However, there is no three dimensional effect, and thus it is difficult to use manually.

Darkfield microscopy

This is also called light field/darkfield microscopy, or by the Leica trade name 'Ultrapak'. The light source comes in from the side and via a half-silvered mirror, and is directed around the outside of the microscope lens system. The final objective lens of the microscope is surrounded by another lens for focusing the light source onto the object. This is excellent for deep firing pin impressions and deeply drilled holes, both of which are extremely difficult to visualise using conventional light sources. The image obtained from such is very similar to that of a contour map and is extremely easy to compare. For normal stria, this light source gives a similar, but far superior, image to a conventional ring light source.

7.1.4 The concept of consecutive matching stria

An evolving concept in striated mark comparisons is the developing study of consecutive matching stria

(CMS) as a quantitative method of describing an observed pattern match. It is a concept that many (including the author) are not comfortable with, but that does not eliminate or reduce the worth of such an approach to quantifying the outcome of striation comparisons.

CMS is simply a means of articulating the best known non-match described and defined by the AFTE Theory of Identification. This topic is dealt with more fully in Chapter 7.2.

7.1.5 Obtaining control samples

When a weapon has been located, it will be necessary to recover 'control' examples of bullets and cartridge cases for comparison with those recovered from the crime scene.

Before firing the weapon, it is necessary to carefully wipe any excess grease, oil or debris from the barrel which might cause additional accidental stria on the fired bullets. The residues obtained on this barrel wipe should be retained for further determination as to whether the weapon has been recently fired.

It is also necessary, if it is a self-loading pistol, to clean any grease or debris from the standing breech face. Such grease could act as a cushion, preventing the transfer of stria onto the cartridge case. In addition, the first round fired could impress the debris into the standing breech face with sufficient force as to leave marks which would be reproduced during subsequent firings.

With self-loading pistols, any oil or grease on the breech face will result in few, if any, breech face marks being impressed into the base of the cartridge case. This will make comparisons difficult, or sometimes impossible.

With rifles, it is essential to remove any oil or grease from the chamber and barrel. Even small amounts of oil in the barrel could effectively cause an obstruction, resulting in a barrel bulge or even a barrel burst.

Oil or grease in the chamber will lubricate the outside of the cartridge case, which can lead to excessive pressures on the standing breech. In extreme circumstances, this could lead to the destruction of a pistol, and it will invariably do so in high-powered rifles.

Before removing any grease or debris, the breech face should be examined under a microscope, as it is often possible to see an imprint in the dirt or oil of the headstamp of the last cartridge fired. This could provide useful information at some later date, and any such impression should be photographed.

After carefully cleaning the weapon, a minimum of four (and preferably more) rounds of ammunition of exactly the same make and type as those from the scene should be fired, and the components collected for examination. These rounds should be collected in sequence and numbered as such, as there could be a progressive change in the barrel due to rusting or some other factor, and this could affect the striation comparison.

It is extremely important for exactly the same type and make of ammunition be used, as minor variations in the hardness of components or pressures produced could seriously affect the appearance of the impressed stria.

The bullets should then be cross-compared until a mental picture is obtained as to what are the salient features and what marks can be disregarded. These cross-comparisons of the control cartridge cases and bullets should, ideally, be photographed, as there could be allegations that the match/non-match was not representative of the whole.

7.1.6   Manufacturing marks on ammunition

Mention has already been made of class characteristics, for example end milling marks on Chinese Type 54 pistols, but one should also be aware of manufacturing marks on the ammunition.

7.1.7   Recovery methods for fired bullets

If a weapon has been recovered, it will be necessary to compare fired ammunition from this weapon with fired ammunition recovered from the scene. Obtaining a series of test cartridge cases from a self-loading pistol presents little difficulty, as they merely have to be picked up. Obtaining fired bullets in a near pristine condition is, however, a little more difficult.

In the past, cotton waste or wadding has been used, but this material can be quite abrasive to soft lead bullets, especially those of .22″ rimfire calibre. This material could easily damage a soft lead bullet to such an extent that a non-match could result. High-grade, long fibre cotton wool is extremely good at preserving the finest stria on the softest of lead bullets. It is, however, very expensive and has to be frequently replaced.

Water tanks

Vertical and horizontal water tanks for bullet recovery are currently very popular, but these also have their own problems:

- With **horizontal bullet recovery tanks**, where the bullet is fired at an angle into one end of the open top of the tank, The problems are mainly concerned with bullet recovery. Once the bullet loses

---

Illustrative Case 2

An example of how confusing ammunition manufacturing marks can be came to light in a laboratory accreditation examination. A number of cartridge cases were submitted and the examiners were asked to determine how many weapons had been used. The problem appeared to be very simple, and everyone returned the same results – four cartridges in one gun and two in another. The examiners had, however, been rather unfair and had obtained two batches of the same make of ammunition, one of which had very pronounced manufacturing marks and the other none. Four cartridges had been fired from one batch and two from the other and, as the breech face marks were extremely faint and the firing pin featureless, the mistake was easy to make. The test was eventually withdrawn, as every participating laboratory returned the same results.

Illustrative Case 3

A newly built US forensic laboratory sited its vertical bullet recovery tank in the corner of the firearms section. After several hundred rounds of ammunition had been fired into the tank, the bulging sides and hammering action on its base had pushed out the walls of the building to such an extent that there was a four-inch (10 cm) gap through the brickwork on either side, through which daylight could be seen.

---

its velocity, it drops to the bottom of the tank and the only practical way of recovering it is with a piece of Plasticine or Blu-Tack on the end of a long stick.

- **Vertical bullet recovery tanks** have to be a minimum of six feet deep to ensure that the bullet loses all its velocity before reaching the bottom of the tank. With a minimum depth of six feet, the tank is often sited on one floor of a building, with the base resting on the floor below.

One problem which all water recovery tanks suffer is the propensity for the bullet to spiral down the tank, eventually hitting the sides and becoming damaged. For some unknown reason, this problem is particularly acute with vertical tanks, and it is commonly referred to as '**bullet progression**'. This, once again, could easily result in a missed positive outcome for a striation comparison.

The bullet progression observed in these tanks appears to be a function of bullet yaw, in which the bullet prescribes a spiral round the axis of its flight due to over-stabilisation of the bullet by the rifling. This spiral around its flight axis is accentuated by the increased density of water compared to air, which sends the bullet into an ever-increasing spiral as it progresses down the tank. If the tank is not of sufficient diameter, the bullet will contact the sides of the tank and become badly damaged. A vertical tank diameter of three feet (one metre) is considered the absolute minimum.

Another problem with vertical recovery tanks is the hydraulic shock produced when a bullet is fired into water. As water is non-compressible, a shock wave is produced when it is struck by a bullet, causing the tank to bulge. When the tank regains its original shape, it rebounds, lifting it off its base and sending large quantities of water out of the top of the tank. The continual hammering action of the tank

---

Illustrative Case 4

Probably one of the most unusual cases involving bullet recovery resulted from the strafing of a fishing boat by a military aircraft. The boat was not sunk, but it was badly damaged. Upon examination of the boat, two 30 mm cannon bullets were found lodged in the smashed engine block and mountings. A microscopic examination of the copper driving bands on the bullets showed that they had been fired through different barrels. Eventually, a number of aircraft were located which could have carried out the shooting, each of which was armed with four 30 mm cannons.

Obviously, Crocell and cotton wool were not going to be the first choice for recovery materials for this type of missile. In the end, a 200 foot trench was dug which was six feet wide and six feet deep. Into a pit at one end of the trench was mounted an action from a 30 mm cannon, onto which the barrels from the suspect aircraft could be attached, one at a time. The pit was filled up with sawdust, which was then soaked in oil. A soldier was positioned every ten feet (3 metres) along the pit and, as the disturbance from the cannon bullet passing through the sawdust was seen, he raised his arm. The last soldier to raise his arm was then given a shovel and told to dig! After much noise and hours of digging, sufficient bullets were located that could be used to determine whose guns were used to strafe the ship.

jumping off its base (even though this might be just a fraction of an inch) and the bulging of its sides can have quite serious consequences for the building in which it is sited.

Probably one of the most convenient and cheap materials for the recovery of bullets goes under the trade name of 'Crocell'. This is a high molecular weight petroleum jelly which is used as a protective coat on high-quality engineering tools. The material, which comes in granulated form, is simply melted and cast into one inch (25 mm) thick slabs. These are placed into a long wooden or steel box. Bullets fired into this material stop in a surprisingly short space (12 inches (29.4 cm) for a .38″ Special and 20 inches (49 cm) for a 9 mm PB), and they can be located quite easily by pulling out the sheets.

Crocell is exceedingly good at preserving fine stria, even for the softest of lead bullets. In addition, after 30 or so shots, the damaged sheets are merely re-cast.

Care should be taken to ensure that, during firing, a piece of card is placed in front of the first sheet of Crocell. If this is not done, unburnt propellant particles issuing from the muzzle of the weapon will accumulate in and on the front sheet of Crocell. After a few re-castings, the quantity of propellant in the Crocell can reach levels where a distinct fire hazard will exist.

7.1.8 Conclusion

As can be seen from the above, obtaining control bullets and cartridge cases and examining them under a comparison microscope is not a straightforward or simple process. Many variables come into play, which can seriously affect the possibility of discovering whether a match exists between a control sample and a crime scene sample or evidential material from the Outstanding Crime Index (Unsolved Crime Index).

Discovery and disclosure must be full and frank, and questions asked as to the following:

- Was the barrel wiped through before test fires were conducted?

- Are the barrel wipes available for examination?

- Do these barrel wipes give any indication as to when the weapon was last fired?

- Was the breech face photographed before test firing?

- What was the recovery medium for the test fires?

- Did the medium used cause any damage to the recovered bullets?

- How many control samples were recovered and examined?

- Which sample was selected?

- Was it the first fifth, tenth etc.?

- Which of the recovered control samples was selected as being representative for comparison purposes?

- If it was not the first control taken, why not, as this would logically be closest to the last round fired during the open fire incident?

- Why was that particular sample selected and the rest rejected?

- Are there photomicrographs of the comparisons between the control samples?

- Are photomicrographs of the match between the scene exhibit and the control available?

- If they are available, do they show the complete comparison or just one part of it? If not, why not?

- If photomicrographs are not available, why not? And if not, can we see the match at first hand on the comparison microscope, either in the court or at the laboratory?

- Is there a video recording of the whole comparison? If not, why not?

- What lighting system was used and why?

- Was the ammunition used for the control samples exactly the same as that used in the shooting incident, and if not, why not?

Further reading

1 Mc Cafferty, J. (1981). The Value of Firearms Examination for the Defence. *Medicine, Science and the Law* 21 (3), 170–174.

2 Samuels, A. (1994). Forensic Science and Miscarriages of Justice. *Medicine, Science and the Law* 34 (2), 148–154.

3 Samuels, A. (1989). Forensic Evidence for the Defence. *Medicine, Science and the Law* 29 (4) 293–297.

4 Steindler, R.A. (1980). Air Gun Pellet Penetration. *Medicine, Science and the Law* 20 (2), 93–98.

5 http://www.neilsands.plus.com/diss1introduction.htm. The Value and Use of Forensic Evidence in Homicide cases

6 http://defence-forensics.co.uk/

7 http://www.forensic.gov.uk/html/media/case-studies/f-31.html.

8 Crocell Hot Dip, Croda Application Chemicals, Churchill Road, England DN1 2TH.

9 Warlow, T. (2004). *Firearms, the Law and Forensic Ballistics* (2nd edition). CRC Press. ASIN: B000Q6ZJAE.

7.2

The Concept of Consecutive Matching Stria

7.2.1 Introduction

An evolving concept in striated mark comparisons is the developing study of consecutive matching stria (CMS) as a quantitative method of describing an observed pattern match. This is a concept with which many, including the author, are not comfortable, but that does not eliminate or reduce the worth of such an approach to quantifying the outcome of striation comparisons.

CMS is considered to be a simple and effective means of articulating the best known non-match described and defined by the AFTE Theory of Identification. Anyone giving evidence in court regarding comparison microscopy should be aware of its existence and be able to integrate its concepts into the observed comparison concordance under review whatever their feelings as to its worth.

7.2.2 Basics

In the 1950s, Biasotti criticised the 'almost complete lack of factual and statistical data pertaining to the problem of establishing identity in the field of firearms identification . . . ' He wrote that, 'if we accept the present apparent state of development as adequate and believe that no objective statistical data for establishing identity can be developed, then the subject of firearms and toolmark identification will

remain essentially an art limited by the intuitive ability of individual practitioners.'

CMS was initially proposed in a paper written by Al Biasotti and published in the *Journal of Forensic Sciences* in 1959. In an extensive analysis of 720 known non-match comparisons of land and groove impressions in fired bullets, Biasotti found no instances in which the CMS exceeded four.

In 1997, Biasotti and John Murdock jointly published their conservative quantitative criteria for identification, as expressed in terms of CMS:

> "In three dimensional toolmarks, when at least two different groups of at least three consecutive matching stria appear in the same relative position, or one group of six consecutive matching stria are in agreement in an evidence toolmark compared to a test toolmark.
>
> In two dimensional toolmarks, when at least two groups of at least five consecutive matching stria appear in the same relative position, or one group of eight consecutive matching stria are in agreement in an evidence toolmark. For these criteria to apply, however, the possibility of subclass characteristics must be ruled out."

Perceived as an alternative to the traditional approach, CMS encountered widespread resistance on the part of firearms and toolmark examiners. According to Stephen G. Bunch, a firearms and toolmark examiner who is one of the most prominent

Forensic Ballistics in Court: Interpretation and Presentation of Firearms Evidence, First Edition. Brian J. Heard.
© 2013 John Wiley & Sons, Ltd. Published 2013 by John Wiley & Sons, Ltd.

critics of CMS: 'Since Al Biasotti conducted his original identification-criteria research in the 1950s, there has been debate over the relative virtues of objective and subjective methods in forensic firearms identification – specifically over the virtues of counting consecutive matching striations on bullets . . . '

In an attempt to downplay the controversy over the relative merits of CMS and the traditional subjective approach (and to defuse the claim that firearms and toolmark identification does not satisfy the Frye or Daubert standards), Nichols has insisted that, 'CMS is not a more objective way of performing examinations, but simply a means by which an examiner can describe what he or she is observing in a striated toolmark comparison'. At the same time, Nichols has described CMS as an attempt 'to standardise the concept of the best-known non-match'.

These two descriptions of CMS cannot both be true, given Nichols's own admission in both testimony and publications that, under the traditional approach, 'differences between examiners as to what constitutes the best-known non-match situation' make it 'not surprising' and 'not necessarily unexpected' for examiners to disagree about whether an inconclusive or an identification is the proper conclusion in a particular case. On the one hand, if CMS is not 'a different method than has been practised throughout the years', the CMS identification criterion must be such a malleable standard that, when examiners disagree as they do under the traditional approach, they each can manipulate CMS to show that they are right. On the other hand, CMS can contribute to standardisation only if the criterion is inflexible enough to settle disagreements that arise under the traditional approach. Nichols fails to realise that unless CMS is more objective than the traditional 'I know it when I see it' approach, there is no justification for using CMS to decide that some, but not other, examiners' conclusions are right.

Nichols stated, to the contrary, that CMS is most favourably viewed as an attempt to use statistical empirical studies to formulate a cut-off point of numbers of consecutive matching stria at which the likelihood that another tool would produce toolmarks that do as good a job at matching the evidence toolmark as the toolmarks produced by the suspect tool is so exceedingly small that, for all practical purposes,

the suspect tool can be identified as the unique source of the evidence toolmark. Viewed in this way, CMS is a step in the right direction in that, by contrast to the traditional subjective approach, it is at least an attempt to establish statistical empirical foundations for firearms and toolmark identification. It is mistake to suggest, however, that the widespread adoption of CMS would solve the scientific problems with firearms and toolmark identification. On the contrary, CMS is a highly imperfect attempt to establish the requisite statistical empirical foundations.

One of the major problems is that the CMS identification criterion is seen by some as applying only to striated, but not impression, toolmarks – that is, scratch marks, not those produced by a firing pin. This is a misconception of the whole concept of CMS, as the impressed marks produced by a firing pin or a breech face mark are simply striated marks reproduced in an impressed mark. A second problem that even proponents of CMS recognise is that the CMS criterion is intended to be applied to individual, rather than subclass, characteristics of toolmarks. Misidentifications will result if, in applying the criterion, examiners mistake subclass characteristics for individual characteristics. CMS does nothing to remedy the lack of strict rules for distinguishing between subclass and individual characteristics, nor to decrease the difficulty of making this distinction.

Although numbers of consecutive matching stria must be counted to apply the criterion, line counting is inherently a subjective process. Very often, two independent experts will get different results concerning the total number of stria and the number of matching stria. The absence of agreement implies that the determination of whether the CMS criterion is met in a particular case is likely to be guided by the individual examiner's subjective sense of whether evidence and test toolmarks match. This tendency is fostered by the attempts of Nichols and others to defuse opposition by insisting that CMS is not an alternative to the traditional approach, but simply a means by which examiners can describe identifications that they have already reached in their mind's eye.

To date, the published studies compare single land impressions on pairs of bullets known to have been fired by different guns to conclude that misidentifications cannot result from the application of CMS to single land impressions. The most the studies can show is that false positives will not result if a match is declared when the number of consecutive matching stria on a single land impression meets the CMS criterion. The studies cannot rule out the possibility that misidentifications will result from the application of CMS to the total number of consecutive matching stria on all of a bullet's land impressions.

Although not necessarily practised by all firearms examiners, these criteria are of growing importance due to the following:

• The expectations of more sophisticated jurors.

• The need for more objective identification criteria.

• The changing environment of the courtroom following Daubert v. Merrell Dow Pharmaceuticals.

• The potential for increased credibility for examiners in the courtroom.

The second of the three principles of the AFTE Theory of Identification indicates that the degree of correspondence which must be exceeded to constitute sufficient agreement for an identification is the best known non-match (by each individual examiner) to have been produced by different tools. Ideally, an examiner would gain experience in this during his or her initial training period, rather than when they begin to perform actual examinations on their own.

The third principle of the AFTE Theory of Identification indicates that, although founded on the scientific method and reproducibility of results, the interpretation is subjective in nature. It is the policy of most laboratories that a second qualified examiner should verify the findings of the first examiner.

Ultimately, sufficient agreement is the product of the examiner's personal training, skills, and experience in:

• recognising corresponding patterns of matching striations;

• recognising corresponding patterns within impressed toolmarks;

• determining the best known non-match in their personal experience;

• comparing striated and impressed toolmarks.

It is incumbent on each examiner to rely on their training and experience to identify and to be able to articulate the process used to determine sufficient agreement and best known non-match.

Typical toolmarks can, for the purpose of CMS comparisons, fall into two broad categories:

• An evidence toolmark from a crime scene is identified as having been made by a particular evidence tool.

• Two evidence toolmarks recovered from the same or separate crime scenes are identified as having been made by a single tool (no tool submitted).

The categories of identification when a tool has been recovered are:

• Identification.

• Inconclusive.

• Elimination.

• Unsuitable for comparison.

The AFTE Glossary defines an identification as:

'Agreement of a combination of individual characteristics and all discernible class characteristics where the extent of agreement exceeds that which can occur in the comparison of toolmarks made by different tools and is consistent with the agreement demonstrated by toolmarks known to have been produced by the same tool.'

This statement reflects the concepts of sufficient agreement and best known non-match. All identifications are based on pattern matching. It is possible to go beyond this qualitative match to the use of quantifiable consecutive matching stria (CMS) to further support identification.

An inconclusive result is noted in the AFTE Glossary as the outcome of a comparison in which there is:

- some agreement of individual characteristics and all discernible class characteristics, but insufficient for identification;

- agreement of all discernible class characteristics without agreement or disagreement of individual characteristics due to an absence, insufficiency or lack of reproducibility;

- agreement of all discernible class characteristics and disagreement of individual characteristics, but insufficient for an elimination.

7.2.3   Arguments for and against the concept of stria comparisons

Countless articles for and against the reliability of stria comparisons have been written. Even to list them here would unfeasible. However, A précis of two very important articles concerning the admissibility of stria comparisons follow.

Dr Adina Schwartz is an Associate Professor with the John Jay College of Criminal Justice and the Graduate Center, City University of New York. In a long paper published in *The Columbia Science and Technology Law Review* in 2005 (see Further Reading section), Dr Schwartz contended the following:

- Despite widespread faith in 'ballistics fingerprinting', because of systemic scientific problems, firearms and toolmark identifications should be inadmissible across the board.

- Those similarities between toolmarks made by different tools and differences between toolmarks made by the same tool imply that a statistical question must be answered to determine whether a particular tool was the source of an evidence toolmark.

- What is the likelihood that the toolmarks made by a randomly selected tool of the same type would do as good a job as the toolmarks made by the suspect

tool at matching the characteristics of the evidence toolmark?

- Firearms and toolmark examiners evade this question by claiming to be able to single out a particular firearm or other tool as the source of an evidence toolmark.

- The absence of statistical empirical foundations cannot be excused on the ground that, regardless of how they do it, firearms and toolmark examiners reach accurate identity conclusions.

- While firearms and toolmark examiners have feared that Daubert would lead courts to exclude their testimony, both before and after Daubert, firearms and toolmark identification testimony has largely been admitted as a matter of course.

- No court, including the two recent courts that have excluded particular identification testimony, has recognised the systemic scientific problems with the field.

- Because of the risk that innocent people will be convicted or even sentenced to death on the basis of erroneous identifications, all firearms and toolmark identifications should be excluded until adequate statistical empirical foundations and proficiency testing are developed for the field.

In an even longer paper, Ronal G. Nichols, in 2007, countered by stating that:

- A careful and thorough review of the literature will demonstrate that the discipline of firearms and toolmark identification is firmly rooted in the application of the scientific method, culminating in the definition of a theory of identification by the relevant scientific community associated with the discipline.

- The great majority of the study in the discipline follows the premise of the scientific method of defining a problem, formulating a hypothesis or tentative explanation, designing and performing an experiment to test the hypothesis, making observations, and interpreting the results to determine the reasonableness of the tentative explanation.

- While Schwartz's criticises the scientific basis of the discipline, she does do without once either referring to or citing the AFTE Theory of Identification.

- The Theory of Identification is the work of the relevant scientific community, a careful reading of which would help answer some of the claims made by Schwartz. It reads:

(a) The theory of identification as it pertains to the comparison of toolmarks enables opinions of common origin to be made when the unique surface contours of two toolmarks are in 'sufficient agreement'.

(b) This 'sufficient agreement' is related to the significant duplication of random toolmarks as evidenced by the correspondence of a pattern or combination of patterns of surface contours. Significance is determined by the comparative examination of two or more sets of surface contour patterns comprised of individual peaks, ridges and furrows. Specifically, the relative height or depth, width, curvature and spatial relationship of the individual peaks, ridges and furrows within one set of surface contours are defined and compared to the corresponding features in the second set of surface contours. Agreement is significant when it exceeds the best agreement demonstrated between toolmarks known to have been produced by different tools and is consistent with the agreement demonstrated by toolmarks known to have been produced by the same tool. The statement that 'sufficient agreement' exists between two toolmarks means that the agreement is of a quantity and quality that the likelihood that another tool could have made the mark is so remote as to be considered a practical impossibility.

(c) Currently the interpretation of individualisation/identification is subjective in nature,

founded on scientific principles and based on the examiner's training and experience.

- That the challenge offered by Schwartz is not as substantiated as an uncritical review of her article would suggest. There are numerous instances in which studies and articles are inappropriately quoted or inaccurately paraphrased.

- During the discussion of some of the scientific issues, there is an apparent lack of understanding of the relative significance as applied to the science of firearm and toolmark identification.

- While the author was apparently aware of the large number of articles available that can be used to address many of these issues, there was no mention of them made in her argument.

- Furthermore, there were instances in which research into some of these primary resources, rather than reliance on some secondary resources, would have been much more enlightening.

Both of these articles (see below for full references) should be read in full.

Further reading

1 Biasotti, A. (1959). A Statistical Study of the Individual Characteristics of Fired Bullets. *Journal of Forensic Sciences* 4 (1), 34–50.
2 Interpol Forensic Science Symposium Reports 2007.
3 http://apps.americanbar.org/abastore/products/books/abstracts/5450051chap1_abs.pdf
4 International Symposium on Setting Quality Standards for the Forensic Community, San Antonio, Texas. May 3–7, 1999.
5 Murdock, J.E. (2011). Scientifically Defensible Criteria for the Identification of Toolmarks. *Workshop seminar at 2011 AFTE Conference*.
6 Schwartz, A. (2005). A Systemic Challenge to the Reliability and Admissibility of Firearms and Toolmark Identification. *The Columbia Science and Technology Law Review* 66, 1–42.
7 AFTE (1998). Theory of Identification as It Relates to Toolmarks. *AFTE Journal* 30 (1) 86–88.
8 Biasotti, A.A. & Murdock, J. (1984). Criteria for Identification or 'State of the Art' of Firearms

and Toolmark Identification. *AFTE Journal* 16 (4), 16–17.

9 Masson, J.J. (1997). Confidence Level Variations in Firearms Identification Through Computerized Technology, *AFTE Journal* 29 (1), 42.

10 Biasotti, A.A. & Murdock, J. (1997). Firearm and Toolmark Identification. In: Faigman, D.L., Kaye, D. K., Saks, M.J.& Sanders, J. (eds.) *Modern Scientific Evidence: The Law and Science of Expert Testimony* Chapter 23, Vol. 2, pp. 140. St. Paul: West. ISBN 0314214100.

11 *United States v. Kain*, Crim. No. 03-573-1 (E.D. Pa. 2004). Subsequently published as "A Challenge to the Admissibility of Firearm and Toolmark Identifications: *Amicus* Brief prepared on Behalf of the Defendant in United States v. Kain, Crim. No. 03-573-1 (E.D. Pa. 2004)." *The Journal of Philosophy, Science & Law* **4**.

12 AFTE Criteria for Identification Committee (1992). Theory of Identification, Range of Striae Comparison Reports and Modified Glossary Definitions – an AFTE Criteria for Identification Committee Report. *AFTE Journal* 24 (2), 336–340.

13 Nichols, R. (1997). Firearm and Toolmark Identification Criteria: A Review of the Literature. *Journal of Forensic Sciences* 42 (3), 466–474.

14 Nichols, R. (2003). Firearm and Toolmark Identification Criteria: A Review of the Literature – Part 2. *Journal of Forensic Sciences* 48 (2), 318–327.

15 Biasotti, A. (1959). A Statistical Study of the Individual Characteristics of Fired Bullets. *Journal of Forensic Science* 4 (1), 37–39

16 Masson, J. (1997). Confidence Level Variations in Firearms Identifications Through Computerized Technology. *AFTE Journal* 29 (1), 42–44.

17 Miller, J. (2001). An Examination of the Application of the Conservative Criteria for Identification of Striated Tool Marks Using Bullets Fired From Ten Consecutively Rifled Barrels. *AFTE Journal* 33 (2), 125–132.

18 Murdock, J. (1981). A General Discussion of Gun Barrel Individuality and an Empirical Assessment of the Individuality of Consecutively Button Rifled .22 Caliber Rifle Barrels. *AFTE Journal* 13 (3), 84–111.

19 Nichols, R.G. (2007). Defending the Scientific Foundations of the Firearms and Tool Mark Identification Discipline: Responding to Recent Challenges. *Journal of Forensic Sciences* 52 (3), 586–594.

7.3

A Statistical Model to Illustrate the Concept of Individuality in Striation Matches

7.3.1 Introduction

Ever since it was first realised that scratch marks produced by a tool, whether it be the rifling of a gun's barrel or that produced by a jemmy on a safe, contained stria which were individual to that tool, a statistical method has been sought to quantify the degree of concordance necessary to prove that individuality. Complicated computer algorithms have been written to recognise repeating series of corresponding lines in two sets of stria and thus assign a likelihood of them having a relationship. However, it has so far proved impossible to assign the degree or percentage of concordance necessary to confirm that common origin.

The following model, developed by the author, does no more than show, via a simple series of boxes (filled, hatched or containing a letter), how remotely unlikely it is for two sets of matching series to occur accidently. The model has found favour among firearms examiners, although one defence expert opined (private communication with the author):

'In my opinion, there is no possible way that such an approach can be valid and I would certainly challenge it if it came up in a case. R v T is an example where I have successfully challenged the use of statistical formula in similar circumstances (footwear marks) . . . The statistical approach, whilst desirable, is neither developed nor validated.'

While these comments are perfectly valid, they are missing the point completely. There is absolutely no way that such a statistical model could be utilised to justify a match. It is simply a method of illustrating the unlikelihood that two accidently occurring sets of conditions with assigned characteristics could match. In a way, it is simply restating the concept of consecutively matching stria (CMS) in numerical terms.

7.3.2 Basics

This probability of two sets of stria accidently being in concordance is difficult to comprehend, due to the statistics involved. As such, when dealing with questions on the subject in court, it is often glossed over with such comments as 'statistically it can be shown but, as I am not a statistician . . . ' or 'empirical studies have shown . . . ' or even 'a match is one which exceeds the best known non-match'.

But how large does an empirical study have to be before it can be determined that a match between two bullets is beyond reasonable doubt? Does an empirical study with one weapon type necessarily have any bearing on other weapon types? And, even more difficult to quantify, what is a 'best known non-match' and how many require observation before one can be recognised?

These are all crucial questions and ones which, if not correctly answered (or, for that matter correctly handled by the prosecution or defence), could lead to misrepresentation of evidence, or even the witness being unnecessarily discredited.

These matters do involve quite difficult statistics, and such mathematical concepts can become very complex. This chapter will attempt to show why no match, no matter how good, will never be one hundred per cent perfect. It will also attempt to handle the statistical side as simply as possible, allowing even the non-mathematically minded to grasp the basics of the subject.

7.3.3   Stria individuality

Many papers have been written with a view to analyse statistically, using idealised computer modelling or digitally enhanced striations marks, the probabilities effecting positive striation comparisons. Amongst these, Tsuneo Uchiyama (1988a, b, c), Biasotti (1955, 1959) and Brackett (1965) are notable. Most of the papers examined have, however, been of a very esoteric nature and only of any real use to theoretical statisticians.

Even so, it is possible to use a very simplified approach and obtain an idea of the probabilities of grooves on bullets from different sources having corresponding stria.

To simplify the matter as far as possible, we can take the analogy of randomly filling a number of boxes. So that the analogy can be translated into matching striations in a rifling groove, there will have to be three conditions:

1. There are 20 boxes, only ten of which will be randomly filled.

2. Each of the filled boxes can be heavily shaded or lightly shaded.

3. Each of the filled boxes can have either an 'X' or a 'Y'.

Taking Condition 1 alone:

In this condition, there are 20, boxes ten of which will be randomly filled, e.g.

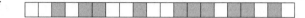

Thus, each of the filled boxes can be lightly shaded or heavily shaded.

The chance that, in a similar 20 boxes, exactly the same combination will be filled is given by the standard statistical formula:

$$_mC_n = \frac{m!}{n!(m-n)!}$$

Where:

C = chance of stria accidentally matching

$_mC_n$ = chance of accidentally matching stria within the parameters 'm' and 'n'.

m = number of boxes

n = number of filled boxes

! = factorial (i.e. $5! = 5 \times 4 \times 3 \times 2 \times 1$)

For this example: $m = 20$; $n = 10$.

$$\text{Chance} = {_{20}C_{10\,10}} = \frac{20!}{10!(20-10)!} = \frac{20!}{10! \times 10!} = 184756$$

Thus, the chance of having two sets of 20 boxes, each having ten randomly filled boxes in the same combination, is a chance of **1 in 184,756**.

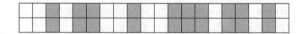

If we now take into consideration Condition 2 in addition to Condition 1:

Condition 2 states that each of the **filled** boxes can be lightly shaded or heavily shaded.

As each box has one of two possible shadings, the chance that the first box will be the same in both sets is $1:2$. The chance that the second box is the same will also be $1:2$. However, as this is dependent upon the first box, the chance that the first two boxes will be shaded exactly the same is $1 : 2 \times 1 : 2$, i.e. 2×2.

Thus, the chance of all ten filled boxes in both sets having the same shade of filling is:

$$2 \times 2 \times 2 \times 2 \times 2 \times 2 \times 2 \times 2 \times 2 \times 2 = 2^{10} = 1024.$$

The chance of ten randomly filled boxes out of 20, each with a randomly chosen fill shading of dark or light is therefore:

$$184,756 \times 1,024 = 189,190,144$$

The chance of the two sets of 20 boxes each with randomly matching ten filled boxes which are either light or dark shading is therefore a chance of 1 in 189,190,144.

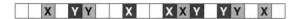

If we now take into consideration Condition 3:
If each of these shaded boxes can then have either an 'X' or a 'Y':

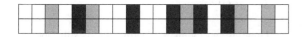

The same probability factor as above is relevant i.e. 2^{10}.

Thus, the figure becomes $189,190,144 \times 1,024 = 193,730,707,456$.

To sum up, then, the chance of two sets of 20 boxes with ten boxes randomly filled with either light or dark shading and either an 'X' or a 'Y' is a chance of **1 in 193,730,707,456.**

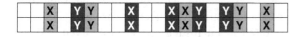

Placing this into the context of a bullet

Let us say that we have a single groove on a bullet, which we divide into 20 longitudinal sections, and in ten of these longitudinal sections are randomly placed ten striations. The chance of two grooves on bullets from different weapons accidentally matching is thus a chance of **1 in 184,756.**

If each of these striations can have one of two profiles (e.g. a pointed shape or a square shape), then the chance of two grooves from different weapons accidentally matching under these criteria are $184,756 \times 1024 = 189,190,144$, i.e. a chance of **1 in 189,190,144**.

If each of these striations can now be one of two widths (e.g. thick or thin), then the chance of two grooves from two different weapons accidentally matching under all three criteria are $189,190,144 \times 1,024 = 193,730,707,456$, i.e. A chance of **1 in 193,730,707,456**

This is, of course, taking a very simple case. In reality, there will be not just 20 possible positions for striations in a groove, but hundreds. There will not just be ten striations but, once again, hundreds – the number only being limited by the resolving power of the microscope. There will not be just two profiles, but tens of possibilities, and the width, once again will have tens of possibilities.

Just taking one groove alone, the number becomes so vast that it must approach infinity. If this is extended to the possibility of finding two bullets where all the grooves match, then the number must be infinitely large and reach a stage where is beyond the realms of possibility.

It can thus be seen that the chance of finding a complete set of accidentally matching stria in bullets from different sources is so infinitesimally small as to be negligible.

This statement is just as viable for other impressed striation marks as it is for the striations found within the rifling of bullets. It thus follows that the pattern of surface contours, comprised of peaks ridges and furrows, found within an impressed toolmark can be considered unique to that tool. It is immaterial whether the tool be the standing breech face of a weapon, a firing pin, the tip of a pry bar or the faces of a bolt cutter – the marks produced will be individual to that tool.

7.3.4 Philosophy

Factors such as the hardness of the materials, pressures produced, build-up of fouling and general debris mean that the striations found on fired bullets and cartridge cases will inevitably exhibit variations from shot to shot. It is thus impossible for two bullets or cartridge cases fired from the same weapon to have absolute concordance in their stria.

Conversely, in bullets and cartridge cases fired from different weapons there will always be some degree of accidental agreement, due to the sheer numbers of stria present.

It has been quoted (Walls, 1968) that up to 25 per cent of the stria in a non-match, and in excess of 75 per cent of the stria in a match, will show concordance. This exceedingly high degree of accidentally matching lines has not, however, been supported by personal observation. There is no dispute that out of the thousands of lines present in any one comparison, a number must show agreement by pure chance alone.

It is by experience alone that the examiner is able to mentally exclude those striations which are not of significance and award the necessary degree of credibility to those which form the basis of a positive match. It is also by experience alone that the examiner is able to ascribe an opinion of common origin, based upon significant agreement between two sets of unique stria. This significant agreement relates to the duplication of a unique pattern of surface contours comprised of peaks, ridges and furrows.

It should be re-emphasised here that it is not the individual stria which form the basis of a match, but the duplication of a series of groups and patterns of stria. In effect, consecutively matching stria (CMS). It is this duplication which enables an expert examiner to determine that a degree of concordance exists that could not happen by chance alone.

Due to the subjective nature of the processes involved in the elimination of insignificant detail, the criteria used by the expert to ascertain the degree of accordance of stria cannot be quantified mathematically. The following principle can, however, be used to quantify the basic concepts used in the assignment of a positive match:

'A positive match between two sets of stria is one in which the extent of agreement exceeds that of the best accepted non-match'.

This is an oft quoted reference, the exact origin of which is unsure. Biasotti (e.g. 1959) quotes this phrase in several of his papers on the subject and could well be the originator.

When positive agreement is said to exceed the best known non-match, it is implying that it must, to some considerable degree, exceed the agreement witnessed in non-matches. What can be ascribed numerically to the statement 'exceed to a considerable degree' is not precisely quantifiable, and once again it comes down to the experience and competence of the examiner.

That the process of assigning a positive match to a stria comparison is an evaluative and thus subjective procedure has been accepted by many. Kind *et al.* (1979) states;

'Much of the knowledge accumulated in the procedure and, used in subsequent comparisons, is of a subjective type, which at present defies numerical classification'.

Biasotti (1959) says:

'Firearms and toolmark identification is still more art (subjective) then science (objective)'.

and Kingston (1970):

'Objective estimates of probability are based upon quantitative experimental data. Subjective estimates are based upon personal knowledge, experience and reasoning. When we know exactly what to quantitate, objective estimates are superior to subjective ones. When we do not know exactly what to quantitate, subjective may be far more realistic than forced objective ones'.

An informative and very interesting paper by Charles R. Meyers, 'The Objective vs. the Subjective Boondoggle' (Meyers, 1987), reviews some of the references dealing with objective and subjective criteria in respect to stria comparisons.

Another interesting paper by Evett (1996) explores the mistaken phrase 'exact science' in relation to the 16 points of comparison used in fingerprint examination and whether forensic science is in fact a 'science'.

The days of the mystical 'all-knowing expert' have, however, long gone. Nowadays, the courts of law demand, very justifiably, a much more scientific approach, and they will not be bulldozed by the 'you must trust me' expert. The competent examiner should always strive to reduce subjectivity to a minimum, while accentuating the objectivity (i.e. the scientific aspects) of his or her examination as much as possible.

The basic difference between an 'expert' and a layman is that due to experience and training, the expert can observe and understand the significance of features and phenomena which the layman would overlook. It is the expert's job to be able to demonstrate to the layman (i.e. the court) the significance of his or her observations. Hiding behind a mask of 'I am the expert, so you will have to trust me' no longer holds sway in modern judicial systems. In this, as in all aspects of forensic science, 'objectivity is everything' – subjectivity alone accounts for nothing.

References

1 Uchiyama, T. (1988a). A Criterion for Land Mark Identification. *AFTE Journal* 20 (3), 236–251.

2 Uchiyama, T. (1988b). Automatic Comparison Model of Land Marks. *AFTE Journal* 20 (3), 252–259

3 Uchiyama, T. (1988c). A Criterion for Land Mark Identification Using Rare Marks. *AFTE Journal* 20 (3), 260–268.

4 Biasotti, A.A. (1955) A Study of Fired Bullets Statistically Analyzed, M. Crim thesis, University of California, Berkeley, CA, USA.

5 Biasotti, A. (1959). A Statistical Study of the Individual Characteristics of Fired Bullets. *Journal of Forensic Sciences* 4 (1), 34–50.

6 Biasotti, A.A. (1981). The Principles of Evidence Evaluation as Applied to Firearms and Toolmark Identification, *Journal of Forensic Sciences* 9 (4), 428–433.

7 Brackett, J.W. (1965). *A Study of Idealised Striated Marks and their Comparison using Models*. Paper presented to 26th Semi-annual Seminar of California Association of Criminalists, Oct. 1965.

8 Walls, H.J. (1974). *Forensics Science*. Sweet & Maxwell. ISBN: 0091099609.

9 Kind, S.S., Wigmore, R., Whitehead, P.H. & Loxley, D.S. (1979). Terminology of Forensic Science. *Journal of the Forensic Science Society* 19 (3), 189–191.

10 Kingston, C.R. (1970). The law of probabilities and the credibility of witnesses and evidence. *Journal of Forensic Sciences* 15, 18–27

11 Meyers, C.R. (1987). Objective v Subjective Boondoggle. *Association of Firearms and Toolmark Examiners Journal* 19 (1), 24–30.

12 Evett, I.W. (1996). Expert Evidence and Forensic Misconceptions of the Nature of Exact Science. *Science and Justice* 36 (2), 118–122.

8.0

Accidental Discharge

8.0.1 Introduction

During the forensic examination of any firearm which has been used in a shooting crime, one should always consider the possibility of an accidental discharge having taken place. It is, however, somewhat rare for a defendant to admit to having shot someone deliberately. All manner of possible reasons will be given for the discharge (or multiple discharges) by the defence counsel, who will be prepared to challenge evidence for the prosecution by way of a defence expert. One must therefore be able to give the fullest account of safety mechanisms present, their functionability, trigger pulls, tests for accidental discharge by jarring, etc., and to be willing and able to back these up in court with non-firing demonstrations. Such illustrative tests are especially convincing when the jury are asked to participate or actually to perform the test themselves.

Such incidents can be roughly divided in to three groups:

- Accidents.

- Accidental discharges.

- Negligent discharges.

Although often overlapping in nature, there are differences in that:

- **accidents** are generally caused by misadventure;

- **accidental discharges** are usually caused by faulty mechanisms;

- **negligent discharges** by criminal negligence.

With accidents, children, hunters, bravado (e.g. Russian roulette) and alcohol are generally involved.

Illustrative Case 1

Two children, one seven years old and the other six, were playing in the study, where their father kept his hunting rifles in a (usually locked) cabinet. Unfortunately, the cabinet was not locked, and the older child retrieved a weapon to play 'cowboys and Indians'. Chasing his sister around the room, he pulled the trigger while shouting 'Bang, bang, you're dead'. Unfortunately, their father had 'forgotten' to unload the weapon and it discharged. The weapon was a Savage Model 99 lever-action rifle in .250-3000 'Savage' calibre. With a muzzle velocity of 3,000 ft/s (910 m/s) and firing a soft-point 87 grain (5.6 g) bullet, this is an extremely powerful weapon. With such a very close range discharge, the damage to the child was devastating, virtually cutting her in half.

Forensic Ballistics in Court: Interpretation and Presentation of Firearms Evidence, First Edition. Brian J. Heard.
© 2013 John Wiley & Sons, Ltd. Published 2013 by John Wiley & Sons, Ltd.

Illustrative Case 2

In 2001, a 21-year-old man was killed[1] while duck hunting, when a shotgun accidentally discharged, shooting him in the head. The loaded weapon, which had been lying on the ground with the safety off and the muzzle pointed toward a river a few feet away, discharged when a hunting dog stepped on the trigger. Scene investigation confirmed that the victim had been standing in the river, planting decoys, with his head approximately level with the adjacent bank. Post-mortem examination and ballistic testing confirmed a range of fire consistent with the witness statements. Examination of the weapon in question documented a light trigger pull but no mechanical defects.

Illustrative Case 3

During a training session of the Royal Bodyguard Unit, one of the more senior members was practising 'quick draws' for shooting at rapidly moving targets. Unfortunately, at one stage, the officer's actions became confused and he fired the weapon before it was clear of the holster. The bullet penetrated his thigh and travelled down the leg, exiting at the ankle. His knee joint was destroyed, the ankle severely damaged and there was extensive muscle damage to the upper and lower leg. Although the Royal Bodyguard is not a military unit, the 'accident' was classified as a negligent discharge.

Illustrative Case 4

During a live ammunition jungle training exercise in Borneo, a soldier shot through a thicket of bamboo, accidently killing a fellow soldier. The soldier claimed that the gun went off accidently, due to his arm being caught on a piece of bamboo. He was found guilty by a military court of negligently discharging a firearm, causing the death of a fellow officer, and was sent to military prison.

With accidental discharges, it is generally either a faulty trigger mechanism or some external influence (e.g. the trigger of a shotgun snagging on a branch) that causes the discharge. The urban myth of a dog or shot bird twitching and pulling the trigger has never, in the author's experience, been shown to be feasible, although it is still regularly reported.

Negligent discharges involve the discharge of a firearm involving culpable carelessness. In judicial and military terms, a negligent discharge is a chargeable offence. A number of armed forces automatically consider any accidental discharge to be negligent discharge, under the assumption that a trained soldier has control of his weapon at all times. This is notably the case in the United States Army, the Canadian Army, the Royal Air Force and the British Army. There is, therefore, a considerable overlap between an accidental discharge and a negligent discharge.

---

[1] *American Journal of Forensic Medicine and Pathology* Sep, 2001: **22**(3), 285–7.

Illustrative Case 5

A nightclub bouncer was charged with murdering a drunk who was attempting to gain entry to the club by shooting him 11 times with a .32″ (7.65 mm) self-loading pistol. His defence was that he only wanted to scare the drunk and he had fired at the ground, but being a 'big strong boy', he must have pulled the trigger too hard and the gun kept going off! The weapon was found to be in full working order and not at all prone to accidental discharge or fully automatic firing. However, what completely destroyed his credibility and defence was the fact that the magazine only held six rounds!

8.0.2 Basics

With the safety mechanisms employed in modern weapons, incidents labelled as 'accidental discharge' have to be treated with some scepticism.

Basically, cases of accidental discharge have to be placed into one of these categories:

1. Faulty lock mechanism.

2. Discharge due to inappropriately low trigger pressure.

3. Failure of the safety mechanism.

4. Inadvertent pulling of the trigger.

5. Inadvertent pulling of the trigger by contact with some object other than the trigger finger.

6. Dropping the weapon.

While there are many designs of lock mechanism, the four illustrated in Figure 8.0.1 show how the basic types work.

8.0.3 Trigger mechanisms

Accepted commercial and military trigger pulls vary tremendously, but generally the following could be considered as acceptable:

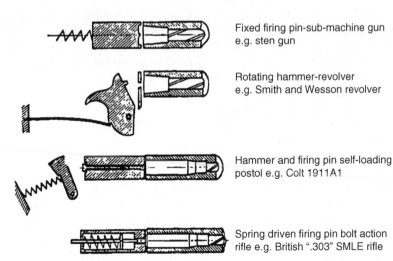

Fixed firing pin-sub-machine gun
e.g. sten gun

Rotating hammer-revolver
e.g. Smith and Wesson revolver

Hammer and firing pin self-loading
postol e.g. Colt 1911A1

Spring driven firing pin bolt action
rifle e.g. British ".303" SMLE rifle

Figure 8.0.1   Basic lock mechanisms.

.22″ Rimfire rifles	3–5 lbs	(1.36–2.25 kg)
Military rifles	4–7 lbs	(1.80–3.15 kg)
Revolvers – single action	4–6 lbs	(1.80–2.70 kg)
Revolvers – double action	10–15 lbs	(4.50–6.75 kg)
Self-loading pistols (SA)	4–8 lbs	(1.80–3.60 kg)
Shotgun	4–5 lbs	(1.80–2.25 kg)

While a 'tuned' trigger pressure as low as 1 lb (0.45 kg) may be totally acceptable in the specialised arena of a target shooting competition, in other circumstances it can be extremely dangerous. Basically, tuning a trigger mechanism involves the polishing of the sear/bent mating surfaces and reducing the contact area between the two. This is an extremely difficult procedure and beyond the scope of anyone other than a highly trained armourer.

Decreasing the strength of the sear spring (which keeps the sear in contact with the bent) and the trigger return spring is also often carried out to improve the trigger pull. If taken too far, this can lead to accidental discharges due to the sear being knocked out of contact with the bent.

One other modification is to reduce the 'trigger back-lash'. This is the continuing rearwards movement of the trigger after the sear has become disengaged from the bent. Once again, if the back-lash is totally removed, the sear and bent can be knocked out of contact via a small impact on the weapon.

Such modifications, even when competently carried out can, even to an experienced shooter in times of crisis, lead to the weapon being inadvertently fired.

Modern target weapons have a huge variety of trigger mechanism types, including the following.

A **set trigger** (sometimes referred to as a **hair trigger**) allows a shooter to have a greatly reduced trigger pull while still maintaining a degree of safety. There are two types: single set and double set.

A **single set trigger** is usually one trigger that may be fired with a conventional amount of trigger pull weight or may be 'set', usually by pushing forward on the trigger. This takes up the creep in the trigger and allows a much lighter trigger pull.

As above, a **double set trigger** accomplishes the same thing, but uses two triggers. One sets the trigger and the other fires the weapon.

Set triggers are most likely to be seen on customised weapons and competition rifles, where a light trigger pull is beneficial to accuracy. Double set triggers can be further classified by phase. A double set, single phase trigger can only be operated by first pulling the set trigger, then pulling the firing trigger. A double set, double phase trigger can be operated as a standard trigger if the set trigger is not pulled, or as a set trigger by first pulling the set trigger. Double set, double phase triggers offer the versatility of both a standard trigger and a set trigger.

Other trigger mechanisms

Electronic trigger

With this type of mechanism, the sear and bent are replaced by an electronic release mechanism. The spring-loaded firing pin can also be replaced with a solenoid-type firing pin.

Electric ignition

In this type of mechanism, there is no sear, bent or firing pin, and the primer is ignited by an electric current. Special ammunition with an electrically fired primer has to be used. This type of ignition system is mainly used in caseless ammunition (see Chapter 4.2) and large calibre weapons. Electrically fired large calibre ammunition can be recognised by the primer having a ring of insulating material between the primer and cartridge case; this is usually black in colour.

8.0.4   Reasons for an accidental discharge

(a) Faulty lock mechanism

Basically, all locks work on the same principle. There is a spring-loaded, rotating (as in a weapon with a hammer) or sliding (as in a bolt action weapon) hammer with a small notch cut in it called a 'bent'. Into this bent fits one end of a pivoting lever which is called the 'sear'. The other end of this lever either forms, or is actuated by, the trigger. When the

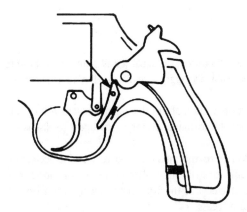

Figure 8.0.2 Sear and bent contact in a revolver trigger mechanism.

lock mechanism is cocked, the sear contacts the bent and holds the hammer or striker in the cocked position until the trigger is pulled (see Figure 8.0.2).

The contact between the bent and sear must be minimal, otherwise the pressure required to disengage the two would be excessive. Likewise, the contact surfaces must be parallel in order to ensure a smooth disconnection. A hooked bent would be all but impossible to disengage, while a rounded surface could slip out of contact under the spring tension of the lock.

Most accidental discharges caused by faulty lock mechanisms can be attributed to a bent/sear fault. Illustrative cases would be appropriate to exemplify this aspect of accidental discharge.

(b) Inappropriately low trigger pressure

For target use, trigger mechanisms are often 'tuned' to give a smoother, lighter trigger pull. It is not unusual to find target pistols and rifles with trigger pulls in the region of 1 lb. With a trigger pressure set this low, the slightest touch will cause the weapon to fire.

(c) Failure of the safety mechanism

One very common fault in shotgun lock mechanisms of the old external hammer type involves a faulty 'rebound safety'. In this type of weapon, there is an

---

Illustrative Case 6: Faulty lock mechanism

In an alleged case of accidental discharge involving a husband/wife dispute, it was claimed that the gun went off accidentally while he was unloading the weapon in the front room. The wife was shot in the head, killing her instantly.

The weapon involved was an extremely expensive Italian side-by-side double-barrelled 12-bore shotgun which had only been used twice before. Trigger pull testing showed that the right and left trigger required a pressure of 4 lbs and $4\frac{1}{2}$ lbs respectively, which is considered acceptable for a weapon of this type.

Tests for accidental discharge consisted of blows with a soft mallet to the heel of the butt, the top and bottom of the lock mechanism and the muzzle end of the barrel. These tests showed that there was no tendency for the weapon to accidentally discharge through jarring. During test firing, it was noted that with each successive pull of the trigger, the pressure required decreased significantly.

Further tests to determine the actual pressure required on the trigger to fire the weapon showed that, after just a few test firings, it had fallen to less than 2 lbs. The gun was also found now to be very prone to accidental discharge by jarring. After just two additional trigger pull tests and two accidental discharge tests, the trigger pull had dropped to less than 1 lb, and then to the point of not being able to cock the mechanism at all.

On disassembling the lock mechanism it was found that, during manufacture, the steel bents of the lock mechanism had not been case hardened. On each pull of the trigger, the much harder sear had stripped metal away from the bent until it no longer existed.

Although the weapon was in good working order and not at all prone to accidental discharge when received, there were doubts as to the changing characteristics of the weapon's lock mechanism and the case was dismissed.

Illustrative Case 7: Gun damaged through poor exhibit handling

One case involved the shooting of a man by a gypsy armed with a .410″ shotgun. As usual, it was claimed that the gun had gone off accidentally while the shooter trying to fend off the (allegedly) aggressive man, and there had been no intention to kill him.

The weapon concerned was a cheap quality single-shot bolt-action weapon of Continental manufacture. It had an excessively high trigger pressure of 12 lbs and there was absolutely no tendency for the weapon to discharge accidentally.

During the trial, the prosecution requested a demonstration as to the method used to test for accidental discharge. The weapon was cocked and, as the gun was turned around to strike the heel of the weapon on the floor, it lightly brushed the top of the witness box. There was a very audible click as the firing pin fell, which at that point sounded like thunder. At that stage, the prosecution asked for a recess.

On disassembling the weapon, it was found that the action had been driven back into the woodwork of the stock to such an extent that the sear was being pushed out of contact with the bent. In addition, the heel of the stock was found to be battered and cracked where it had been repeatedly hammered onto the floor.

Obviously, nobody was going to accept responsibility for this damage, but it was suspected that everyone involved in the case had to convince themselves that the weapon was not prone to accidental discharge. This was explained to the jury and, as the prosecution counsel did not object, the case was allowed to continue on the evidence as to what condition the weapon was in when originally received.

---

additional bent, in the form of a hook rather than a notch, called the 'half cock' or 'rebound bent'. As the bent is hook-shaped, the sear is firmly locked into place and it should not be possible to push the hammer forward manually or to pull the sear out of contact with the bent via the trigger. When in this half cock or rebound position, the only way of releasing the sear is by pulling the hammer back to the full cock position and then pulling the trigger. The internal springing of the lock mechanism is so arranged that, when the hammer is in the down or uncocked position, a spring will pull the hammer slightly to the rear into this half cock notch. In this position, the hammer will be unable to reach the striker.

In cheaper weapons, where the manufacturing tolerances are larger and the materials are not always of the best quality, it is not unusual for there to be sufficient 'play' in the mechanism, enabling the hammer to be pushed forward. This 'play' is often sufficient for the firing pin to touch the primer. Dropping the weapon, or inadvertently striking the hammer, will often discharge such a weapon accidentally, when it is in this half cock safety position.

Illustrative Case 8: Weapon accidentally fired, killing a burglar

Being awakened by the sound of breaking glass, a house owner armed himself with an old double-barrelled shotgun. On confronting the burglar, a fight ensued, during which the house owner was violently thrown back against a door frame. At that stage, the weapon discharged, removing most of the burglar's head. The house owner claimed that the weapon was in the safety or rebound position, and that the gun had discharged accidentally on hitting the door frame.

On examining the scene, a deep impression of one of the weapon's hammers was found in the woodwork of the door frame. This, and the fact that the half cock bent was worn to the extent that the firing pins actually rested on the cartridge primer, was enough to show that there was no intent on the part of the house owner.

Illustrative Case 9

The Hong Kong and Singapore police were, from 1932, issued with Webley Mk III and Mk IV revolvers. These were of WWII vintage and, due to wartime manufacturing tolerances being somewhat greater than those in peacetime, they did have a tendency for the rebound safety to be ineffective. As a result, weapons were carried with an empty chamber under the firing pin.

Many self-loading pistols and revolvers have a 'half cock' safety so that the gun may safely be carried with a live round in the chamber. Unless the weapon is of very low quality, it is very unusual to find a faulty half cock safety mechanism in a modern pistol.

(d) Inadvertently Pulling the Trigger

In general, this is very difficult if not impossible, to prove one way or another. Numerous cases are on record of a violent fight during which a person holding a weapon has been violently thrown back against a wall, with a claimed clenching of the hand holding the weapon resulting in an inadvertent discharge of the weapon.

Hundreds of tests have been carried out, using volunteers under controlled conditions[2] to test the probability of this happening. In the majority of these tests, it was found that for self-loading pistols and revolvers in the single action mode, there was little tendency for the trigger to be pulled unless the trigger pressure was exceptionally low. If anything, the person holding the weapon generally released the trigger. For revolvers in the double action mode, it was found that there was no tendency at all for the trigger to be pulled to the extent that an accidental discharge will occur.

That said, these were controlled tests, of course, and what happens when there is a violent confrontation or one person fears for his or her life is completely another matter.

One area where one can be a little more definitive in respect to the accidental pulling of the trigger is when the weapon is violently pulled away from the person holding it. It is easy to simulate the unexpected snatching of a weapon, and persons both experienced and inexperienced in weapon handling can easily be tested as to their likely response. These tests[3] have shown that there is a far greater likelihood of the trigger being released when the weapon is snatched away. In fact, trained shooters almost invariably react in this way. Figures show that there is an approximately 75 per cent chance that an experienced shooter will inadvertently release the trigger if an attempt is made to pull their gun away. With inexperienced shooters, the probability drops to about 65 per cent, but this is still quite significant.

One again, these were controlled tests, and what happens when there is a violent confrontation or one person fears for his/her life is another matter.

Illustrative Cases 10 and 11 describe two incidents that exemplify this type of 'accidental discharge' quite well.

(e) Inadvertent pulling of the trigger by some object other than the trigger finger

This is probably the cause of more hunting accidents than all the other causes added together. There are numerous recorded cases of twigs snagging on the trigger of loaded shotguns and rifles, and I am sure that many of them are genuine accidents. Less likely are those incidents allegedly involving inquisitive dogs, rabbits twitching in game pockets and even shot pheasants landing on the trigger guard!

---

[2] Unpublished work by author.

[3] Unpublished work by author.

Illustrative Case 10: Accidental discharge while holstering a weapon

The first of these cases involved a police officer who was inserting his gun into a holster which was held in his left hand. The weapon discharged, with the bullet taking a large portion of the holster through the palm of his left hand. A careful examination of the internal surface of the holster and a gun handling test (see Chapter 15, 'Gun Handling Tests') on the officer's right hand showed that the index finger had been on the trigger at the time of firing, and that the weapon was almost fully holstered. For some reason, he had his finger in the trigger guard while he was holstering the weapon. The act of trying to force the weapon into the holster while his finger was snagged on the top of the holster must have fired the weapon. Further testing did show, however, that it was all but impossible for the weapon to be discharged in this way if the hammer had not been first cocked into the single action mode.

Illustrative Case 11: Quick draw accidental discharge

The second case involved another police officer who was found in a toilet with a hole in his right foot. His statement said that he had taken his gun out of the holster to disentangle his lanyard and when he re-holstered the weapon, it went off, shooting him in the foot. His explanation was that the lanyard had caught on the trigger and fired the weapon. Muzzle discharge residues inside the holster showed that the weapon must have been almost completely out of the holster at the time the firing occurred. In that position, it was impossible for the lanyard to have pulled the trigger. From the examination it was plainly obvious that he had been practising 'quick draws' in front of the mirror and had inadvertently pulled the trigger.

Illustrative Case 12: Fingerprint expert inadvertently discharging a shotgun

It would be highly unlikely for the soft touch of a fingerprint dusting brush to have sufficient force to discharge a weapon while the trigger was being searched for prints. There was, however, an incident where the fingerprint officer, having found nothing on the trigger, proceeded to use it to steady the weapon while he was dusting the butt stock. Sufficient force was applied to the trigger to discharge one barrel of the shotgun. The shot went straight through the ceiling and into the room above, much to the consternation of the police officers who were searching there for evidence.

Illustrative Case 13: Tractor driver shot by his own gun

This involved a farmer who kept his shotgun behind the seat back of his tractor just in case he saw the odd rabbit. While he was backing the tractor up to a hedge, prior to starting a ploughing run, the gun became entangled in some brambles. When the tractor started forward, one barrel discharged, completely removing the back of his head.

8.0.5 Negligent discharges

The common phrase of 'I didn't know the gun was loaded' is a strong indicator of a negligent discharge.

Such discharges usually occur when the trigger of the firearm is deliberately pulled for a purpose other than shooting, for example dry-fire practice, demonstration or function testing. Alcohol is also often associated with such negligent discharges.

Unintentionally leaving a firearm loaded is more likely to occur when the individual handling the gun is poorly trained. It may also happen with removable, magazine-fed firearms, as the magazine may be removed, giving an unloaded appearance even when a round remains chambered.

A second common cause of accidental discharges is when the gun handler places his finger on the trigger before deciding to shoot. With the finger so positioned, many activities may cause the finger to compress the trigger unintentionally.

Testing for accidental discharge

Any test to determine whether a weapon is prone to accidental discharge must exceed the strains and pressures normally expected to be placed on a weapon, but not to the extent that the weapon is damaged. The tests must also attempt to replicate, as far as possible, the conditions under which the weapon is alleged to have accidently discharged.

The first test must always be to determine the pressure required on the trigger to fire the weapon. While this would seem to be quite straightforward, only a slight deviation from the correct method will give widely different results.

Many people still use and recommend testing the trigger pull via the use of weights. This is both difficult in practice and inaccurate. Basically, it involves clamping the gun in a suitable stand, with the muzzle pointing vertically upwards. A cradle of known weight is hung over the trigger, and weights added until the hammer drops. This is not a particularly accurate method, as the exact weight at which release occurs is unknown.

A far better method is via the use of a spring or digital balance. This must have a hooked bar so that the pressure is exerted in exactly the same plane as the trigger finger (see Figure 8.0.3). At least ten results should be taken. With each test, it is essential that the direction of pull should be in line and parallel with the barrel.

The most basic tests for accidental discharge are carried out with a soft or nylon-nosed hammer of about 1 lb (0.45 kg) weight. The weapon is then

---

Illustrative Case 14

A case which was categorised as an accidental discharge, but could just as easily be called a negligent discharge, occurred in a prestigious forensic laboratory during the examination of a self-loading pistol. The weapon had been dry-fired for trigger pressure testing and it had been subjected to the normal range of accidental discharge tests, all of which were satisfactory. However, instead of test-firing the weapon firstly with a single round of ammunition, a full magazine was inserted. The slide was pulled back and released and, without the trigger being touched, the weapon proceeded to fire fully automatically until the magazine was empty. Although no one was injured, the resulting ricochets severely damaged many of the instruments in the laboratory.

On examining the weapon, it was found that at some stage, the firing pin tip had broken off and had become lodged in the firing pin hole, leaving sufficient protrusion for it to reach the primer of a chambered round. When the first round was chambered, there was sufficient force to discharge that round and all subsequent rounds. Firing pins that break and lodge in the firing pin hole are not unknown, and the author has encountered several during his career.

This could be classified as a negligent discharge, as the weapon should have been fired with a single round in the magazine several times before more than one round was loaded.

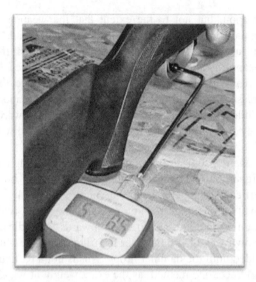

Figure 8.0.3   Digital trigger pull tester.

struck with increasing severity on the muzzle, the butt, under the trigger guard, on top of the weapon, on the hammer spur and on the front of the trigger guard.

After the hammer tests, it is most important that attempts are made to duplicate what is alleged to have caused the accidental discharge. This could

include dropping the weapon on the floor, striking the butt against a wall, 'punching' the muzzle of the weapon into surfaces of varying hardness, etc. Great care must be taken not to damage the weapon in any way by being by being overzealous with these tests.

During the above tests, it is preferable to have a live primed case in the weapon's chamber. This is due to the fact that, in some circumstances, the hammer may drop but the weapon's inbuilt safety mechanism might prevent the firing pin striking the primer and causing a discharge. This would only be apparent if a live primer was present and it did not discharge.

Further reading

1 http://firearmsid.com/a_firearmfunction.htm
2 Heard, B.J. (2008). *A Handbook of Firearms and Ballistics, Examining and Interpreting Forensic Evidence* (2nd Edition). Wiley-Blackwell. ISBN: 978-0-470-69460-2.
3 Warlow, T. (2004). *Firearms, the Law and Forensic Ballistics* (2nd edition). CRC Press. ISBN: 781439818275.
4 http://www.forensicsciencecentral.co.uk/firearms.shtml
5 Greener, W. (1835). *The Gun; or, A Treatise on the Various Descriptions of Small Firearms*. Longman.

9.0

Identification of Calibre from the Bullet Entry Hole

9.0.1 Introduction

Determination of the bullet entry hole can be vital in bullets that completely penetrate (often referred to by firearms examiners as 'through and through penetrations'), especially when there has been an exchange of fire. Determining whether an innocent bystander was shot by a police bullet or one from the perpetrators' weapons can be vital.

On light-coloured clothing, there is often a ring of blackening which can give a very approximate diameter of the bullet, although this is virtually impossible if the clothing is dark. This bullet wipe mark, as it is generally referred to, results from a

---

Illustrative Case 1

A shoot-out occurred between police and armed robbers occurred at lunchtime in the centre of a city. The robbers were part of the Dai Hunge Jai (Big Circle Gang), most of whom were ex-military and absolutely ruthless. The police were armed with .38″ Special calibre revolvers loaded with plain lead bullets, and the robbers had 7.62 × 25 mm calibre Type 54 self-loading pistols loaded with fully jacketed bullets. Firing into the crowds at will, the robbers eventually made their escape, leaving a dead newspaper seller lying on the pavement. He had been shot in the chest, with the bullet completely penetrating his body. As he was wearing a dark coloured T-shirt, the question was, 'Who shot him − police or robbers?'

A sodium rhodizonate test confirmed the presence of lead and gave the approximate diameter of the bullet as 0.35″. This was, however, too close to both the police bullets' diameter of 0.357″ and the robbers' 7.62 mm (0.32″) to be able to differentiate between the two. A lift of the area was taken and examined via the SEM/EDX (See Chapter 14). This showed that the gunshot residues adhering to the edges of the hole were lead, barium and antimony, and that the bullet was a lead/tin alloy. There being no trace of the jacketed material from the robbers' bullets, nor the mercury, antimony and tin associated with 7.62 × 25 mm ammunition, the conclusion was that the fatal bullet had been fired by the police.

Such bullet hole and associated residue examinations could be 'conveniently' omitted from an investigation. These tests are, however, quick and easy to conduct and there is absolutely no justification for them not being performed. Excuses such as 'the laboratory does not have an SEM/EDX' cannot be condoned, as simple chemical spot tests will suffice (Chapter 14).

Forensic Ballistics in Court: Interpretation and Presentation of Firearms Evidence, First Edition. Brian J. Heard.
© 2013 John Wiley & Sons, Ltd. Published 2013 by John Wiley & Sons, Ltd.

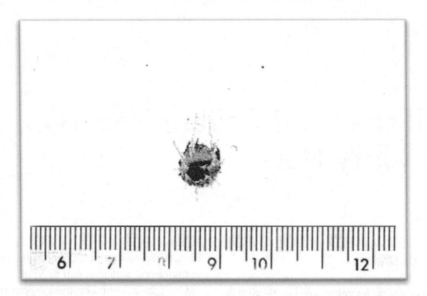

Figure 9.0.1   Bullet wipe mark on paper.

combination of debris picked up from inside the barrel, discharge residues escaping past the bullet as it passes down the bore, case mouth sealant (from military ammunition) and/or bullet lubricant (usually from plain lead revolver ammunition) (see Figure 9.0.1).

9.0.2   Basics

Skin and fabric

In skin and fabrics, it is, unless a Wadcutter type bullet is used, all but impossible to determine the calibre of a missile from its entry or exit hole. Wadcutter bullets, as discussed earlier, are intended for target practice. As such, they are designed to cut a clean hole through the target to facilitate the determination of the shooters accuracy.

When round-nosed or even hollow-point bullets are used, the hole produced by the bullet is very much smaller than its calibre. In skin this is caused by the skin's natural elasticity, which allows the bullet to force apart the cell structure. After passage of the bullet, the skin regains its original shape, exhibiting only a very small entry hole surrounded by a bullet wipe mark which is much smaller than the original calibre of the bullet.

In fabrics, it is the weave that separates, allowing the bullet to pass. Often, torn fibres will be visible, but these indicate little other than the direction in which the bullet was travelling.

Wood

With wood, the bullet entry hole is, once again, much smaller than the diameter of the bullet. The wood fibres stretch and eventually tear as the bullet passes through. After passing through the wood, most of the fibres spring back, making it extremely difficult to determine the calibre.

When dealing with wood, there is, however, a little known method of determining the calibre with a reasonable degree of accuracy[1]. If a piece of fairly strong white paper is placed over the wood surrounding the hole, and a soft lead pencil is carefully rubbed over the surface (much as in the way brasses are rubbed), a circle very closely approximating the diameter of the bullet will appear.

---

[1] Unpublished work by Beta TAM Chi-kung, Ballistics Officer, Royal Hong Kong Police.

Vehicle tyres

Vehicle tyres are almost self-sealing, and it is often impossible to determine even the point of entry without immersing the tyre in water.

Metal

The determination of calibre from a bullet hole in a vehicle's body can also be extremely difficult. For example, semi-jacketed hollow-point bullets can expand on impact, giving the impression of a much larger calibre. At other times, the jacket material can be stripped off, leaving the lead core to penetrate and giving the impression of a much smaller calibre.

Conversely, extremely high-velocity bullets, such as the .223″ (5.56 mm) AR15 bullet, can leave an extremely large entry hole. Often, there will also be a 'splash back' effect, where metal flows back out of the hole, giving the impression it is an exit, not an entry, hole. Identification just of the entry/exit holes in these circumstances can require considerable experience.

Bullets fired through short barrels

When high-pressure handgun cartridges, loaded with plain lead bullets, are fired through short-barrelled weapons, there is an additional problem. Here, as the bullet emerges from the barrel, the gases that follow are still at an extremely high pressure. Once the bullet is freed from the constraints of the barrel, the pressure of the gases on its base are so great that it will expand. Sometimes, this base expansion can increase the diameter of the bullet by 50 per cent or more, giving rise to a much larger entry hole than one would normally expect. In addition, the bullet can become unstable, as the base expansion is not always constant. This can, in extreme cases, cause the bullet to tumble in flight.

In handguns, this phenomenon is only of any consequence with plain lead bullets fired in .357″ and .44″ Magnum weapons with a barrel length of less than three inches Figure 9.0.2.

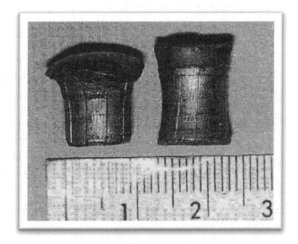

Figure 9.0.2 .357″ Magnum bullets fired through a 6″ and 2″ barrel.

Rifles which have had their barrels shortened can exhibit this bullet base expansion with fully jacketed bullets as well.

9.0.3 Determination of bullet type

As a bullet passes down the barrel, the rifling will tear off small fragments of the bullet. Some of these fragments will remain in the bore, while others will be blown out of the bore by the gases following the bullet. Some of these fragments do, however, remain attached to the bullet in the form of sub-microscopic pieces of swarf. As the bullet passes through any material – whether it is human flesh, fabric or wood – these fragments can be transferred to the medium through which it is passing.

Such fragments are exceedingly small but, if an adhesive taping is taken from the periphery of the bullet entrance hole, they can be recovered. Examination under an electron microscope will enable these fragments to be qualitatively analysed and the bullet type and, possibly the country of origin, identified.

It is important, in the interpretation of these results, to distinguish between volatilised lead from the bullet base and fragments from the bullet driving surface. Volatised lead from the base of a bullet can come from either a jacketed bullet, where

---

Illustrative Case 2: Police exchange of fire

During a particularly bad shoot-out with a gang of armed robbers, five innocent bystanders were injured and two were killed by gunfire. The police were using semi-jacketed .38″ Special + P calibre revolver ammunition and the robbers 7.62 × 25 mm Chinese ammunition. There was a bullet fragment in the wound of one of the victims, and this proved to be a very small piece of copper/zinc jacket from a police round. From its appearance, it had obviously ricocheted before striking the bystander. The rest of the victims all had fully penetrating wounds.

It was obviously of some importance to show whether any of the other bystanders had been accidentally shot by the police. Tapings were taken from the entry holes, and an analysis of these revealed the presence of copper-coated steel fragments in all instances. This proved beyond reasonable doubt that they had all been shot by the robbers, not by the police.

---

the lead core is exposed at the base, or a plain lead bullet. Non-volatised lead can only come from the surface of a plain lead bullet. Volatilised lead can be recognised by being spheroidal or having smooth contours, while lead from the bullet's surface will be rougher and swarf-like.

Likewise, it is important to distinguish between copper/zinc alloys from contamination and those particles torn from the bullet's jacket by the rifling. Size and morphology is one identifier; the other is from quantitative analysis, if this is possible.

Examples would include the identification of lead and copper/zinc alloy as coming from a semi-jacketed bullet. Another would be the identification of copper-coated steel from 7.62 × 25 mm ammunition of Chinese manufacture.

With larger fragments, accurate quantitative analysis will often enable the make of ammunition to be determined. The fragments recovered from the periphery of bullet entry holes are, however, invariably too small for this type of analysis. The problem here is that for accurate EDX (energy dispersive X-Ray) analysis via the SEM, a very flat surface is required.

With larger fragments (0.25 mm or greater), which can be seen under an optical microscope, it is possible to crush them between microscope slides to give the mirror-like surface required. The rough, irregular swarf-like shape of the particles torn from the bullet's driving surface are normally too small for

manipulation and, therefore, are unsuitable for this type of analysis.

Further reading

1 Fisher, B.A.J. (2004). *Techniques of Crime Scene Investigation*. CRC Press.
2 Vandiver, J.V. (1983). *Criminal Investigation – A Guide to Techniques and Solutions*. Metuchen, NJ and London, The Scarecrow Press, Inc.
3 Sinha, J.K. (1999). Evaluation of Bullet Holes in the Absence of Bullets and Smoothbore Firearms, *Proceedings IAFS* 118, 87–88.
4 Kijewski, H. (1979). Determining Caliber, Bullet Type, and Velocity from the Morphology of the Wound in the Skull. *Archiv fuer Kriminologie* 164 (3,4) 107–121.
5 Bergman, P. & Springer, E. (1987). Bullet Hole Identification Kit: Case Report. *Journal of Forensic Sciences* 32 (3), 802–805.
6 Cook, C.W. (1983). Bullet Hole Size Information. *AFTE Journal* 15 (4), 53–55.
7 Garrison, D.H. (1996). The Effective Use of Bullet Hole Probes in Crime Scene Reconstruction. *AFTE Journal* 28 (1), 57–63.
8 Haag, L.C. (2005). *Shooting Incident Reconstruction* (2nd ed.).
9 Nennstiel, R. (1986). Forensic Aspects of Bullet Penetration of Thin Metal Sheets. *AFTE Journal* 18 (2), 18–48.
10 Trahin, T.L. (1987) Bullet Trajectory Analysis. *AFTE Journal* 19 (2) 124–150.

10.0

Ricochet Analysis

10.0.1 Introduction

The number of times that 'it must have been a ricochet' has come up in defence must outweigh all the other excuses added together. But what is a ricochet? At what angle will a bullet ricochet from a solid substance and how does that compare with a ricochet from water? What distinguishing features on a fired bullet can indicate that it did in fact ricochet? Will a ricocheting bullet travel further than one that has not? These are all very important questions which the following will, in some way, assist in answering.

10.0.2 Basics

When a bullet strikes any surface, there is a critical angle at which the bullet will bounce off or **ricochet** from the surface, rather than penetrate. After ricocheting from the surface, the missile will lose a considerable amount of its velocity (anything up to 35 per cent in test firings[1]) and, invariably, lose its stability. Thus, its range will be considerably shortened. This is contrary to the popular belief that a ricocheting bullet will carry further than one fired at the elevation for maximum range.

Illustrative Case 1

This was a case of an armed police officer allegedly attempting to extort money from a criminal. It involved the possibility of a shot having been fired at the victim while he was sitting on the balcony of his house.

The victim could point out where he thought the accused was standing when the shot was fired. This was in deep vegetation and it should have been easy to determine whether a shot was fired from holes in the leaves. It was, however, somewhat complicated, as there were many leaf-cutter wasps in the area which had cut neat holes in most of the leaves. Eventually, by eliminating those holes which were too small or too large for a .38″ Special bullet to have caused, a trajectory for the bullet was established. This coincided with a lead smear on the balcony floor and an impact mark on the wall behind.

An SEM/EDX analysis of the lead smear and impact mark showed the lead alloy to be similar to that in the ammunition issued to the police at that time. There was, however, insufficient evidence to pin the crime down to a particular officer, as no bullet was ever recovered.

---

[1] Unpublished work by author.

Forensic Ballistics in Court: Interpretation and Presentation of Firearms Evidence, First Edition. Brian J. Heard.
© 2013 John Wiley & Sons, Ltd. Published 2013 by John Wiley & Sons, Ltd.

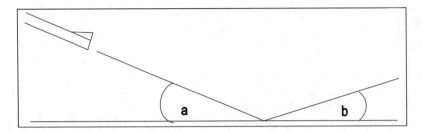

Figure 10.0.1   Angle of ricochet. a = incident angle, b = ricochet angle.

10.0.3   Variables influencing the liability of a missile to ricochet

Bullet

Bullet construction is a major factor in determining both the likelihood of ricochet, as well as where the bullet will travel afterward. Hard bullets have a greater tendency to penetrate than do softer ones. Bullets that break up, such as high-velocity, thin-jacketed hunting bullets, have a low risk of ricochet.

Velocity

Ricochets are often more common with low-power calibres such as .22″ or .25″ (6.35 mm) calibre, which can have trouble penetrating some materials. A ricochet can, however, occur with any calibre. Higher velocity projectiles have a tendency either to penetrate the target or to break up on contact with it.

Target material

Bullets are more likely to ricochet off flat, hard surfaces such as concrete or steel, but a ricochet can occur on almost any surface, including grassy soil, given a flat enough angle of impact. Materials that are soft, that give easily or can absorb the impact, such as sand, have a lower incidence of ricochet. Bullets ricochet easily from water.

Angle

The angle of departure, both vertically and horizontally, is difficult to calculate or predict due to the many variables involved, not the least of which is the deformation of the bullet caused by its impact with the surface it strikes. Ricochets will almost always continue on a somewhat diagonal trajectory to their original trajectory, unless the impact is against a flat surface perpendicular to the angle of incidence (or approach), in which case the angle of ricochet depends on the other variables involved.

The actual degree at which a bullet will ricochet from a surface is called the **critical angle**. Predicting this critical angle for any bullet/surface configuration is, however, extremely difficult.

Considering the number of times in the investigation of armed crime that incidents of ricocheting bullets are encountered it is surprising how little literature there is on the subject. Probably the most authoritative work was by Lucien Haag[2]. Several other papers[3,4,5,6] have also investigated the

---

[2] Haag, L.C. (1975). Bullet Ricochet: An Empirical Study and a Device for Measuring Ricochet Angle. *AFTE Journal* **7**(3), 44–51.

[3] Hartline, P., Abraham, G. & Rowe, W.F. (1982). A Study of Shotgun Ricochet from Steel Surfaces. *Journal of Forensic Sciences* **27**(3), 506–512.

[4] McConnell, M.P., Triplett, G.M.& Rowe, W.F. (1981). A Study of Shotgun Pellet Ricochet. *Journal of Forensic Sciences* **26**(4), 699–709.

[5] Jauhari, M. (1969). Bullet Ricochet from Metal Plates. *Journal of Criminal Law, Criminology and Police Science* **60**(3) 387–394.

[6] Rathman, G.A. (1987). Bullet Ricochet and Associated Phenomena. *AFTE Journal* **19**(4), 374–381.

Illustrative Case 2

This case involved a taxi in central London being shot at by a terrorist group. The weapon involved was a .357" Magnum revolver, which was loaded with semi-jacketed bullets, some of which had a hollow point, while others had a solid round nose.

The front windscreen of a British taxi is only angled back by approximately 15° and, under normal circumstances, such a low angle would not be expected to support a bullet ricochet. However, the first round fired at the front windscreen had a hollow-point bullet, which cleanly ricocheted from the screen, leaving a stripe of lead up the glass. This bullet was located at a later stage and was found to have a mirror-like flat surface on the lead portion of the nose. The second bullet fired was a round-nosed, fully jacketed bullet, which cleanly penetrated the glass, narrowly missing the driver.

In this instance, the angle of the screen was clearly insufficient to support a ricochet with a round-nosed bullet. The hollow-point nose did, however, collapse on impact, effectively increasing the angle and allowing the bullet to ricochet from the glass.

effects of shotgun pellets ricocheting from steel and concrete.

The parameters affecting the potential to ricochet are so diverse, however, that it is difficult to lay down any firm and fast rules as to ricochet potential. Empirical studies need to be carried out for each individual case. There are, though, a few generalisations that can be applied.

1. In most cases of bullets ricocheting from a hard surface, the angle of ricochet is considerably less than the angle of incidence.

   As can be seen from Tables 10.0.1 and 10.0.2, with hard-jacketed, high-velocity missiles striking a frangible material such as stone or concrete, it is

not always the case that the angle of ricochet is less than the angle of incidence.

It would appear that if sufficient cratering of the surface occurs on bullet impact, the exit plane of the crater will be of greater angle that the incidence angle. This equates to the bullet striking the surface at a greater incidence angle and, therefore, a greater ricochet angle.

2. The critical angle for a soft or hollow point bullet is lower than that for an equivalent fully jacketed bullet. In this instance, it would appear that the collapsing hollow-point bullet nose increases the incident angle, thus increasing the propensity for ricochet.

Illustrative Case 3

While up a ladder painting his house, a man received a bullet wound in his upper back. The bullet passed between the ribs and destroyed his heart, killing him almost instantly. The bullet, a .30" Carbine calibre, was found to have spiral scratches, with the degree of twist almost perfectly matching those of the rifling. These spiral scratches were present from the nose to the base of the bullet.

Approximately one mile (1.7 km) away from where the man was shot was a civilian range. At this range was a 'Running Deer' competition for M1 carbine assault rifles. The sand butts at the end of the range were found to be far too shallow and to contain too many large stones for such a construction. Behind the butts were found numerous spent bullets, all of which had obviously passed through the sand and gravel butts.

Obviously, one bullet had ricocheted from the sand at such a high angle that it was travelling almost straight down when it hit the man on the ladder. The terminal velocity of such a missile was such that, had it hit a bone of any size, it would have been stopped.

Table 10.0.1   Ricochet Angles vs. Incident Angle for Various Bullets on Smooth Concrete

Calibre	Bullet Type	Velocity	Ricochet Angle at Incident Angle of:	
			10°	30°
.22″ LR	RN	1,100 ft/sec	1.33	1.88
.22″ LR	HP	1,100 ft/sec	1.3	1.19
.38″ Special	RN	650 ft/sec	1.02	1.5
.357″ Magnum	SJHP	850 ft/sec	1.3	1.7
7.62 × 25 mm	FMJ	1300 ft/sec	2.0*	12 to 35*
7.62 × 39 mm	FMJ	2700 ft/sec	3.5*	2 to 25*

*Indicates severe cratering, leading to variable results and, in some cases, disintegration of bullet.

Table 10.0.2   Ricochet Angle for .45 ACP FMJ Bullets From Various Surfaces

Material	Calibre	Ricochet Angle at Incident Angle of:	
		15°	25°
Glass	.45″ ACP	Broke glass	Broke glass
Concrete	.45″ ACP	2°	3°
Steel Plate	.45″ ACP	2.5°	4°
Wood	.45″ ACP	17°	17°
Sand	.45″ ACP	Penetrated	Penetrated

Table 10.0.3   Critical Angle vs. Velocity for Various Calibres Fired at Water

Calibre	Velocity (RN bullet)	Critical Angle
.22″	850 ft/sec	8°
.22″	1,000 ft/sec	8°
.22″	1,250 ft/sec	7.5°
.38″ Special	650 ft/sec	6°
.38″ Special	800 ft/sec	7°
.357″ Magnum	900 ft/sec	6°
.357 Magnum	1,050 ft/sec	7°

NB. Some of the bullets used in this test were hollow-point. The nose was, however, filled with epoxy resin and shaped to give the desired round-nosed profile.

3. The critical angle for a given bullet type/target medium is not velocity dependent. This effect is illustrated by Table 10.0.3.

4. Bullets will invariably lose their gyroscopic stability and tumble after ricocheting. This tumbling gives rise to a distinctive whine or whirring noise, as the tumbling bullet passes through the air.

5. Bullets which have ricocheted from glass, steel, concrete or wood have a very distinctive flat spot which is characteristic of the material where the contact has been made (Figure 10.0.2.) This contact point will often have paint, wood fibres or concrete adhering to it for easy identification. If the material was glass or polished steel, the mirror-like surface is quite distinctive. This is not, however, the case with a bullet which has

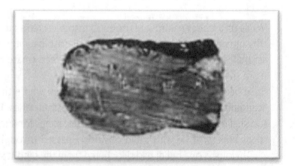

Figure 10.0.2   Typical appearance of a plain lead bullet after ricocheting from a rough, hard surface.

Illustrative Case 4

While being chased by pirates, a fisherman was shot with a 7.62 × 39 mm Type 54 assault rifle (Chinese version of the AK47 Kalashnikov). At the post-mortem, only one small entry hole in the upper rear right leg was observed, and the femur was found to be fractured but not broken. No exit wound could be found on the body, and an X-ray of the lower torso did not reveal any signs of a missile. However, when an X-ray of the upper torso was taken, a complete 7.62 mm bullet was located in the upper chest area. Eventually, after much dissection, a wound track up though the body was located, showing that the bullet had, in fact, ricocheted from the femur. Witness statements from others on the boat revealed that at the time of the shooting, the deceased was lying down on the deck of the boat. The angle of entry was sufficiently low for the bullet to have ricocheted, rather than passing straight through the leg.

---

ricocheted from water. Even with hollow point bullets, it is unlikely that it will be possible to differentiate between a bullet which has ricocheted from water and one that has not.

6. Wounds produced by bullets ricocheting from hard surfaces will generally be easy to identify, due to the bullet's tumbling action. If the bullet does happen to strike point-first, the misshapen bullet will leave a distinctive entry hole, generally with ragged edges. Once it enters the body, the bullet will, due to its inherent unstable condition, tumble end over end, leaving a large, irregular wound channel. Jacketed bullets tend to break up on ricocheting, peppering the skin with jacket and lead core fragments.

7. High velocity bullets with a thin jacket (e.g. .223″ or .220″ Swift) will invariably break up before ricocheting. This applies even to water.

Not all ricochets occur in the environment. It is quite feasible for a bullet to ricochet from a bone while travelling through a body.

It is interesting to note that when round shot was used by naval vessels, ricocheting missiles from the water was a recognised form of tactics in sea warfare. By skipping a missile across the water at hull height, it was much easier to hit an enemy ship than to try and calculate the correct elevation for the missile to strike the ship during its trajectory. This method worked well with round shot, where the angle of incidence and the angle of ricochet were approximately the same. However, modern projectiles, which are spin-stabilised and have an aerodynamic shape, do tend to rise at a greater angle after ricocheting from water, and the technique was found to be of little use.

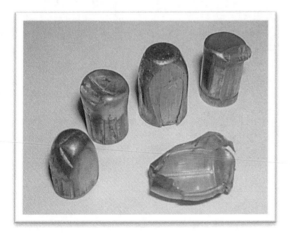

Figure 10.0.3 Typical appearance of jacketed bullets after having ricocheted from various surfaces.

Further reading

1 Burke, T.W. & Rowe, W.F. (1992). Bullet Ricochet: A Comprehensive Review. *Journal of Forensic Sciences* 37 (5), 1254–1260.
2 Haag, L.C. (1979). Bullet Ricochet from Water. *AFTE Journal* 11 (3) 27–34.

3 Nennstiel, R. (1984). Study of Bullet Ricochet on a Water Surface. *AFTE Journal* 16 (3), 88–93.

4 Jauhari, M. (1970). Approximate Relationship Between the Angles of Incident and Ricochet for Practical Application in the Field of Forensic Science. *Journal of Criminal Law, Criminology and Police Science* 62, 122–125.

5 Federal Bureau of Investigation (1969). Bouncing Bullets. *FBI Law Enforcement Bulletin* 38, 1–6.

6 Garrison, D.H. (1998). Crown & Bank: Road Structure as it Affects Bullet Path Angles in Vehicle Shootings. *AFTE Journal* 30 (1), 89–93.

7 Gold, R.E. & Schecter, B. (1992). Ricochet Dynamics for the Nine-Millimetre Parabellum Bullet. *Journal of Forensic Sciences* 37 (1), 90–98.

11.0

Bullet Penetration and Trajectory through Glass

11.0.1   Introduction

The list of general misconceptions over the penetration of window glass, toughened, plate and bullet-resistant glass is huge and, of course, these have been used as excuses for all manner of shooting incidents. Some of the more recognisable are as follows:

1. After penetrating glass the bullet will experience a large deviation from its original path.

2. The bullet will fragment into numerous non-lethal pieces.

3. Low velocity BBs (5.45 mm steel balls) will not damage glass.

4. Soft lead air gun pellets will not penetrate glass.

5. From the bullet hole, it is impossible to determine from where the missile was fired.

6. It is perfectly safe to stand behind 'bullet-proof glass' while it is being fired at.

In one way or another, all the above – and many more – are incorrect.

Here, it should be stated that nothing is truly 'bullet-proof' whether it be glass, 'bullet-resistant vests' (BRV) or any other material. There will always be some missile that can defeat the material, either due to its velocity, its construction and/or its weight. Products designed to defeat bullets are therefore best described as '**bullet resistant**'.

Before delving into the subject, a description of the various types of glass, bullet resistant glass and glass substitutes is in order.

11.0.2   Glass types and glass substitutes

Flat glass, sheet glass, or plate glass

This is a type of glass, initially produced in plane form, that is commonly used for windows, glass doors and transparent walls. The flat glass is sometimes bent after production of the plane sheet. Most flat glass is soda-lime glass, composed of about 75 per cent silica (SiO_2) plus Na_2O and CaO, together with several minor additives, and it is produced by the float glass process.

Normal window or plate glass is a hard but fragile material, which is easily broken into sharp shards.

Forensic Ballistics in Court: Interpretation and Presentation of Firearms Evidence, First Edition. Brian J. Heard.
© 2013 John Wiley & Sons, Ltd. Published 2013 by John Wiley & Sons, Ltd.

Toughened or tempered glass

This is a type of safety glass, processed by controlled thermal or chemical treatments to increase its strength compared with normal glass. Tempering creates balanced internal stresses which cause the glass, when broken, to crumble into small granular chunks instead of splintering into jagged shards. The granular chunks are less likely to cause injury.

As a result of its safety and strength, tempered glass is used in a variety of demanding applications, including passenger vehicle windows, shower doors, architectural glass doors and tables, refrigerator trays and as a component of bullet-proof glass.

Toughened glass is physically and thermally stronger than regular glass. The greater contraction of the inner layer during manufacturing induces compressive stresses in the surface of the glass, balanced by tensile stresses in the body of the glass.

The toughened glass surface is not as hard as annealed glass and is therefore somewhat more susceptible to scratching. To prevent this, toughened glass manufacturers may apply various coatings and/or laminates to the surface of the glass.

Toughened glass is used when strength, thermal resistance and safety are important considerations. The most commonly encountered tempered glass is that used for side and rear windows in automobiles. The windscreen or windshield of a car is made of laminated glass.

Laminated glass

This is a type of safety glass that holds together when shattered. In the event of breaking, it is held in place by an interlayer, typically of polyvinyl butyral (PVB), between two or more layers of glass. The interlayer keeps the layers of glass bonded even when broken, and its high strength prevents the glass from breaking up into large sharp pieces. This produces a characteristic 'spider web' cracking pattern when the impact is not enough to pierce the glass completely.

Laminated glass is normally used when there is a possibility of human impact or where the glass could fall if shattered – for example, in automobile windshields.

Bullet-proof glass

Also known as **ballistic glass, transparent armour** or, more correctly, **bullet-resistant glass**, this is a type of strong but optically transparent material that is particularly resistant to being penetrated when struck by bullets. Like all known materials, however, it is not completely impenetrable. It is usually made from a combination of two or more types of glass – one hard and one soft. The softer layer makes the glass more elastic so that it can flex instead of shatter. Bullet-proof glass varies in thickness from three-quarter inch to three inches (1.8–7.5 cm).

Even the best glass has a faint greenish tinge to it and, as the glass becomes thicker, the green colouration deepens. This colouration somewhat restricts the practical limits of such glass.

Bullet-resistant glass is usually constructed using polycarbonate and layers of laminated glass. The polycarbonate layers usually consist of products such as Armormax, Makroclear, Cyrolon, Lexan or Tuffak.

The laminated glass layers are built from glass sheets bonded together with polyvinyl butyral, polyurethane or ethylene-vinyl acetate, and the end product is typically thick and very heavy.

One of the design elements of bullet-resistant glass is that it must have a layer of polycarbonate on the non-strike face to prevent spalling of the glass. Spalling in bullet-resistant glass is when shards of glass are knocked off the non-strike surface. These shards can be lethal for anyone on the non-strike side of the glass.

Security laminates

Another construction which is becoming popular is the use of security laminates as a film on the inner surface of ordinary glass. This, when bonded with the application of a pressure-sensitive adhesive and cured fully, also provides a protection similar to multi-layered bullet-resistant glass.

One-way glass

A recent innovation is the use of one-way bulletproof glass, especially for 'cash in transit' vehicles. This glass resists incoming small arms fire striking the outside, but it will allow those on the other side, such as guards inside the vehicle, to fire out through the glass at the exterior threat.

One-way bullet-proof glass is usually made up of two layers – a brittle layer on the outside and a flexible one on the inside. A bullet fired from the outside hits the brittle layer first, shattering an area of it. This absorbs some of the bullet's kinetic energy and spreads it on a larger area. When the slowed bullet hits the flexible layer, it is stopped. However, when a bullet is fired from the inside, it hits the flexible layer first. The bullet penetrates the flexible layer because its energy is focused on a smaller area; the brittle layer then shatters outward, due to the flexing of the inner layer, and does not significantly hinder the bullet's progress.

Recent advances

Transparent armour

US military researchers are developing a new class of transparent armour incorporating aluminium oxynitride (Trade name: ALON) as the outside 'strike plate' layer. This is much lighter and performs much better than traditional glass/polymer laminates. Aluminium oxynitride 'glass' can defeat extreme threats such as .50 calibre armour-piercing rounds, using material that is not prohibitively heavy.

Spinel ceramics

Certain types of ceramic spinel (a class of mineral) can also be used for transparent armour, due to their properties of increased density and hardness when compared to traditional glass. These new types of synthetic ceramic transparent armours can allow for thinner armour with equivalent stopping power to traditional laminated glass.

Polycarbonates or polymethyl methacrylate (PMMA)

This is a transparent thermoplastic, often used as a lightweight or shatter-resistant alternative to glass. It is sometimes called 'acrylic glass'. Chemically, it is the synthetic polymer of methyl methacrylate and goes under the trade name of Plexiglass.

11.0.3 Deviation of missile after penetrating glass

Generally speaking, there is much confusion over this topic, with published papers reporting extremes one way or the other.

A paper by Harper (1939) reported a relatively small deviation, as does Rathman (1993) while Thornton (Thornton & Cashman, 1986) reports a much larger deviation. Papers by Haag (1987) describe the measurement of deflection, Garrison (1995) the penetration of car body parts in general and Bell (1993) the effects on bullets fired through tempered (toughened) glass.

Mostly, however, they generally add little to the understanding of the mechanics involved. The authors' experience, involving many hundreds of test firings (unpublished papers), have shown that after penetrating glass there is, generally speaking, very little deviation from the bullet's normal path.

11.0.4 Penetration of normal window glass

Very low velocity steel BBs (4.45 mm) will generally case a very small hole, often no more than 0.1″ (2.45 mm) in diameter. This hole penetrates the glass, ejecting a large cone of glass (called *spalling*) from the side opposite the impact site. If the cone is not uniform in circumference, it can give an indication from which direction the shot was fired. For $^1/_4″$ (6.2 mm) glass, the required velocity can be as low as 200 ft/sec (61 m/sec).

For lead air gun pellets, which are soft and readily deformable, a velocity of over 400 ft/sec (122 m/sec) is required to produce the same effect. To penetrate the same glass, the velocity must be increased to at least 550 ft/sec (168 m/sec). With these easily deformable missiles, it is very difficult to estimate the calibre of the missile from such damage to glass.

With higher velocity missiles, the diameter of the hole through the glass can give an approximation of the calibre. The degree of shattering around the hole can give some indication as to the velocity of the missile. There are, however, so many variables that empirical testing is the only way that this estimation can be achieved.

11.0.5 Penetration of laminated and bullet-resistant glass

When struck by a bullet, laminated glass will first bulge away from the site of impact. This causes a series of radial cracks. As the glass continues to bulge, concentric cracks are produced, the quantity of which are determined by the energy given up by the bullet to the glass (Saferstein, 1982). The quantity of crushed glass around the periphery of the impact site is also a function of the transferred energy.

Easily deformed, low-velocity bullets, such as the .32″ S&W or the .38″ S&W, will generally have insufficient energy to penetrate a laminated windscreen or bank teller glass, and give up all their energy on impact.

As a result of the energy transfer, glass around the impact site will be crushed and, depending upon the thickness of the laminate, crushed glass may spall off the remote face with considerable force. Crushed glass will also be projected some way back, depending once again on the energy transferred, from the impact site towards the firer. Often, the plastic laminate will have been stretched beyond its elastic limit and will have torn in the process. The torn laminate and the quantity of crushed glass seen on the non-impact side of the glass will often give the impression that the glass has been penetrated when, in fact, it has not.

Laminated glass lends itself well to the determination of the sequence of multiple shots. In laminated glass the radial cracks from the first shot will spread out from the impact site in a straight line, while those from the second will stop when they reach a radial

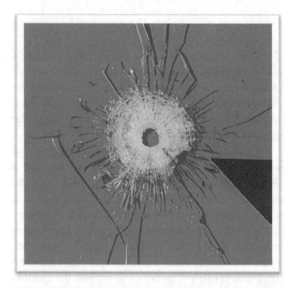

Figure 11.0.1   Hole in laminated glass produced by a 9 mm Parabellum bullet.

crack from the first shot. With some care, this sequence can be established for several shots.

Figures 11.0.1 and 11.0.2 (scale × 0.5) illustrate the difficulties in estimating the calibre of bullet from a penetrating hole in laminated glass.

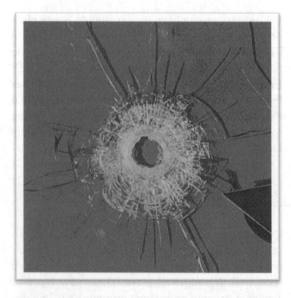

Figure 11.0.2   Hole in laminated glass produced by .22″ long rifle hollow-point bullet.

11.0.6 Penetration of tempered or toughened glass

The penetration mechanism for tempered glass is somewhat different as, once the surface is punctured, the glass shatters into tiny pieces. Radial crack lines spread out from the site of impact to the very edges of the glass, cross-linking as they go. This cross-linking can take many hours – even days – to accomplish fully. Depending on the velocity of the missile, the missile type, the thickness of glass and even ambient temperature, this cross-linking can give an indication as to a time frame for the impact. With so many variables, empirical testing is the only way that this time frame can be estimated.

At the instant of impact, there is a bulging away from the impact side, which results in the production of peripheral crushing of the glass, rather than concentric rings.

Provided the glass has not disintegrated, it is possible to tell the sequence of multiple shots in toughened glass. The radial cracks from the first shot will spread out to the edges of the glass, while those from the second will stop when they reach a radial crack from the first shot. With some care, this sequence can be established for several shots,
although the situation does become somewhat confused due to the number of crack lines involved.

Determination of the impact site, calibre of weapon and type is often rendered impossible with this type of glass, due to the disintegration of the glass round the bullet entry site. If the hole, or part of it, is still intact, the site must be preserved with clear adhesive sheets so that a later laboratory examination can be performed.

Even after the impact site has disintegrated, an approximation of its position can be obtained by following the radial cracks back to their point of origin. This is best done, after preserving what remains of the glass, over a sheet of white card, marking the continuation of the lines in pencil.

It should be noted here that tempered glass can take heavy impacts if spread over a large area. A low-velocity steel ball will, however, have a sufficiently high point of impact energy transfer to craze completely even very thick tempered glass. Here, the mechanism is one of a non-deforming steel ball transferring all its energy over an exceedingly small impact area. The resulting energy transfer per unit area is sufficiently high to defeat the integrity of the tempered glass, causing it to craze.

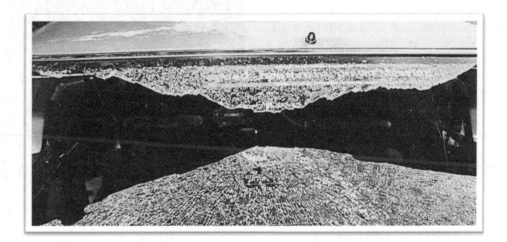

Figure 11.0.3 Typical results of a .38″ Special + P hollow-point bullet hitting the rear screen of a car.

Illustrative Case 1

During the early 1970s, there were numerous protests outside the US Embassy in London. On several occasions, the huge front doors, which were constructed from very thick tempered glass, were found to be completely crazed. The initial belief was that this had been caused by a high-velocity rifle. However, the small impact site, with no penetrating missile, was typical of that caused by a small-calibre steel ball bearing. Although they could not be proved to be the missiles which had caused the damage, several steel BBs were located close to one of the smashed glass doors. It could not be conclusively proved, but the final conclusion was that it was either a steel ball fired from a catapult or a BB fired from a low-powered air weapon that had been used. Today, with the use of a scanning electron microscope, copper or nickel traces at the site of impact could make the identification somewhat more certain.

11.0.7 Determination of bullet type from the entry hole

Determination of the bullet calibre from the resulting hole and degree of concentric cracking can be made, although the variables make this a difficult task.

In *laminated glass*, the degree of concentric cracking is directly proportional to the quantity of energy given up by to the glass as it passes through.

The amount of energy given up will depend upon the bullet's calibre, its construction and its velocity. The easier it is for the bullet to deform, the greater the concentric cracking. The greater the deformation of the bullet, the larger the transfer of energy. As the deformation increases, so does the diameter of the penetration site. The resultant bullet hole thus represents the actual size of the bullet after deformation. Figures 11.0.1 and 11.0.2 are illustrative of this, whereby the soft plain lead .22″ LR HP (long rifle calibre, hollow point) bullet has expanded, giving a much larger hole than the 9 mm PB (Parabellum) round, which has a hard jacketed bullet.

In *tempered glass*, the situation is somewhat different, as any penetrating missile will cause radial and concentric cross-linked cracking over the whole of the glass. The degree of crushing round the periphery of the entrance hole can give an indication of the calibre, but this is extremely difficult in practical situations due to the disintegration of the glass.

In tempered glass, to differentiate between a non-penetrating bullet hole and something caused by a stone requires a great deal of experience. Often, with something like a small sharp-pointed stone, small

fragments of glass will spall off the inside surface, and this could be confused with a low-velocity steel BB. The difference here would be that a hard spherical object will tend to produce a spall with a regular cone shape, while a stone will produce an irregularly

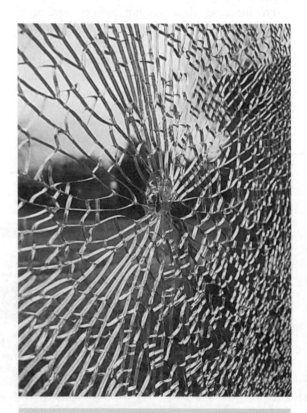

Figure 11.0.4 Penetrating hole in toughened glass caused by sharp stone.

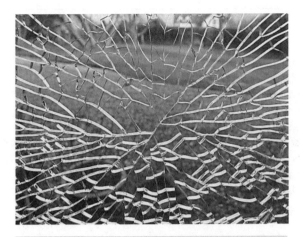

Figure 11.0.5   Non-penetrating damage caused by sharp stone.

Table 11.0.1   Deflection of Bullet from its Intended Path at Three Different Impact Angles

| | Angle of Impact | | |
Calibre	0°	25°	45°
.22″ LR HP	0°	20°	50°
.25″ ACP	0°	0°	5°
.38″ Special	0°	2°	2°
9 mm PB	0°	0°	0°

LR HP = Long rifle calibre, hollow point bullet
ACP = Colt automatic pistol
PB = Parabellum calibre

shaped spall (Figure 11.0.4 .) Non-penetrating damage can be a great deal more difficult to identify, as there is no point of damage (Figure 11.0.5). In these cases, it is best to err on the side of caution.

11.0.8   Deflection of bullet by glass

A series of controlled test firings (unpublished papers by the author), with various calibres of weapon, were fired at a laminated windscreen glass held at varying angles. The results from these limited tests indicated that there was little deviation of the bullet from its intended path. These tests are shown in Table 11.0.1.

Illustrative Case 2

Several windows in a very expensive flat were found to have been holed by a missile of some description. There were some concerns as to the exact type of missile that caused the damage, as the flat was situated on the tenth floor and the damaged windows looked out onto a very steep hillside covered in dense tropical undergrowth. On examination, it was discovered that the damage had been caused by a small, round (BB) steel ball and that the cone of glass had spalled from the outside surface of the glass. This was irrefutable evidence that the missile had been fired from the inside of the flat and not the outside.

Illustrative Case 3

This case illustrates how unpredictable the results of glass penetration by bullets can be. During an exchange of fire in which one police officer was shot and severely injured, the culprits attempted to make their escape by car. With the vehicle driving away at considerable speed, one officer managed to hang onto the open driver's side window. In an attempt to stop the car, the officer's two colleagues fired at the driver through the rear window.

One of the rounds fired at the rear of the car split into two on penetrating the rear window. One piece of the bullet fatally wounded the driver, while the other hit the passenger in the neck penetrating his carotid artery. The question was, 'Did anyone from inside the car fire at the officers?' By preserving what remained of the rear screen, it was possible to show the sequence of shots and prove that no shots were fired from inside the vehicle.

Illustrative Case 4

A case in the early 1970s involved a bank robbery in which the tellers had recently been protected with laminated 'bandit/bullet-proof' glass screens. These were an early type of laminated glass with no anti-spall laminate on the non-strike face. After being given the money from all the tills, the robber, who was armed with a sawn-off 12-bore shotgun, calmly walked up to one of the tellers and shot her through the security glass. Although the pellets did not penetrate the laminated glass, the spalling from the teller's side of the glass was so severe that several of the larger shards completely penetrated her body, killing her almost immediately.

The glass in this case was one laminated with three sheets of glass and two layers of plastic. To reduce scratching, both outside layers were glass. In more modern bullet-resistant glass, the non-strike face always consists of a sheet of clear acrylic plastic of some description, bonded to the last layer of glass. This almost completely eliminates spalling.

From Table 11.0.1, it can be seen that a bullet such as the plain lead hollow-point .22″ LR bullet easily deforms and is easily deflected from its intended path. The .38″ Special lead bullet is less deformable than the hollow point bullet and is only slightly deviated. The two jacketed bullets have not deformed at all, and are not affected at all by the glass. It must be noted that these constitute a limited number of tests carried out under laboratory conditions, and the results may not viably translate into real-world shooting incidents.

Figure 11.0.6 shows the degree of spalling from the rear face of laminated glass of the same type as used in Illustrative Case 4. As can be seen, the back-splash of glass from the strike face is also quite considerable and, in the above case, the robber sustained severe lacerations to his left hand due to this splash-back.

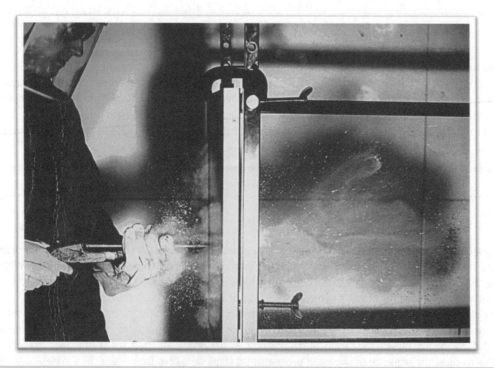

Figure 11.0.6   Test firing of 12-bore shotgun against bullet-proof glass without non-strike face anti-spalling layer.

Illustrative Case 5

In another bank robbery, this time there was a more modern type of laminated bullet-resistant glass with anti-spall layers on the non-strike side of the glass. The gun used by the robber was a cheap quality .380″ calibre revolver and, this time, the teller just happened to have his .22″ target pistol (illegally, it should be said) in a shoulder holster. The robber demanded the money, at which point the teller pulled out his gun. Not to be outdone, the robber started to fire at the teller, who replied with his gun. When the smoke cleared, there were eight very flat .22″ bullets on the teller's side and six equally flat .38″ bullets on the robber's side. The teller was unharmed but, after being arrested, the robber was taken to hospital with a severely lacerated right hand and a missing eye. The teller did not get off completely free, as he lost his firearms licence and his job!

Further reading and references

1 Greener, W.W. (2003 reprint). *The Gun.* New York: Bonanza Books.

2 Thornton, J.I. & Cashman, P.J. (1986). The Effect of Tempered Glass on Bullet Trajectory. *Journal of Forensic Sciences* 31 (2), 743–746.

3 Harper, W.W. (1939). The Behavior of Bullets Fired through Glass. *Journal of Criminal Law, Criminology and Police Science* 29. (1)

4 Stahl, C. J., Jones, S. R., Johnson, F. B. & Luke, J. L. (1979). The Effect of Glass as an Intermediate Target on Bullets: Experimental Studies and Report of a Case. *Journal of Forensic Sciences* 24 (1), 6–17.

5 Rathman, G.A. (1993). Bullet Impact Damage and Trajectory Through Auto Glass. *AFTE Journal* 25 (2), 79–86.

6 Haag, L.C. (1987). The Measurement of Bullet Deflection by Intervening Objects and the Study of Bullet Behaviour After Impact. *AFTE Journal* 19 (4), 382–387.

7 Garrison, D.H. (1995) Examining auto body penetration in the reconstruction of vehicle shootings. *AFTE Journal* 27, 209–212.

8 Bell, P. (1993). *Characteristics of bullets fired through automobile window glass.* Paper presented at the California Association of Criminalistics Seminar, 1993.

9 Saferstein, R. (1982). *Forensics Science Handbook.* New Jersey, USA: Prentice-Hall.

10 Bertino, A.J. & Bertino, P.N. (2008). *Forensic Science: Fundamentals and Investigations* (p. 407). Cengage Learning.

11 Lundin, L., Air Force Research Laboratory Public Affairs (October 17, 2005). *Air Force testing new transparent armor.*

12 Walley, S.M., Field, J.E., Blair, P.W. & Milford, A.J. (2004). The effect of temperature on the impact behaviour of glass/polycarbonate laminates. *International Journal of Impact Engineering* 30, 31–52.

13 Shah, Q.H. (2009). Impact resistance of a rectangular polycarbonate armor plate subjected to single and multiple impacts. *International Journal of Impact Engineering* 36, 1128–1135.

14 Company specifications from Total Security Solutions and/or Pacific Bulletproof, accessed 9 May 2011.

15 Chandall, D. & Chrysler, J. (1998). A numerical analysis of the ballistic performance of a 6.35 mm transparent polycarbonate plate. Defence Research Establishment, Valcartier, Quebec, Canada. DREV-TM-9834.

16 Gunnarsson, C.A., Ziemski, B., Weeressoriya, T. & Moy, P. (2009). Deformation and Failure of Polycarbonate during Impact as a Function of Thickness. *Proceedings of the SEM Annual Conference June 1–4,* Albuquerque, New Mexico, USA

17 Cros, P.E., Rota, L., Cottenot, C.E., Schirrer, R. & Fond, C. (2000). Experimental and numerical analysis of the impact behaviour of polycarbonate and polyurethane liner. *Journal de Physique IV* 10, Pr9-671–Pr9-676.

18 Haag, L.C. (2012). Behavior of expelled glass fragments during projectile penetration and perforation of glass. *American Journal of Forensic Medicine and Pathology* 33 (1), 47–53.

12.0

Range of Firing Estimations and Bullet Hole Examinations

12.0.1 Introduction

If there is one area of forensic firearms examination that produces more confusion and incorrect identification than any other, it is range of firing estimations. There are a vast number of factors which can influence the resultant close range deposition of discharge residues or the pattern produced by shotgun pellets. These can range from the material upon which the residues are deposited upon, to the wind strength and direction, the make and age of ammunition used and the length of barrel through which the round had been fired (Figure 12.0.1).

12.0.2 Basics

On discharge of a firearm, a large volume of 'smoke' or, more correctly, **gunshot residue** (GSR – also called **firearms discharge residue** (FDR)), is discharged at high velocity from the muzzle. This gunshot residue consists of a mixture of unburnt and partially burnt propellant, amorphous sooty material, a mixture of incandescent gases, primer discharge residues and, depending on the type of bullet used, volatilised lead from the base of the bullet.

Of these components, the primer residues form only a minute part of these firearms' discharge

---

Illustrative Case 1

An inexperienced examiner came to the conclusion that in a police open fire incident, the officer was at a distance in excess of three feet (0.92 m) from the victim. This was based upon the lack of visible residues on the deceased T-shirt and the fact that at distances greater than three feet, residues from a two-inch (5 cm) barrelled .38″ Special are no longer visible on the target. This, however, did not tally with the witness statements. They all said that before firing, the police officer pulled the victim towards him by grabbing his T-shirt. The T-shirt was badly bloodstained, which would have obscured any residues which may have been present. However, infra-red photography, which reduces the effect of the bloodstaining, revealed that the revolver had been fired while in close contact with the T-shirt, which had, in fact, been pulled towards him by the officer (see Figures 12.0.2, 12.0.3 and 12.0.4).

Forensic Ballistics in Court: Interpretation and Presentation of Firearms Evidence, First Edition. Brian J. Heard.
© 2013 John Wiley & Sons, Ltd. Published 2013 by John Wiley & Sons, Ltd.

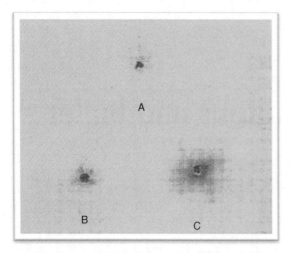

Figure 12.0.1 Discharge residue patterns for the same make of ammunition fired at the same distance through different barrel lengths: (A) 6″ barrel. (B) 4″ barrel. (C) 2″ barrel.

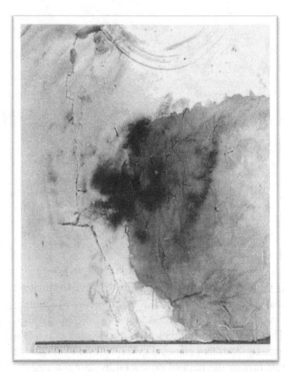

Figure 12.0.3 T-shirt photographed under infra-red lighting.

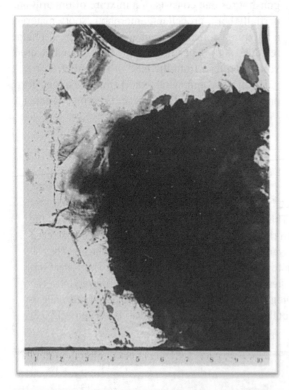

Figure 12.0.2 T-shirt photographed under normal lighting.

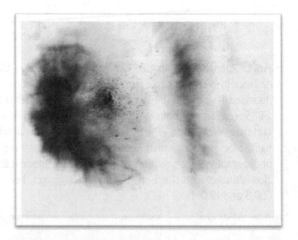

Figure 12.0.4 GSR distribution reconstructed by having muzzle of revolver in light contact with T-shirt while pulling the vest towards the firer.

residues. This component is, however, of fundamental importance in determining whether a person has fired or has been in the vicinity of a weapon being fired. This aspect will be fully dealt with in Chapter 14, titled 'Gunshot Residue (GSR) Examination'.

As the bullet passes through any material, some of the surface of the bullet will be rubbed off onto the margins of the bullet hole. More of this lead or jacket material will be rubbed off the bullet on the entry side of the hole than on the exit. Chemical tests, especially when dealing with jacketed bullets, can often be inconclusive as to which side of a garment the bullet entry hole is situated. Examination, using the SEM/EDX, of a simple adhesive lift taken from the periphery of each side of the hole, will quickly reveal which side of the hole has the greater quantity of bullet material, and thus from which side of the garment the bullet entered.

If the bullet has passed through a body and exited from the rear, there will be a similar, but far smaller, transfer of bullet lead and jacket material on the inside of the garment than on the outside.

12.0.3   Range of firing estimations for pistols and rifles

At close ranges, up to two feet (60 cm) in a handgun and six feet (approx. 2 m) in a rifle, the impact of these discharge residues on the target enable the range of

firing to be accurately determined. However, when the muzzle of the weapon is in very tight contact with the skin, the discharge residues from these firearms may be completely absent. Due to the lack of discharge residues and its appearance, the wound is often, in fact, mistaken for the exit rather than the entry hole.

In this situation, the discharge residues follow the bullet into the tissue, often leaving no trace around the margins of the wound. In areas of the body where the skin and subcutaneous tissue covers bone (e.g. the skull, scapula or sternum), the gases become trapped between the subcutaneous tissue and the bone. The gases expand with extreme rapidity and immediately attempt to exit from the same hole through which they entered. As the gases now form an exceedingly large volume, the only way they can exit is by bursting back out through the tissue surrounding the bullet entry hole. The result is a gaping **stellate tear**, with blood, tissue and often bone being ejected some distance backwards towards the firer.

Although stellate tearing is generally only seen where the skin covers bone, it can also be observed where the underlying tissue consists of rigid muscle (e.g. the pectorals or the upper thigh region). In this case, the gases become trapped in the subcutaneous fat which occurs between the surface skin and underlying muscle. This is relatively uncommon and, when it does arise, the stellate tearing is far less pronounced.

The degree of stellate tearing depends upon the volume of gas produced and the firmness with which

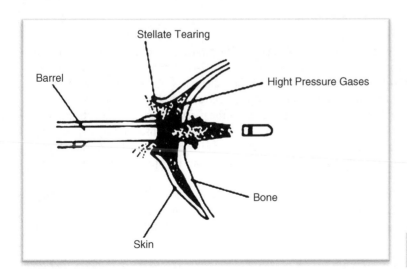

Figure 12.0.5   Stellate tearing in contact wound over bone.

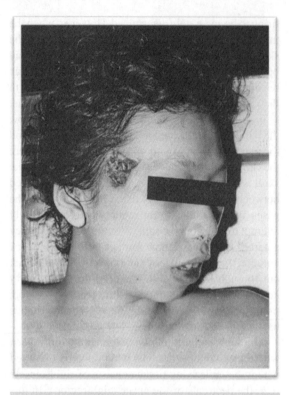

Figure 12.0.6   Stellate tearing resulting from a contact wound with a .38″ Special revolver.

the weapon is held against the skin. Thus, a .32″ ACP held loosely against the temple would probably cause very little stellate tearing, but a 12-bore shotgun held tightly against the pectoral muscle would produce massive tearing.

Without careful examination, a poorly defined stellate wound can easily be mistaken for an exit wound. To identify the wound correctly, it is necessary to excise the wound when partially burnt and unburnt propellant particles should be easily located within the tissues. The identification of the range of firing as tight contact can then be made.

At ranges greater than tight contact, the impact of the discharge residues on the target can be used to accurately determine the range at which the shot was fired. The method employed for the detection of these components is generally a simple visual examination under a low-powered microscope. The observed distribution of the firearms' discharge residue particles can then be compared with test-fired samples.

It should be stressed that the test firings must be made with exactly the same ammunition and in the same type of weapon, with the same length barrel. Different types of ammunition can give vastly variable discharge residue patterns. Likewise, the longer the barrel, the more complete the burning of the propellant and the fewer discharge residues (see Figure 12.0.1).

Illustrative Case 2

A fisherman's boat was boarded by pirates in the South China Sea. The pirates did not believe his claim that he had nothing of worth on the boat and shot him in the chest with a 12-bore shotgun. Witnesses on the boat confirmed that the shotgun had been pushed hard against the fisherman's ribs as it was fired. Figures 12.0.7 and 12.0.8 clearly show the imprint of the unfired, top, barrel of the shotgun and the 'winged' foresight. The imprint of the unfired barrel was formed as a result of the gases following the pellets into the wound, causing the tissues to bulge out against the unfired barrel. As this was an unsupported area of skin, the discharge gases did not accumulate under the skin with sufficient pressure to cause stellate tearing. There was, however, sufficient to cause the skin to bulge outwards, causing the imprint of the second barrel to be formed.

Several weeks after the incident, the pirates were apprehended and found to be in possession of a Chinese military style 'over and under' 12-bore shotgun with a folding stock and a winged foresight. An examination of the internal surfaces of the barrel showed only the lower barrel to have been recently fired, and that the top barrel contained blood and tissue which was matched to that of the deceased.

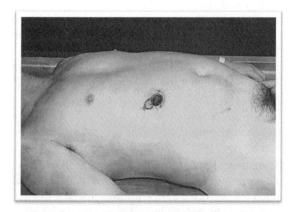

Figure 12.0.7   12-bore shotgun held in tight contact with the fisherman's chest.

It is also advantageous, when conducting the range of firing estimations, to select a target material as similar as possible to that under examination. It is of little use trying to compare, for example, test patterns made on a smooth material made from a man-made fibre with those on a thick woolly material. Likewise, for range of firing estimations on skin, a much more meaningful result will be obtained if tests are carried out on pigskin rather than on a fine-weave sheet of cotton.

The appearance of the discharge residue components will vary depending on the range, weapon type, barrel length, propellant type and ammunition used.

These observed effects can conveniently be split into three main groups:

Scorching

This is caused by the incandescent gases as they emerge from the muzzle of the weapon. Although they initially leave the barrel at a temperature of around 2,000 °C, they rapidly cool and, at a distance of no more than a few centimetres, their scorching effect will be insignificant. The affected area is also highly localised, being no more than half a centimetre around the periphery of the bullet entry hole.

The scorching effect of these gases is generally not visible on skin, due to its high water content. Even

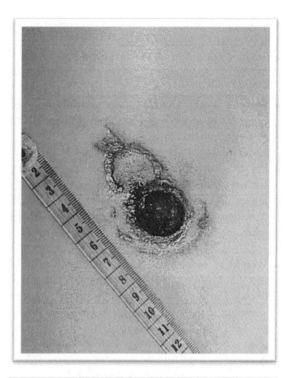

Figure 12.0.8   Close-up of wound in Figure 12.0.7.

when scorching is present, it is often difficult to discern beneath the amorphous sooty layer which occurs at short ranges.

Hair can exhibit a scorching effect, being generally identifiable by the crinkled nature of the individual hairs. Similarly, the finer fibres encountered in materials made from wool display the effects of scorching much more readily. The fibres are often shrivelled up to a fraction of their normal length and are completely blackened.

In man-made fibres, the effect is very pronounced, with the ends of the fibres being melted into globules. This, however, must not be confused with the surface finish applied to many of the cheaper man-made fabrics. This finish is accomplished by quickly running a hot gas flame over the surface of the fabric, causing the ends of the individual fibres to melt into globules and resulting in a much harder-wearing fabric. It is these globules that can be easily mistaken for the scorching effect of the discharge gases. The potential confusion can easily be overcome by examining fibres from remote areas of the garment.

The degree of scorching is also dependent upon:

- **Surface condition of the target**. If it is wet, the degree of scorching will be very much reduced.

- **Powder type**. Double-based propellants (see Chapter 4.7), for example, burn much hotter than single-based propellants.

- **Pressure produced**. A high-pressure cartridge, such as a Magnum, will produce a correspondingly higher degree of scorching than a non-Magnum cartridge, due to the higher temperature of the gases produced.

- **Weight of propellant**. The greater the weight of propellant, the greater the volume of gases produced. Thus, a rifle calibre will produce far more scorching than the same calibre in a pistol cartridge.

Blackening

This is caused by carbonaceous material in the discharge residues, mainly resulting from incomplete combustion of the propellant. It can also result from excessive quantities of bullet lubricant, or even from the bitumen sealant used between the bullet and cartridge case in military ammunition. It is composed mainly of amorphous carbon, although fine particles of partially burnt propellant can also be present.

This effect really begins where scorching finishes, and it can be up to ten inches (25 cm) from the muzzle in rifles and five inches (12.5 cm) in pistols.

The weight of propellant obviously effects the degree of blackening in the same way as scorching, i.e. the greater the charge, the greater the blackening. The effects of pressure and propellant are, however, exactly the opposite. A lower pressure means less efficient combustion, which gives rise to a greater proportion of carbonaceous materials. Likewise, the lower the temperature of burning, the less efficient the propellant.

This blackening is only a light surface coating and it is very easily removed with water or by rubbing with a cloth. Hospital blankets and rain are particularly efficient at removing this type of discharge residue. The absence of blackening should not, therefore, be considered conclusive proof as to the range of firing.

Blackening is often more obvious to the naked eye than it is through a low-powered microscope.

Unburnt and partially burnt propellant particles

Being much heavier than the carbonaceous material, the propellant particles can be found on the target at much greater distances. With low-powered microscopy, these particles can be located on the target at ranges up to three feet (0.92 m) for a handgun and to over four feet (120 cm) for a rifle. With three feet (0.92 m) being the approximate arm length for an adult, the presence or absence of propellant particles can be extremely important in determining the sequence of events in a shooting case, e.g. was it a deliberate act, or did the weapon fire due to the gun being pulled away from the grasp of the firer?

Factors influencing the quantity of this particulate matter found on the target are very similar to those for carbonaceous material. That is, the more efficient the cartridge and the longer the length of the barrel, the fewer the number of propellant particles that will found on the target.

Unlike carbonaceous material, the propellant particles adhere much more strongly to fabrics. Often, the particles will melt the fabric and weld themselves into place.

With skin, the particles will, at very close range, often enter the epidermal layer and take the form of '**tattooing**' which is all but impossible to remove.

12.0.4   Extended range of fire estimations

Using a scanning electron microscope to examine adhesive lifts taken from the surface surrounding the bullet entry hole, the range of firing can be estimated up to a distance of 16 feet (5 metres). This type of examination is, however, concerned with the search for the metallic components of the primer residues, not for burnt and unburnt propellant particles.

This is a specialised and extremely laborious technique. It will be covered at greater length in the chapter on gunshot residues.

12.0.5   Range of firing estimations on badly decomposed bodies

Unless a shotgun has been used, estimating the range of firing on a badly decomposed body can prove to be extremely difficult. The putrefying tissue either masks the presence of the residues, or they are removed as the outer layers of skin slough off.

12.0.6   Bullet wipe marks

Bullet lubricant, bullet/case mouth sealant, and gases which have squeezed past the bullet on it passage through the bore, all leave the outside of the bullet coated with a layer of black sooty material. If the barrel of the weapon had not been cleaned since it was last fired, the bullet will also pick up these residues as well.

Illustrative Case 3

A case where the range of firing was of considerable importance involved the shooting and subsequent dismembering of a young insurance sales woman.

After being shot and dismembered, the body parts were placed in several black plastic bin liners and dumped on a hillside. The ambient temperature was in excess of 35 °C and, in the two days it took for the body to be discovered, it had become severely decomposed.

An examination of the body revealed the presence of two bullet entry holes, of approximately .22″ (5.4 mm) calibre, in the skull (Figures 12.0.10 & 12.0.11). It was noted that the skin surrounding one of these entry holes had a mushy khaki appearance, while the other had the normal blackened appearance of decomposing tissue.

Inside the skull were found two badly damaged home-made lead bullets of approximately .22″ calibre. A microscopic examination of these bullets did not reveal the presence of any rifling, and what stria were present indicated that the bullets had been fired through different barrels.

A suspect was eventually arrested, and in his flat was found a double-barrelled, blank-firing pistol which had been converted to fire .22″ calibre ammunition (Figure 12.0.9).

An examination of the internal surfaces of the barrels showed them both to have been recently fired. A microscopic comparison of bullets fired from the pistol with those recovered from the victims head showed them to have been fired from the converted pistol.

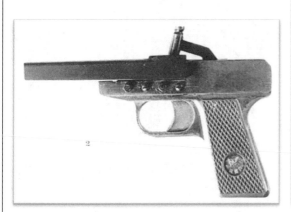

Figure 12.0.9   Blank-firing pistol converted to fire .22″ ammunition.

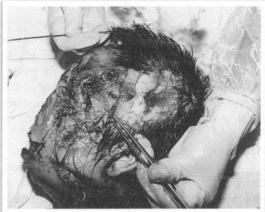

Figure 12.0.10   Discolouration around wound near temple area.

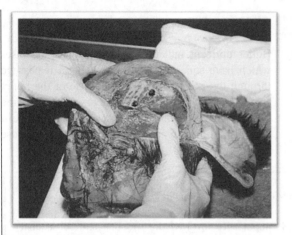

Figure 12.0.11   Two .22″ calibre entry wounds on right side of head.

The pistol had a single, non-selective trigger. A non-selective trigger is one in which, when both hammers are cocked, the first pull on the trigger will always fire the right barrel and the second pull on the trigger will always fire the left barrel (i.e. it is impossible to select which barrel will be fired first).

Test firings revealed that while the trigger pulls were excessively heavy, the weapon was somewhat prone to firing both barrels together. It was therefore necessary to determine, from the body, the range of firing, in order to eliminate any defence of accidental discharge during a struggle.

It was assumed that the difference in appearance between the two bullet entry holes could have something to do with one shot being fired closer to the head than the other, and that the discharge residues were having some effect on the rate of decomposition of the surrounding skin.

A number of pieces of pigskin were shot at varying ranges with exactly the same weapon and ammunition as that used in the crime. The skin was then sealed in black plastic bags of the same type that the body parts had been found in. These bags were then placed on the rooftop of Police Headquarters and opened at half-day intervals. It was found that the pappy khaki colouration to the skin could be exactly duplicated in the pigskin when the rounds were fired at close proximity. The test was then carried out on pieces of human skin and the results were exactly the same.

These tests showed that the first shot was fired at a range of about 2″ (5 cm) and that the second was fired at a distance in excess of 12″ (29.5 cm). As such, this could not have been an accidental discharge with both barrels discharging together.

As the bullet passes through an object, whether it be cloth, skin or some solid object, this black material is deposited on the periphery of the bullet entry hole. This black ring is often referred to as the 'bullet wipe' and, where no discharge residues are present, it is a very useful identifier of the bullet entry hole.

The quantity of material left on the 'bullet wipe' mark is dependent on the quantity of carbonaceous material left in the barrel from previous shots and then, subsequently, picked up by the bullet during its passage through the bore.

Assuming that the first shot fired was through a clean, unfouled barrel, the bullet wipe mark should

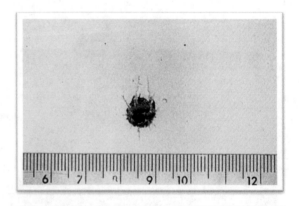

Figure 12.0.12   Bullet wipe mark on white card.

be easily distinguishable from the second bullet that had been fired through the barrel which had been fouled by the first bullet. In this instance, the first bullet wipe mark will contain less carbonaceous material than the second, and will thus appear much fainter than the one from the second shot. In cases where multiple shots have been fired, it is thus possible to determine, with a reasonable degree of accuracy, which was the first shot to strike the target. After the second shot, however, there is no change in the degree of carbonaceous material deposited around the entry hole.

12.1

Chemical Tests for Range of Fire Estimations and Bullet Entry/Exit Hole Identification

12.1.1 Introduction

In any-well funded forensic laboratory, chemical spot tests for bullet entry/exit hole determination are, generally, a thing of the past. The vast majority of chemical tests used for such purposes can be carried out with a far higher degree of precision using a scanning electron microscope (SEM) with an energy dispersive X-ray analyser (EDX).

At close distances, the range of firing estimations are normally carried out by visually estimating the density of partially burnt propellant particles on the surface being examined. However, this can be difficult, if not impossible, on dark-coloured materials.

For practical purposes, at ranges in excess of 20 inches (50 cm), the residue particles that issue from handguns become too small to visualise. The presence of these discharge residues can, however, be picked up with a SEM/EDX at ranges of 15 feet (5 metres) or more.

The process is very laborious and involves taking tapings from control firings at a set distance, usually four inches (10 cm) from the bullet hole. From these tapings, a GSR particle density is calculated for each range. These particle densities are then compared with tapings taken from the garment in question, and a range of firing estimation is obtained.

As the GSR distribution will be different for each type of ammunition/barrel length combination, it is essential that these parameters are known before range of fire estimations can be calculated from the GSR particle density distribution tables. This technique does, however, enable range of fire estimations to be made at distances which cannot be accomplished by any other method.

The importance of range of firing determination cannot be emphasised enough. Even though no-one in the legal profession would be expected to understand the chemistry behind the following chemical tests for discharge residues, the use, possible misuse and limitations of these tests must be understood.

12.1.2 Chemical tests for range of firing estimations

In cases where an SEM is not available, the tests described below can still be used. Great caution should be used with the interpretation of any results obtained from these tests, as none are specific. At

Forensic Ballistics in Court: Interpretation and Presentation of Firearms Evidence, First Edition. Brian J. Heard.
© 2013 John Wiley & Sons, Ltd. Published 2013 by John Wiley & Sons, Ltd.

best, the results could be presumptive – and at worst, only indicative.

Sodium rhodizonate test

The most valuable of the available spot tests is the sodium rhodizonate test for lead. This test is a rapid and very cheap method for determining the entry and exit holes in those cases where a microscopic examination is ambiguous.

The test relies on the specificity of this reagent, in acidic conditions, to give a positive reaction to lead. It also relies on the bullet being either plain lead or, if it is a jacketed bullet, having picked up some lead primer residues on its passage through the bore.

When passing through cloth, the residues and/or some of the bullet lead will be transferred from the bullet to the impact side of the target. Thus, if we are dealing with a bullet which has completely penetrated a body, the outside surface of the bullet entry hole on the outer garment will give a positive reaction to lead, as will the inside surface of the bullet exit hole.

This test is also used for range of fire estimations, to identify particles of lead from the lead styphnate or lead peroxide contained in the primer residues.

Method for lead

The test is carried out by firmly pressing a clean filter paper which has been lightly moistened with 0.1N hydrochloric acid (HCl) over the bullet hole. The filter paper is then dried using a hot air blower and is carefully spotted with a saturated solution of sodium rhodizonate in water. The filter paper will eventually take on an orange colour from the sodium rhodizonate. The filter paper is then warmed once again with the air blower, but not dried. The solution of 0.1N HCl is then lightly spotted, or preferably sprayed, onto the paper until the orange colour disappears. If there are any lead particles present, they will remain as a purple coloration.

This test can also be used for the detection of barium, one of the components of GSR, although it is not as sensitive as the test for lead. It can, however, be used in conjunction with the test for lead, giving a more specific identifier for GSR.

Method for barium

After spotting with the 0.1N HCL solution and noting (or preferably photographing) any purple-coloured spots, hold the paper over a solution of 880 ammonia solution. This will, with care, make the liquid on the filter paper mildly alkaline (preferably about pH 8). This will remove the purple colouration due to the lead and leave the liquid in a condition where the sodium rhodizonate will react with barium is present. Any barium that is present will give red/brown-coloured spots. These should be in the same position as the purple-coloured spots, showing that the particles giving these results contain lead and barium, which is highly indicative of being GSR. If the spots are not in the same position, then they could be due to environmental contamination.

Walker test for nitrites

This is used for the detection of nitrites in the partially burnt and unburnt propellants. These nitrites come from the nitrocellulose propellant, not the primer. On darkly coloured clothing, the test can indicate the distribution of such particles, thus enabling the range of firing to be estimated.

The test uses the slightly sticky, gelatinous surface layer of desensitised photographic paper to pick up the particles from the cloth. Any nitrites present are then converted to a diazo dye compound. depending on what chemicals are used, these diazo compounds will be brightly coloured red/orange dyes that can easily be seen and photographed.

It should be noted that many compounds other than nitrocellulose propellants can give a positive result to this reaction (e.g. urine, face powder, fertilisers). Nitrocellulose is also found in many other readily available products, including table tennis balls, guitar coatings, guitar picks, aircraft dope and as a coating for playing cards. It has also been used in certain automobile paints. As such, a positive result from this test should be treated with great caution.

Greiss test

This is identical to the Walker test, except for the main reagent, which is naphthylamine instead of 2-naphthylamine-4,8-disulphonic acid. This reagent gives orange spots. Once again, this is mainly used for detection of propellant particles in range of firing estimations. Positive results to this test should be treated with the same degree of caution as those from the Walker test.

Marshal Test

Once again, this is a modified Walker test for nitrites, using a 0.5 per cent solution sulphanilic acid and 0.5 per cent solution of N-α naphthyl-ethylenediamine hydrochloride in methanol.

Again, positive results to this test should be treated with the same degree of caution as those from the Walker and Greiss Tests.

Tewari test

As above, but with antazoline hydrochloride (2-N-benzylanilinomethyliminazoline hydrochloride) as the reagent.

Positive results to this test should, once again, be treated with the same degree of caution as those from the Walker, Greiss and Marshal tests.

Lunge Reagent

This was the original 'dermal nitrate test' used for proof of firing a weapon. This test is often referred to as the standard test for discharge residues, but it is virtually useless as it gives positive results for a very wide range of chemicals. The method is, however, included here for historical reasons.

In this test, paraffin casts were made of the shooter's hands and this reagent sprayed onto the cast. However,

so many chemicals other than nitrocellulose can give a positive to this test that it is now never used for identification of gunshot residues on hands.

The original reagent consisted of a 0.25 per cent solution of diphenylbenzidine in concentrated sulphuric acid. This was dropped carefully onto the suspected particle. A deep blue coloration is a positive for this reagent. Diphenylbenzidine is, however, very carcinogenic and so is now no longer used. Diphenylamine gives exactly the same results.

Great care should be exercised when using this test, as concentrated sulphuric acid is exceedingly corrosive.

Harrison and Gillroy Reagent

While this reagent is really intended for the identification of GSR on hand swabs, it can be used just as well for range of firing estimations, once the particles have been removed from the garment via the desensitised photographic method.

The reagent used in this test is a ten per cent solution of triphenylmethylarsonium iodide in alcohol. An orange coloration is positive for antimony. If dried and then sprayed with a saturated solution of sodium rhodizonate, red spots will be positive for barium or lead. If this is then dried again and then sprayed with dilute hydrochloric acid, any purple spots will be positive for lead. If the spots are then exposed to 35 per cent ammonia solution, any particles containing barium will give a red coloration. As this test can identify antimony, barium and lead, it is a good identifier for lead-based primer residues. However, the constant wetting, drying and wetting again does render the test rather insensitive.

12.1.3 Range of firing estimations on heavily bloodstained garments

Although it may still be possible to see unburnt propellant particles under low-power microscopy, the, the sooty deposit from close-range discharges may be completely obscured by the blood.

In instances such as these, the only recourse is to use of infra-red photography. By the use of various

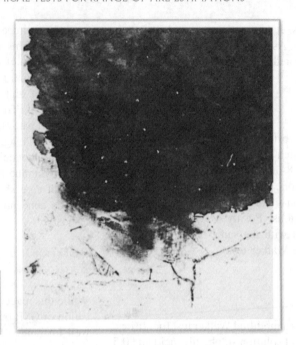

Figure 12.1.1 Pin heads indicating position of propellant particles on bloodstained clothing for range of fire estimation.

filters and different wavelengths of infra-red (IR) light, the colour of the garment and any bloodstaining can be eliminated, leaving the sooty deposit. This can then be photographed, using IR-sensitive film, and compared to test firings in the normal way (see Figure 12.1.1).

Alternative method for the visualisation of propellant particles on bloodstained garments

Even with heavily bloodstained garments, it should be possible to locate, microscopically, partially burnt propellant particles. The problem is that it is difficult to obtain visually an accurate picture of the distribution of these particles.

Without recourse to elaborate and time-consuming chemical tests, and especially if IR photography is not available, there is, however, a simple method of overcoming this problem.

The position of each particle, located under a low-powered microscope, is indicated by sticking a pin through the garment and into the backing board. By viewing (or even better, by photographing) the garment from directly above, the pin heads can clearly be seen against the bloodstaining. This can

then be compared directly with test firings as previously mentioned.

12.1.4 Range of firing estimations for non-toxic non-lead primers

In general, it has been noted that, when estimating ranges of firing from discharge residue dispersion, those from non-toxic primers do not tally well with those from lead-based primers[1]. This disparity is probably due to the quantity of partially combusted materials present, as well as the higher organic content of non-toxic primer compositions. Lead, which is a major component of so-called 'toxic' primers, has a high specific gravity and, as such, it will carry further than non-inorganic residues from non-toxic primers.

In very general terms, the spread of discharge residues from non-toxic primers will be less than that from lead-based primers, and the range at which

---

[1] Gundry, R., & Rockoff, I. *Comparison of Gunshot Residue Patterns from Lead-Based and Lead-Free Primer Ammunition.* www.gwu.edu

they can be detected will be correspondingly shorter. As an example, if we take a .38 Special round of ammunition fired from a six-inch (14.7 cm) barrel, a GSR spread of three inches (7.5 cm) is witnessed around the bullet entry hole. With a lead-based primer, this will indicate a range of 16 inches (39.2 cm) while a Sintox round under the same conditions will indicate a range of 13 inches (32 cm).

As there are so many different non-toxic compositions in use, range of firing estimations must be made with exactly the same ammunition as that used in the case under review.

A complicating factor is that non-lead-based primer compositions can give what appears to be a positive reaction with sodium rhodizonate. This is probably due to the presence of barium which, in a mildly alkaline (pH 8) solution, gives a red/brown colouration, while lead gives a purple colouration in acidic (pH 2.8) conditions. If the correct pH is not selected, the test results can be confusing to the inexperienced.

Further reading

1 Dalby, O., Butler, D. & Birkett, J.W. (2010). Analysis of Gunshot Residue and Associated Materials –A Review. *Journal of Forensic Sciences* 55 (4), 924–943.

2 Grima, M., Butler, M., Hanson, R. & Mohameden, A. (2012) Firework displays as sources of particles similar to gunshot residue, *Science and Justice* 52 (1) 49–57.

3 Meng, H.H. & Caddy, B. (1997). Gunshot residue analysis – review. *Journal of Forensic Sciences* 42 (4), 553–570.

4 Mosher, P.V., McVicar, M.J., Randall, E.D. & Sild, E.H. (1998). Gunshot residue-similar particles produced by fireworks. *Journal of the Canadian Society of Forensic Science* 31 (3), 157–168.

5 Romolo, F.S. & Margot, P. (2001). Identification of gunshot residue: a critical review, *Forensic Science International* 119 (2), 195–211.

6 Schwoeble, A.J. & Exline, D.L. (2000). *Current Methods in Forensic Gunshot Residue Analysis*. CRC Press LLC.

7 Wallace, J.S. (2008). *Chemical Analysis of Firearms, Ammunition, and Gunshot Residue*. CRC Press LLC.

12.2

Range of Fire Estimations for Shotguns

12.2.1 Introduction

As shotguns fire cartridges loaded with pellets, rather than a single missile, the range of firing can be estimated with considerable accuracy up to 20–30 yards. This estimation relies on the fact that the pellets do not fly through the air as a single cohesive mass, but begin to disperse as soon as they leave the muzzle. The dispersion is caused by air pressure within the pellet mass, forcing the individual pellets apart.

In addition to the air pressure causing dispersion of the shot, any deformation of the individual pellets will also influence the dispersion. This deformation could come about through poor manufacturing tolerances, especially in low cost ammunition, but it is more likely to occur either during the initial stages of firing or the pellets' passage down the bore. The initial force on the shot column as it accelerates down the bore crushes the pellets together, causing irregular dimpling. In addition, once the shot column reaches the barrel choke, the pellets are squashed together, causing more deformation. While these problems can be eliminated to a certain extent by use of mono-wads and packing the inter-shot spaces with a lightweight inert substance, such as expanded polystyrene, there will always be some resultant deformation of the pellets. In extreme cases, this will result in pellets outside of the normal shot pattern, which are called 'flyers' (see Figure 12.2.3).

There are so many factors which can influence this dispersion of shot that each and every case must be carefully examined as to the exact circumstances surrounding the incident. These would have to include:

- shotgun bore size;

- whether the shot is lead or non-toxic;

- if non-toxic, the particular type of non-toxic shot;

- wad column type, i.e. traditional felt type or mono-wad;

- if mono-wad, the type and construction of mono-wad;

- length of cartridge;

- weight of shot;

- size of shot;

- velocity of shot;

- length of barrel;

- barrel choke.

There are, naturally, many misconceptions as to what will influence the spread of shot. Some of the

Forensic Ballistics in Court: Interpretation and Presentation of Firearms Evidence, First Edition. Brian J. Heard.
© 2013 John Wiley & Sons, Ltd. Published 2013 by John Wiley & Sons, Ltd.

most common misconceptions would include the following:

- The distance, in inches, from the centre of the pattern to the point where the wads hit the target gives the range in yards. This is totally untrue and should never be used for estimation of range of firing.

- With sawn-off shotguns (i.e. shotguns that have had their barrel(s) considerably reduced in length to aid concealment), the shot spread is many times that of a full length barrel. While there is some increase in the spread of shot, it is only marginal.

- In heavy rain, the pellets will be disrupted by the raindrops, which increases the spread of pellets. Once again, this has, for all practical purposes, been found to be false, due to the relative weight and velocity of the pellets compared to that of raindrops.

With the importance of range of fire estimation in crime investigations, each and every one of the above must be taken into account when interpreting the results of the firearms expert's findings. Everything must be done to establish that the expert took every precaution possible to ensure that the test conditions matched, as closely as possible, those of the incident under investigation.

12.2.2   Basics

Degree of shot dispersion

The degree of dispersion of the shot is dependent on many factors, the most important of which are:

(a) Cartridge pressure

(b) Wad type

(c) Barrel choke

(d) Barrel length

(a) Cartridge type

The higher the pressure generated by the cartridge, the more the shot will be disrupted as it emerges from the barrel by the following gases. This effect is largely offset by the wads used in modern cartridges, but it is a factor which does effect the dispersion of shot.

(b) Wad type

The wadding in traditional shotgun cartridges consisted of an over powder wad, a series of filler wads and an over shot wad (see Figure 12.2.1).

A.   Overcharge card wad
B.   Undershot wad
C.   Overshot wad
D.   Cushion wads
E.   Shot column
F.   Rollover crimp
G.   Propellant
H.   Base wad

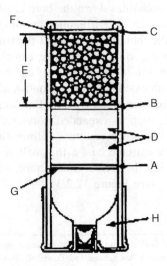

Figure 12.2.1   Older style shotgun cartridge with felt wads.

The over powder wad was intended to act as a gas seal to prevent the high-pressure gases from escaping up into the shot column during firing. The filler wads were to cushion the shot against the rapid acceleration during its progress down the barrel, and the over shot wad was to retain the shot in the cartridge case.

This construction, however, suffered from a number of drawbacks. On firing, hot gases could escape pass the over powder and filler wads into the shot charge. This could result in pellets becoming partially melted and fused together. Likewise, the filler wads did not provide sufficient cushioning of the shot to prevent distortion due to inter-shot contact or, in extreme cases, the cold welding together of small clumps of shot due to the pressures produced.

Also, during the shot's passage through the barrel, severe distortion could occur through contact with the inside surface of the bore. Shot which had become so distorted would not fly in a predictable manner, resulting in distorted and enlarged patterns.

Modern wads tend to be of the plastic cup type, with an integral shock absorber and gas seal (Figure 12.2.2). The shock absorber consists of a semi-collapsible section which very effectively cushions the shot column at the moment of acceleration. The integral plastic cup protects the shot during its passage through the bore, and the plastic gas seal prevents the leakage of hot gases into the shot column.

Cartridges loaded with this type of one-piece wad (monowad) will give much a much more controlled spread of shot than one loaded with the old-type wad column.

It should be noted that with a more 'green' approach to the environment, there is a shift

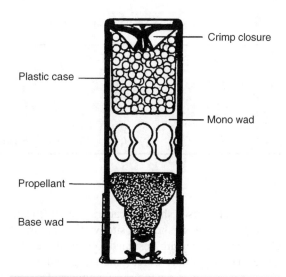

Figure 12.2.2 Modern monowad type shotgun cartridge.

away from plastic-cased ammunition and plastic monowads. The more traditional materials, such as paper cases, felt wads and card separators, are being increasingly used once again in modern shotgun ammunition.

(c) Barrel choke

Except for a few very unusual weapons, shotguns have smooth-bored barrels. Most sporting weapons have a constriction applied to the muzzle end of the weapon's bore to control the spread of the shot. This constriction is called 'choke'.

Illustrative Case 1

An example of how shot that is unprotected by a modern cup type monowad system can become cold welded involved the jilted boyfriend of a girl who was a very keen horse rider. The ex-boyfriend was so upset that he decided to teach the girl a lesson. Hiding in a clump of trees close to a bridle path where the girl normally went riding he lay in wait with a .410" shotgun loaded with very fine (dust) shot. His plan was to fire at the horse, which would feel the prick of the dust shot and bolt thus 'teaching the girl a lesson'. Unfortunately, the dust shot cold-welded and came out of the barrel as a solid lump. Instead of hitting the horse, it went straight through the neck of the girl, virtually decapitating her.

Table 12.2.1 Common Shotgun Choke Sizes

Constriction (mm)	Constriction (Inches)	British Designation	European Designation	US Designation
0.00	0.00	Cylinder	CL	Cyl
0.25	0.01	$^1/_4$	++++	Improved Cyl
0.50	0.02	$^1/_2$	+++	Modified
0.75	0.03	$^3/_4$	++	Improved Mod
1.00	0.04	Full	+	Full

There are also shot spreaders, or diffusion chokes, which work the opposite way from normal chokes in that they are designed to spread the shot more than a cylinder bore, generating wider patterns for very short range use. A number of recent spreader chokes, such as the Briley 'Diffusion', uses rifling in the choke to spin the shot slightly, creating a wider spread. The Briley Diffusion uses a 1 in 36 cm twist, as does the FABARM Lion Paradox shotgun. Oval chokes, designed to provide a shot pattern wider than it is tall, are sometimes found on combat shotguns, primarily those of the Vietnam War era.

As the column of shot passes through the choked part of the barrel, the diameter of the shot column is reduced, thus elongating it. This reduction in diameter results in the outer layers of shot in the column being given an inward acceleration. This delays the spreading of the shot once it leaves the barrel, thus reducing its degree of dispersion.

The tighter the degree of restriction, the tighter the pattern of shot at the target. The usual degrees of choke in the British system are called Full, Three Quarters, Half, Quarter, Improved Cylinder and True Cylinder.

The degree of constriction is, irrespective of the bore of the weapon, as follows:

- Full Choked barrels have a constriction of 0.004″;

- Half Choked barrels 0.002″;

- Improved Cylinder 0.0005″;

- True Cylinder have no restriction at all.

One important thing to notice from these figures is that all bores should give the same spread of shot with a given 'choke' at a given distance, the only variation being that as there is less shot in a .410″ bore cartridge than a 12-bore cartridge, the density of shot at the target will be less.

Table 12.2.1 shows the most common choke sizes.

The degree of choke is based upon the percentage of the total pellets in a cartridge that will be within a 30″ circle at any given range.

The following tables show the effect of choke on pattern measured by percentage of shot in a 30″ circle and the spread of shot at various ranges.

The **spread** of shot is the diameter of a circle which contains the majority of the shot charge at any

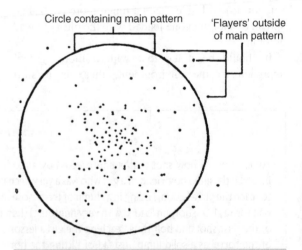

Figure 12.2.3 Typical shotgun pattern showing flyers.

Table 12.2.2   Table Showing the Percentage of Total Pellets in a 30″ Circle for Various Chokes

Barrel Choke	Range in Yards							
	20	25	30	35	40	45	50	55
True cylinder	80	69	60	49	40	33	27	22
Improved	92	82	72	60	50	41	33	27
Quarter	100	87	77	65	55	46	38	30
Half	100	94	83	71	60	50	41	33
Three quarters	100	100	91	77	65	55	46	37
Full	100	100	100	84	70	59	49	40

Table 12.2.3   Table Showing Spread of Shot, in Inches, for Various Chokes

Barrel Choke	Range in Yards						
	10	15	20	25	30	35	40
True cylinder	20	26	32	38	44	51	58
Improved	15	20	26	32	38	44	51
Quarter	13	18	23	29	35	41	48
Half	12	16	21	26	32	38	45
Three quarters	10	14	18	23	29	35	42
Full	9	12	16	21	27	33	40

given range. Factors such as irregularly shaped shot, shot that has contacted irregularities in the bore, pellets which become imbedded in the wads, etc. can all give rise to what are called 'flyers'. These are pellets that do not fly true with the rest of the charge, falling outside of the main body of shot at the target. Deciding which pellets constitute flyers, and should thus be excluded from the main spread, requires much experience with the examination of shot patterns and is something that cannot be explained in a book.

The figures given in the following tables are for cartridges loaded with a modern monowad. All of these figures have been left in the Imperial system, as giving the metric conversions would render the tables extremely difficult to interpret. All the tables are for lead pellets and monowad cartridges.

Using Tables 12.2.3 and 12.2.4, it is possible to determine the actual number of pellets in a 30″ circle in any of the six borings of a gun at the stated ranges.

(d) Barrel length

Shortening the barrel by sawing off the muzzle end does have some effect on the spread of shot, though not as great as popular tradition has it. What effect exists is mainly due to the high-pressure gases disrupting the shot column as it exits from the barrel.

Shotgun propellants are very fast burning, giving rise to a very sharp rise in pressure during the first few moments of ignition. In full-length barrels, the overall pressure within the barrel drops very considerably as the shot nears the muzzle and the volume of gas between the over powder wad and the standing breech of the weapon increases.

As the barrel is progressively shortened, the pressure being exerted on the base of the shot column as it exits the barrel become progressively greater. These pressures can lead to a destabilisation of the shot column and a 'blown' pattern. This

Table 12.2.4   Actual Number of Pellets for Various 12-bore Shotgun Cartridge Loadings that will Strike in a 30″ Circle

Weight of Shot	Number of Pellets in Shot Load					
	Shot Size					
	3	4	5	6	7	8
$1\frac{5}{8}$ oz	228	276	358	439	552	732
$1\frac{1}{2}$ oz	210	255	330	405	510	675
$1\frac{1}{4}$ oz	175	213	275	338	425	562
$1\frac{3}{16}$ oz	160	202	261	321	404	534
$1\frac{1}{8}$ oz	157	191	248	304	383	506
$1\frac{1}{16}$ oz	149	181	234	287	361	478
1 oz	140	170	220	270	340	450
$\frac{15}{16}$ oz	131	159	206	253	319	422
$\frac{7}{8}$ oz	122	149	193	236	298	394
$\frac{13}{16}$ oz	113	138	179	219	276	366
$\frac{5}{8}$ oz	87	106	138	169	212	282
$\frac{9}{16}$ oz	78	96	124	152	191	254
$\frac{7}{16}$ oz	61	75	97	118	149	187
$\frac{5}{16}$ oz	44	53	69	84	106	141

Example: Number of pellets striking within a 30″ circle at 40 yards for a $\frac{1}{2}$ choked barrel with a charge of $1\frac{1}{16}$ oz No. 6 shot. Total pellets in $1\frac{1}{16}$ oz shot are 287. This is multiplied by 60 (percentage in circle at 40 yards) divided by $100 = 172$.

effect can be identified by an irregular shot pattern and a larger spread than would normally be expected.

The effect is, however, much less than popular tradition would have us believe, and is only marginally greater than that for a full-length cylinder-bored barrel.

12.2.3   Shotgun cartridges fired in revolvers

A number of manufacturers produce shotgun cartridges for most calibres of revolver. These are intended for very short-range vermin destruction or equally short-range personal defence. The

---

Illustrative Case 2

During a cash in transit robbery, the guard was shot twice — once in the face and then in the mouth — with what was, according to the driver of the security van, a large revolver. During the post-mortem, two .410 shotgun card wads, a quantity of No. 6 pellets and some candle wax were recovered from the deceased's face and throat. The pellet pattern on the face had a distinct spiral pattern to it, which was typical of that caused by shot fired through a rifled barrel.

A suspect was arrested, and in his possession was a WWI Webley .455″ calibre revolver. together with a number of .410″ shotgun cartridges. The wads, with the exception of a thin card wad, had been removed, and the case length reduced, enabling the cartridges to be chambered and fired in the .455″ revolver. To prevent the shot falling out of the cartridge case, molten candle wax had been poured over the top to seal it in place. When fired, these cartridges produced the distinctive spiral pattern seen on the face of the deceased. Due to the fact that most of the shot still remained in the cartridge, they were very effective, with only a slight reduction in kinetic energy when compared with a full length cartridge.

cartridges are invariably loaded with small quantities of very small shot and are often enclosed in a plastic shell. These can often be recognised by the spiral pattern produced as a result of the weapon's rifling.

Suggested further reading

1 Greener, W.W. (1967) *The Gun and its Development* (9th ed.). New York, Bonanza Books.

2 Di Maio, V.J.M. (1985). *Gunshot Wounds, Practical Aspects of Firearms, Ballistics and Techniques*. Elsevier.

3 Fatteh, A. (1976). *Medicolegal Investigation of Gunshot Wounds*. J.B. Lippincott Co.

4 Hatcher, J. (1935). *Textbook of Firearms Investigation, Identification and Evidence*. Marines, NC, USA, Small Arms Technical Publishing Company.

5 Jauhari, M. & Chatterjee, S. (1972). Statistical Treatment of Pellet Distribution Data for Estimating Range of Firing. *Journal of Forensic Sciences* 17 (1), 141–149.

6 Rowe, W.F. & Hanson, S.R. (1985). Range-of-fire estimates from regression analysis applied to the spreads of shotgun pellet patterns: results of a blind study. *Forensic Science International* 28 (3–4) 239–250.

7 Moreau, T.S., Nickels, M.L., Wray, J. L, Bottemiller, K. W. & Rowe, W.F. (1985). Pellet Patterns Fired by Sawed-Off Shotguns. *Journal of Forensic Sciences* 30 (1), 137–149.

13.0

The Use of X-ray Photography for Projectile Identification

13.0.1 Introduction

The use of X-rays in the investigation of gunshot wounds can provide invaluable information to the forensic investigator and the courts. X-ray photography can assist by:

- determining whether part or all of a bullet is still within the body;

- locating the exact position of the bullet;

- determining the type of bullet and an approximation of its calibre in those instances where the bullet cannot be surgically removed;

- determining the bullets paths through the body;

- determining the position of the pellets and wads in shotgun wounds prior to surgery;

- locating bullet fragments where the bullet has broken up.

Illustrative Case 1

This case concerned a Hong Kong fisherman that had been illegally fishing in the fish-rich waters off Vietnam. A Vietnamese gunboat gave chase and, when the fisherman refused to stop, the crew of the gunboat opened up with everything they had on board, including TT33 7.62 × 25 mm pistols, a 12.7 mm DShK heavy machine gun and several Kalashnikov AK47 7.62 × 39 mm assault rifles.

The fishing boat took numerous hits from both the AK47s and the DShK. In addition, the captain was hit with a 7.62 × 39 mm bullet and died almost immediately. Eventually, the fishing boat reached international waters and the Vietnamese gun boat gave up the chase.

The captain's body was buried in ice along with the fish in the hold, to preserve it for burial back in Hong Kong.

At the post-mortem examination, it could be seen that the front of the body, where it had been completely immersed in the ice, was perfectly preserved, while the back was black and in a state of advanced decomposition. Only one bullet wound was visible, which was in the centre of the chest area. This wound had every characteristic of being a bullet exit hole, but the pathologist, most unusually, begged to differ, insisting it was an entry hole. As such, he opined, the bullet must still be in the body.

Forensic Ballistics in Court: Interpretation and Presentation of Firearms Evidence, First Edition. Brian J. Heard.
© 2013 John Wiley & Sons, Ltd. Published 2013 by John Wiley & Sons, Ltd.

No X-ray equipment was forthcoming, and an extremely messy and tedious dissection of the body was undertaken, following imaginary bullet wound tracks. At the conclusion of this dissection, during which no bullet was found, the body was turned over, revealing the decomposed skin on the back. It was then noticed that this thick, blackened layer had separated from the underlying layers and was quite mobile and had slipped from its correct position.

When the blackened layer of skin was moved back into its correct position, a bullet entry hole was discovered in the centre of the chest area, just to the right of the mid line. This entry hole had been completely covered up by the wrinkled-up layer of decomposed skin.

The bullet had obviously entered the fisherman's back and passed straight through the body, exiting from the front. A simple X-ray of the body would have shown the bullet track and the complete absence of a missile, saving hours of unnecessary dissection.

13.0.2 Estimation of calibre from X-ray photographs

Although X-rays can be used to accurately locate a bullet and determine its trajectory through the body, they cannot be used to determine precisely its exact calibre. The problem here is that, due to the way X-rays are taken, the image of the missile will always be magnified to some extent; as the distance from X-ray plate to missile increases, so does the magnification. Thus, a bullet that is lodged just below the surface of the skin at the front of a body will seem much larger on an X-ray plate than a bullet lodged just under the skin at the rear of the body – that is, assuming the body is lying on its back when the X-ray is taken (see Figure 13.0.1).

This problem can be off-set to some extent by taking two X-ray images, one face on and one from the side. These can then be used to estimate the depth of the missile in the body. A number of bullets of varying calibres can then be placed alongside the body at the approximate depth of the bullet in the body and another X-ray taken. This X-ray can be used to estimate the bullet's calibre; see Figures 13.0.2, 13.0.3 and 13.0.4 (all by permission of Evan Thompson).

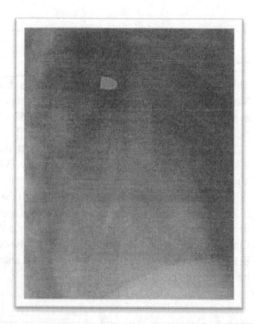

Figure 13.0.2   Bullet lodged deep in body.

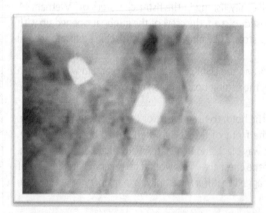

Figure 13.0.1   X-ray photograph showing identical projectiles with different apparent dimensions due to the magnification effect.

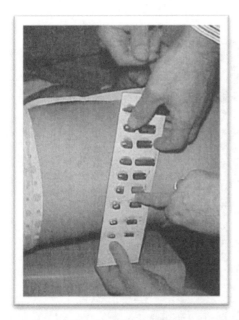

Figure 13.0.3 Bullets being placed in approximate position.

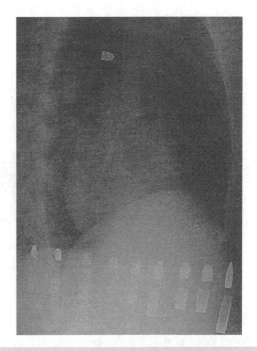

Figure 13.0.4 Comparison of bullet calibre.

An alternative method is to use a micrometre with its jaws set to a known measurement, place this alongside the body at the same position as the embedded bullet and then take the X-ray.

One of the most characteristic X-ray photographs is that from a high velocity soft-pointed hunting bullet. In such a an X-ray, a snowstorm of lead fragments can be seen along the wound track.

One area where X-ray photographs can be confusing is where Winchester Silvertip ammunition has been fired. These bullets have a jacket made of aluminium rather than the usual copper/zinc alloy.

Illustrative Case 2

An interesting case, for once not involving a dead body, involved the identification of missile holes in a vast 18-foot (5.5 metres) diameter table which was reputed to be that of the famous King Arthur, a legendary fifth-century British king (Biddle, 2000) (see Figure 13.0.5). The table had been hanging on the wall of the great banqueting hall of Winchester Castle, Hampshire for an unknown number of years, and it was not until it was taken down for restoration that a number of missile holes were discovered.

An examination of the table's surface showed there to be a total of 45 complete penetrations (see Figure 13.0.6). X-ray photographs revealed the presence of a further five missiles still imbedded in the thick oak timbers of the frame. Unfortunately, preservation restrictions prevented me from removing any of these still imbedded missiles.

Using X-rays at 90° to the table's top surface, I was able to determine the exact depth of the missiles and their calibre ranged between 0.6–0.9″ (1.52–2.3 cm). It was also noted that the missiles were of an irregular, but basically spherical, shape. This suggested that they were not mould cast bullets of the conventional type.

History tells us that in the early part of the 17th century, the military forces in England were armed with a wide variety of firearm weapons, ranging from 0.5″ to 1.0″ (1.27–2.45 cm) bore diameter. The foot soldiers were almost

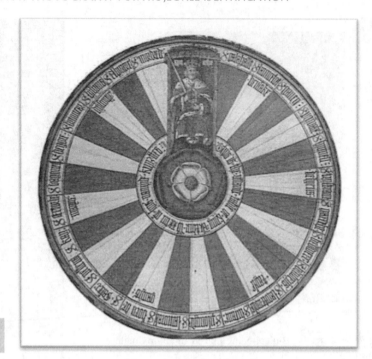

Figure 13.0.5 'King Arthur's Round Table' in Winchester Castle.

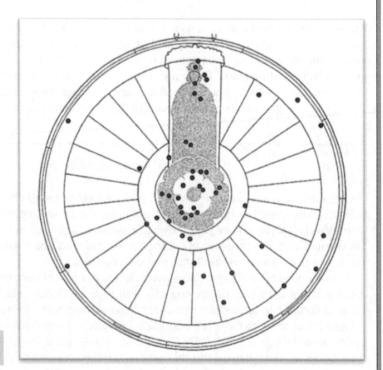

Figure 13.0.6 Missile entry holes in table.

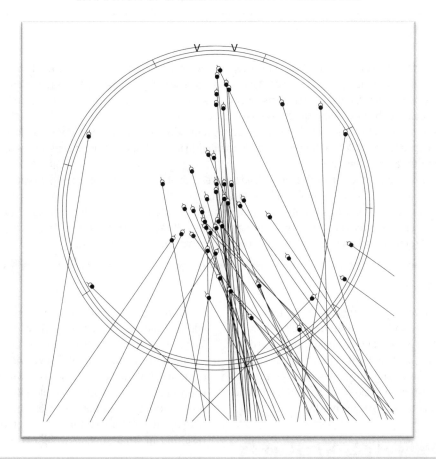

Figure 13.0.7 Trajectory of missiles from entry and exit holes.

always armed with a simple smooth-bored matchlock musket, and cavalrymen with a wheel-lock pistol or carbine. The missiles used in these weapons were, at that time and especially in times of battle, just lumps of lead which were crudely hammered into a rough shape and size to fit the bore of the weapon being carried. This situation was standardised by an order in 1673, where the calibre of service muskets was fixed at 12-bore (0.7292″ = 1.85 cm).

If the damage to the table was inflicted by military troops, then this probably took place before the last quarter of the 17th century, as witnessed by the type and size of missiles.

Historical records revealed that the castle was taken by Oliver Cromwell's Parliamentary forces in 1642. The castle and town were regained by the King in 1643 but were taken again by Parliamentary forces, directly under Cromwell's command, in 1645.

The trajectories of the missiles were found by comparing the positions of the entry and exit holes and side on X-rays of the large beams under the table (see Figure 13.0.7). Although these trajectories would appear to be somewhat confusing, historical records show the position of the dining table in the Great Hall during the 17th century. From this, it can be ascertained that the majority of the shots were fired from either side of the banqueting table, while those directed at the painting of King Arthur came from the head of the take.

Obviously, the missile holes were nothing to do with King Arthur, and the table was eventually dated, via dendrochronology, to the 14th century (all images of table courtesy of Prof. Martin Biddle).

Illustrative Case 3

Another illustrative case of the use of X-ray photographs concerns an old man who dropped dead on the streets of Hong Kong. There were no suspicious circumstances but, to ensure that no pacemakers or anything else were present in the body which could cause problems with a cremation, the body was X-rayed. It was at this stage that the shadow of a bullet embedded in the spine was seen.

At the post-mortem, the bullet was found to be deeply imbedded in calcified material surrounding the bullets location. On removal, the bullet was found to possess no rifling marks at all, and the jacket material was so thin that it crumbled to dust at the slightest touch.

A close examination of the old man's skin revealed the presence of a very old and almost imperceptible puckered wound inside his navel. This was typical of a long-healed bullet entry wound.

The bullet was easily identified as having been fired from a 7.7 mm Arisaka rifle which had obviously been fired at the old man when he was very much younger, during the 1941–1945 Japanese occupation of Hong Kong. A case of attempted murder by the Japanese military, possibly, discovered over 50 years too late?

The aluminium readily separates from the core when entering the body and the aluminium jacket does not show up well on X-rays and can easily be missed. As the lead core will exhibit class characteristics impressed by the rifling during its passage through the bore, this can be mistaken for a plain lead bullet with non-characteristic rifling marks.

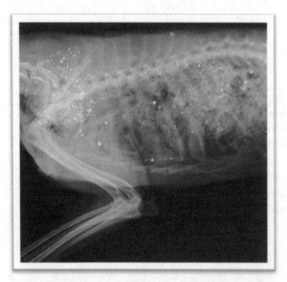

Figure 13.0.8 X-ray photograph of a wild dog shot with a .25-3000 rifle showing a snow storm of lead fragments.

Another possible area of confusion over the missile and the number of shots fired could arise over Winchester 0.25″ ACP (6.35 mm) cartridge loaded with a hollow-point bullet. The cavity of this bullet contains either a steel or lead ball, which is intended to ensure expansion of the bullet in this low-powered round. Rarely does the bullet expand on striking a body, and the ball simply falls out of the cavity, resulting in what appears to be two missiles on the X-ray.

Fibre, and occasionally plastic, shotgun wads can be seen on X-ray photographs, despite the fact that they contain no metallic elements that would be opaque to X-rays. The reason for this is that they pick up lead deposits from previous shots as they pass down the barrel, and these are visualised on the X-ray as faint opaque circles (see Figure 13.0.8). With the move towards more eco-friendly paper cartridges containing felt wads, these could be seen more frequently in the future.

Further reading

1 Brogdon, B.G. (1998). *Forensic Radiology*. CRC Press. ISBN: 0-8493-8105-3.
2 Biddle, M. (2000). *King Arthur's Round Table*. Boydell Press. ISBN: 0-85115-626-6.

14.0

Gunshot Residue Examination

14.0.1 Introduction

When attempting to prove that a person has fired a weapon, the detection of gunshot residues (GSR) on the hands of a suspect can be of great significance.

The use of the scanning electron microscope (SEM) with associated energy dispersive X-ray analyser (EDX) for this analysis is probably the most important advance in the field of forensic firearms examination since the invention of the comparison microscope. It is important, however, that one has an understanding of the limitations of such evidence: the possibility of environmental contamination or cross-contamination; the requirement for minimum particle counts for positive findings; and the importance of associated GSR particles. An overview of the history of the subject will assist in placing the significance of this advanced analytical technique into its true perspective, as well as the shortcomings of some of the other methods which are still in use today.

Even the identification of GSR via the SEM is not without its difficulties. With particles that are often no more than 0.5 microns (also called micrometres; symbol 'μm', $1\,\mu\mathrm{m} = 0.0001\,\mathrm{cm}$ or 3.93×10^{-5} inches) in diameter, the possibility of airborne contamination is very real. With even a light wind, contamination from the exhaust system at a firing range, even if it is a considerable distance away from a scene of a crime, is a very real possibility. Even more likely is cross-contamination from an arresting officer's equipment, even if he or she had not fired a gun for several months.

By observing the strictest of anti-contamination collection procedures, minimum positive particle counts and associated particle ratios, however, the chance of false positive results through contamination can be all but eliminated.

The *FBI Bulletin* of 2011 states:

'In a GSR case, the submitting agency, attorneys, judge, and jury all want to know if the suspect fired a gun. Unfortunately, the presence or absence of GSR on a person's hands cannot answer that question. Rather, as the accepted practice, all positive gunshot residue reports include a qualifier, such as "The presence of primer residue on a person's hand is consistent with that person having discharged a firearm, having been in the vicinity of a firearm when it was discharged, or having handled an item with primer residue on it." Conversely, negative GSR reports often contain a qualifying statement, such as "The absence of gunshot residue on a person's hands does not eliminate that individual from having discharged a firearm." And, when GSR is found on an inanimate object, like clothing, a qualifier could be, "The presence of primer residue on an item is consistent with that item sometime having been in the vicinity of a firearm when it was discharged or having come in contact with primer residue on another item." A forensic GSR report also may list the instrumentation used (e.g. SEM/EDS) and the criteria employed to define the gunshot residue (e.g. elemental composition and morphology). GSR testimony can be challenging because of the difficulty in interpreting the results.'

Forensic Ballistics in Court: Interpretation and Presentation of Firearms Evidence, First Edition. Brian J. Heard.
© 2013 John Wiley & Sons, Ltd. Published 2013 by John Wiley & Sons, Ltd.

14.0.2   Basics

Formation of discharge residue

When a weapon is fired, a great volume of incandescent ($\approx$2,000 °C) gaseous material is produced. This is mainly combustion products from the propellant and consists of carbon dioxide, carbon monoxide, water as steam, and oxides of nitrogen. In among this vast cloud of gases are also partially burnt and unburnt propellant particles and combustion products from the priming compound. These solid particles are collectively called **gunshot residue (GSR)** particles (see Figure 14.0.1). Less frequently, they are also referred to **firearms discharge (FDR)** residues.

One of the most important aspects concerning the primer discharge residues is the mechanism of their formation. The importance of this will become clear in the section dealing with the identification of GSR particles using the scanning electron microscope.

At the moment when the firing pin strikes the primer and the priming compounds violently explode, the temperature in the primer cap rises to approximately 2,500 °C. The metallic components in the residue are volatilised and emerge from the primer pocket as vapour. This cloud of vaporised metallic components rapidly condenses forming exceedingly small spherical and spheroidal particles in the size range 0.1 μm to 5 μm (where 1 μm = 1×10^{-6} metres).

As the vapours produced within the primer pocket are tightly confined, the resulting spheroidal particles will contain various combinations of the elements present. Some will obviously only contain one element, some two, and others all of the metallic elements present. It is the particles containing all of the elements that, together with their morphology, makes them unique to GSR.

Distribution of GSR particles

During the firing of a handgun, the vast majority of gunshot residue particles exit at great velocity from the muzzle of the weapon and are projected away from the firer.

In *self-loading pistols*, some of the remainder escape from the ejection port to settle on the hand holding the weapon. In *revolvers*, some of the particles escape from the gap between the rear of the barrel and

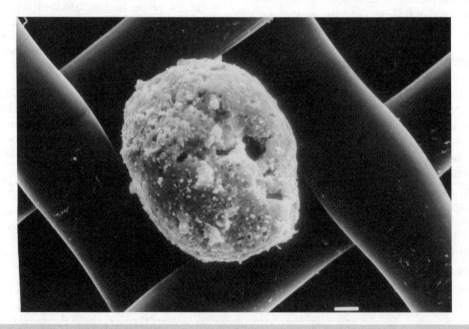

Figure 14.0.1   Large GSR particle. Scale bar = 1 μm.

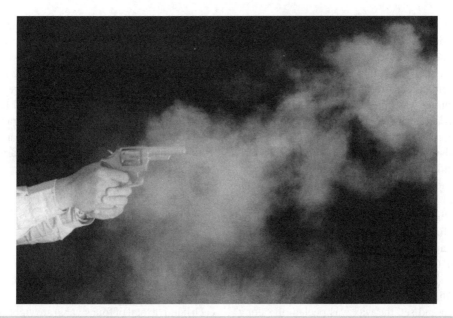

Figure 14.0.2 GSR cloud from firing a revolver.

the front of the cylinder (see Figure 14.0.2). While this gap is somewhat further forward than the ejection port in self-loading pistols, the gases are at a substantially higher pressure and still settle on the firing hand.

In *rifles and shotguns*, the situation is a little different. If the weapon is of the self-loading variety, then gases will escape from the ejection port, as with a self-loading pistol. In this case, residues could be deposited on the hands of the firer, depending on the position of the ejection port. If, however, the weapon is of the bolt-action or locked breech variety, as in a normal break barrel-action shotgun, then there will be virtually no gas escape from the breech end of the barrel until the action is manually opened. In this case, the deposition of GSR on the hands of the firer will only occur if the action is opened immediately after firing.

As well as the GSR particles that escape from the muzzle and breech end of the weapon, some are also left in the fired cartridge case and in the barrel and chamber of the weapon.

The vast majority of the GSR particles produced during the firing of a cartridge consist of partially burnt and unburnt propellant particles, which are mainly organic in nature. The rest consist of the metallic compounds left over from the discharged priming compound. In addition to these, some

particles of plain lead which have volatilised from the base of the bullet, or copper and zinc particles from the inside surface of the cartridge case, are also often found amongst the GSR particles.

With non-toxic ammunition, it is unlikely that material will be volatilised from the base of the bullet, as the materials used in the construction of this type of bullet require a much higher temperature than 2,500 °C.

14.0.3 Identification of GSR Particles

Organic components

The quantity of organic compounds left over from the burning of the propellant is obviously vast in comparison to those from the priming compound. As a result, early attempts at detecting gunshot residues were directed towards the recovery and identification of the organic components. These included the identification of nitrites and nitrates in partially burnt propellant particles, using chemical spot tests.

One very popular test was the **Walker test** (Walker, 1940), which used desensitised photographic paper as a medium to pick up and retain the particles. After picking up the particles, these were then visualised using a chemical spot test for the nitrites present. The technique was, however, mainly intended for recovery of GSR particles from clothes, and was of little use in discovering whether a person had fired a weapon.

The technique was quite long, but was very efficient at picking up partially burnt propellant particles from clothing for range of firing estimations.

The **Greiss**, **Marshal and Tewari tests** were merely variations on the Walker test using different chemicals to produce other coloured diazo compounds.

Probably the most infamous test, and one which is routinely referred to even today, was the **dermal nitrate** or **paraffin test**, which was first introduced by Teodoro Gonzalez of the Mexico City Police laboratory in 1933. This involved taking a cast from the back of the suspects hand using hot paraffin wax. When cooled and set, the wax was peeled off, along with any imbedded GSR particles. The cast was then sprayed with **Lunge reagent**, which is a 0.25 per cent solution of diphenylbenzidine in concentrated sulphuric acid. Later variations of the test used diphenylamine in concentrated sulphuric acid. Both of these reagents gave a deep blue coloration with nitrates from the partially burnt and unburnt propellant particles.

Unlike the Walker, Greiss and Marshall tests, which merely indicated the presence of these particles on the hands, the paraffin test did give a distribution pattern for the particles.

As particles are only deposited on the back of the hand during firing, the palm being wrapped around the weapon's grip and thus protected, the presence of these particles only on the back of the hands is highly indicative of a person having fired a weapon.

While it gave good information regarding the distribution of these particles, the test itself was not only indicative of nitrates. Fertiliser, rust, face powder, sugar, paint and even urine were also found to give a positive reaction to the Lunge reagent. In 1935, the FBI indicated that the test was not specific and cautioned against its further use[1].

Thin layer and gas chromatography were also used at this time to detect the nitrocellulose component of propellants. While these were quite

---

[1] *FBI Law Enforcement Bulletin*, Vol. 4, No.10 (1935) and Vol. 9, (1940).

successful, nitrocellulose is not a desirable analyte for GSR analysis due to its presence in many consumer products such as nail polish, wood finishes, paints and even the surface of playing cards.

Gas chromatography and high-pressure liquid chromatography have also been used for the identification of propellant particles (Andrasko, 1992).

As the identification of propellant particles is less specific than that of the primer discharge residues, such methods have found little favour.

Inorganic or metallic component identification

In the 1950s, a test was developed (Harrison & Gillroy, 1959) for the identification of lead, barium and antimony, the main metallic components of primer discharge residues. In this test, the back and palm of each hand (a total of four swabs) are vigorously rubbed with a swab moistened with dilute hydrochloric acid. This physically removes any GSR particles and places them into an acidic environment. The swab is then dried and treated with a solution of triphenylmethylarsonium iodide. Any orange spots indicate the presence of antimony. After drying, a solution of sodium rhodizonate is added. Any red spots indicate barium; if these turn purple on the addition of dilute hydrochloric acid, this indicates the presence of lead.

The great advantage of this test over the dermal nitrate test was the low incidence of false positives. Its shortcomings, however, included a relatively low sensitivity and the fact that it only showed the presence of the individual elements on the hands. What was required was to show the presence of all three elements in discrete particles, as occurs in GSR particles. Merely identifying the presence of the individual elements leaves open the interpretation as to whether they originated from the discharge of a firearm or from the general environmental and occupational contaminants.

In 1966, the use of **neutron activation analysis** (NAA) for the identification of GSR was reported (Ruch *et al.*, 1964). In this, the samples are placed in a nuclear reactor and bombarded with neutrons, making the various elements present radioactive. By analysing the energy distribution and intensity of the radioactive emissions, it is possible to identify the elements present and the amount of each. This is a highly sensitive method of analysis for most elements but it is, of course, not applicable to lead, the main component of GSR. Another problem is that not everybody has a convenient nuclear reactor.

In 1970, Bashinki, Davis and Young of the Oakland Police Laboratory, USA, reported on the use of sodium rhodizonate for the detection of GSR. This test is only useful for the identification of lead and barium but, because of its sensitivity and simplicity, it is still a commonly used test. While it is of little use in determining whether a person has fired a gun, it is still very useful for range of firing estimations on dark clothing and the identification of entry and exit holes in clothing.

In 1972, a technique was reported for the analysis of GSR by **atomic absorption spectroscopy** (AAS; Green & Sauve, 1973). Atomic absorption derives its name from the fact that the atoms of an element will absorb light at a wavelength which is particular to that element. Also, the quantity of light absorbed is proportional to the quantity of that element present.

Basically, a solution of the chemical under test is aspirated into a flame which is sufficiently hot to vaporise the element into its free atoms. If light of the appropriate wavelength is shone through the flame, a portion of the light will be absorbed by the free atoms present. It is the wavelength of the light absorbed that identifies the element present, and the quantity of light absorbed that reveals the quantity of the element.

Heated graphite tubes were later used instead of a flame, as this was found to give a greatly enhanced sensitivity. This technique was called **flameless atomic absorption spectroscopy** (FAAS). While this is an extremely sensitive and accurate analytical technique for lead, barium and antimony, it still lacks the specificity required. The results only show that the three elements are present – it can not show that they are all in a single particle. As such, the elements could be environmental contaminants picked up separately (e.g. antimony as a surfactant on most fibres to give them lustre, barium from face make-up powders and lead from battery terminals or innumerable other sources).

Many other techniques have been tried, including proton-induced X-ray emission (Sen *et al.*, 1982), anodic stripping voltammetry (Brihaye *et al.*, 1982) and auger electron microscopy (Hellmiss *et al.*,

1987). For one reason or another, none of these has ever gained any great deal of credibility. The most that can be said for any of them is that they provide presumptive evidence for the presence of GSR particles. This lack of certainty can reduce the value of this type of scientific evidence in a court of law to near zero.

14.0.4 The use of the scanning electron microscope (SEM) with energy dispersive X-Ray analysis (EDX) for the detection and analysis of GSR particles

The most successful technique to date for the analysis of GSR particles is without a doubt the scanning electron microscope with an energy dispersive X-ray analyser (SEM-EDX). Basically, this is a microscope which uses a beam of electrons to visualise the object under observation, rather than visible light as in a conventional optical microscope. As the beam of electrons is focused by a series of magnets rather than glass lenses, the control is infinitely finer. The electron beam scans the sample in a raster pattern, which is picked up, after reflection from the object under examination, by a video camera. The image is then manipulated electronically and the result visualised on a high-definition monitor.

With a depth of field in the region of two hundreds times greater than an optical microscope and an extremely high resolution, magnifications in excess of 1,000,000× are possible. With this depth of field, images appear to be almost three-dimensional.

In addition, on striking the sample, the electrons give up some of their energy to the elements present and this energy is then re-emitted as X-rays, the wavelength of which is particular to the elements present. These X-rays are analysed via the EDX for wavelength and intensity, and a qualitative and quantitative analysis of the object under examination can be obtained. It should be emphasised here that for GSR analysis, a quantitative (i.e. the quantities or percentages of each element present in a sample) analysis is not applicable, as the GSR particles are formed from a gaseous cloud containing an imperfect mixture of the primer residues.

With most of the other techniques used for GSR analysis, the sample is destroyed during its examination. With the SEM-EDX, however, the sample is virtually unaffected by the analysis and can be re-examined, if necessary, many times. This is very relevant for defence examinations and should be taken advantage of.

Probably the earliest researches into the use of the SEM/EDX for GSR analysis were carried out in the Metropolitan Police Forensic Laboratory in New Scotland Yard, London, around 1968 by the author and Dr Robin Keeley. However, it was not until 1978 that the first paper was published as a Metropolitan Police Forensic Laboratory Report. This was a general introduction to electron microscopy, with GSR examination forming only a small part. It did, however, lay down the basic techniques for the collection, examination and identification of GSR tapings taken from the hands of suspects.

In 1977, Metracardi & Kilty of the FBI laboratory produced an extensive paper on the subject (Matricardi & Kilty, 1977). Without doubt, the most extensive work on SEM/EDX for GSR analysis was a paper by Wolten et al. (1977). This was a contract paper sponsored under the Law Enforcement Administration and its findings probably did more to advance this subject than any other. The paper is in three parts and covers everything from primer compositions, particle formation, distribution during firing, collection, analysis and interpretation, to environmental considerations.

Other papers followed in profusion (DeGaetano, 1992; Zeichner et al., 1992; Gunaratnam & Himber, 1994; Zeichner et al., 1989; Wallace & McQuillan, 1984), all of which have added more to the science.

The basic techniques for obtaining the samples and examining them on the SEM have, however, remained the same.

It should be noted at this juncture that the commonly held belief that GSR particles must be spherical is completely wrong. At best, they are spheroidal, and they are most usually amorphous. However, angular-shaped objects cannot be GSR, as GSR particles have condensed from vaporised primer residues. One infamous paper described in great detail, with associated photographs, how spherical GSR particles had been recovered from numerous suspects. Unfortunately, the photographs showed perfectly circular impressions on the tapings where the particles had been shaken out of a fired cartridge case.

It should also be emphasised that any particle recovered from the hands of a suspect over $5\,\mu m$ in diameter should be viewed with great suspicion. GSR particles are not stuck to the hands by some 'magic super glue' type material – they are simply lying on the surface or trapped in the hair follicles and minute folds in the skin. Large particles will fall off extremely rapidly, and any found on a hand taping could, at best, result from contamination.

14.0.5   Sample collection

The methodology for sample collection for GSR analysis is simplicity itself. The most commonly used technique employs a 1 cm × 1 cm strip of double-sided adhesive tape stuck onto a thin acetate strip. The acetate strip allows the adhesive surface to be manipulated conveniently without any fear of contact with the sampler's hands. One of these tapes is used to take samples from each of the four areas, as illustrated below.

During the taking of the samples, the skin must be stretched as far as possible to ensure that any GSR particles that may be hidden within the folds of the skin or inside the hair follicles are removed. It is absolutely essential that the sampler wears a different pair of disposable gloves for each sample taken.

It is important to cover the sampled area at least three times, even if the adhesive has lost its tackiness. The adhesive is quite soft and particles can still be pressed into the surface even if there is no discernible stickiness left.

It is also important to be consistent in the number of times the area is covered, to ensure constancy for interpretation of the results.

Alternative sampling technique

Although a 1 cm × 1 cm square of double-sided adhesive tape on a strip of acetate is an effective and cheap way of collecting samples for GSR examination, it does have a number of disadvantages. Of these, the most serious is the requirement for it to be carbon-coated and the concomitant possibility of contamination.

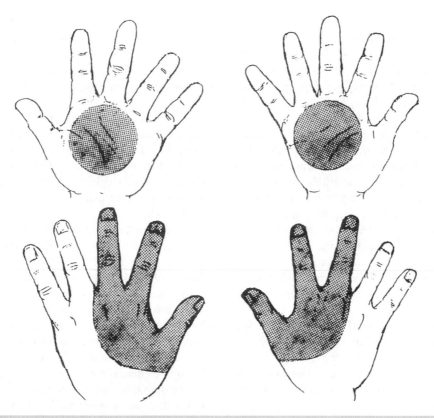

Figure 14.0.3 Sampling areas for GSR taping.

The carbon coating must be applied to prevent the sample charging while it is being scanned by the SEM electron beam. This is an essential stage in the sample preparation when using this type of sampling technique and it cannot be skipped.

For carbon coating, the sample must go through the following procedures:

- Removal of acetate strip containing sample from the protective tube.

- Removing the 1 cm × 1 cm sample from the acetate strip.

- Sticking the sample onto an SEM stub with double-sided tape.

- Placing the stub in a multiple stub holder for coating.

- Sputter-coating the sample in a near vacuum.

- Re-pressurising the coater to ambient conditions.

- Transfer of the sample from the coater to the SEM.

Each and every step involves the possible contamination of the sample, with the two most serious being:

1. Placing the sample alongside other samples and, more seriously, control GSR samples in the sputter coater while air is drawn across the sample as the coating chamber is evacuated.

2. Re-pressurising the coater chamber, where a large volume of potentially contaminated air from outside is drawn across the sample.

This whole process can, however, be simplified, and the number of procedures where the sample is exposed to the outside air can be reduced to an absolute minimum. This involves the use of pre-carbon-coated adhesive discs.

These adhesive discs are similar to double-sided tape, but the adhesive material, which is specially formulated for SEM use, is pre-impregnated with carbon dust. This completely eliminates the requirement for carbon-coating of the sample.

These discs are available from SEM supply companies, who can pre-apply these to SEM stubs. These stubs are then individually placed in clean, sealed SEM stub tubes under ultra-clean conditions. The tubes have special stub holders in the cap, which enables a tube to be removed simply from the cap for sampling. Once the tube is replaced over the cap, it self-seals, preventing any chance of the sample being tampered with.

With this sampling technique, the tube is simply taken off the cap and the adhesive disc is dabbed over the relevant part of the hand and then replaced back in the tube.

When it comes to the SEM examination, the SEM stub is removed from the cap with a pair of SEM stub tweezers and is transferred to the SEM stub holder and into the SEM chamber. It can then be examined directly in the SEM without any further treatment.

Sampling precautions

If the hands being sampled are wet or have been sweating, they should be allowed to dry naturally. Blow-drying the hands must *not* be used, since it will remove all GSR particles. There is also the additional problem of the blow dryer itself being contaminated, or airborne contamination being blown onto the hands.

Sampling from areas of the hand that are covered with blood should be avoided at all costs, as the imaging technique used during the searching for the particles (back-scattered imaging) is completely overloaded by the iron content of haemoglobin in blood.

It is extremely important that any chance of contamination be avoided. There will, in all probability, be only a few particles of GSR deposited on the hands after firing a round of ammunition. Contamination by a single particle of stray GSR from the sampler would be extremely difficult to detect and could easily be construed as a false positive result.

If the sampler has any contact at all with firearms they should, before taking the samples, change their clothes, shower and wash their hair thoroughly. During the taking of samples disposable gloves, boiler suit and hair cover should also be worn. The gloves should be changed after each sample has been taken, even if the sampler has had no contact with a weapon. The disposable suit should be changed for each suspect examined. It should also be stressed that, if the suspect has to be handcuffed, new disposable nylon restraints should be used, rather than police-issue handcuffs, which may well have been contaminated either from range courses or from a gun that the officer might be wearing.

A control blank taping should also be submitted with the samples. The tapings should be placed in individual bottles and sealed; the individual bottles should be placed in sealed bags, and the sealed bags placed in another sealed bag. All disposable gloves and suits must be retained and sealed in separate bags, in case there is any question of cross- or airborne contamination.

Illustrative Case 1

The following case gives a rather extreme example of how easy it is to contaminate GSR samples. During conversations with the firearms examiners at a particular laboratory, it was discovered that all their shooting incidents were with .22″ weapons. The officers were also proud to point out that they had never had one negative case with respect to GSR, and that they always found lead, barium, antimony and aluminium on their hand tapings. This was a little surprising, as the vast majority of .22″ priming compounds contain only lead and barium. It transpired that the officers, who did all the sampling themselves, were also firearms instructors, firing anything up to 200 rounds a day. The ammunition they fired, unsurprisingly, contained lead, barium, antimony and aluminium in the primer.

14.0.6 GSR retention

Gunshot residue particles deposited on the hands as a result of firing are not stuck there by some 'magic' glue like property, and neither are they imbedded in the skin. They are merely lying on the surface of the skin and are, therefore, readily removed by everyday activities.

If there is anything in their favour for being retained on the surface of the skin, it is their exceedingly small size. Being in the range of 0.1–5.0 μm, they readily become trapped in the microscopic folds of the skin or drop down into hair follicles. Even so, for all practical purposes, all GSR particles will be removed from the hands by everyday activities within three hours of a weapon being fired.

Washing the hands will immediately remove all the GSR particles. Great care should also be taken if a suspect requests to be allowed to go to the toilet as urine is also very effective at removing GSR particles. Likewise, if the suspect requires medical treatment and is covered in a rough hospital blanket, the GSR particles will also be immediately removed. This is most important.

Insertion of drips into the back of the hand by the hospital should also be discouraged, as the insertion point is usually scrubbed with a disinfectant. The medical profession are usually more than willing to assist, and other sites for drip needles are easily located.

If it is raining or the suspect is sweating heavily at the time of firing, the result will, once again, be negative.

In the case of a deceased person, the problem of removal of GSR particles by everyday activities is not relevant. Assuming the GSR particles are not removed by some external means, they should remain on the hands of the deceased indefinitely. If, however, the body has been placed in the mortuary refrigerator, the skin does become clammy and it is very difficult to take the samples. If possible, it is preferable to take the GSR tapings from the body at the scene or, if not, as soon as possible after the body has arrived at the mortuary.

Conservation of GSR particles

On arrest, every attempt should be made to preserve what residues may be on the hands and to prevent any contamination until the samples can be taken. The only way to do this is to cover each hand, either with paper bags or with large, clean envelopes. Being porous, the paper bags will reduce sweating and the likelihood for either contamination or the accidental or purposeful removal of GSR particles.

Any attempt at conserving any GSR particles that may be on the hands by placing them in polyethylene bags is very detrimental to recovery rates. The

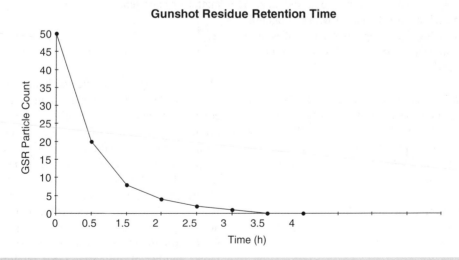

Gunshot Residue Retention Time

Figure 14.0.4   GSR retention vs. time.

problem here is that the hands sweat profusely in the bags, and any residues that may be present will very soon end up in the bottom of the bag. There is also a problem with static electricity attracting the particles from the hands onto the surface of the bag.

GSR distribution

When interpreting GSR distribution results from an SEM analysis of the four tapings taken from hands, the following points must be considered:

- The gases issuing from the muzzle are projected at great velocity away from the firer. Unless there is a very strong wind blowing towards the firer, these GSR containing gases will not be deposited on the hands.

- The gases issuing from the breech end of the barrel, whether it is a revolver or a self-loading pistol, are of much lower velocity than those from the muzzle. Unless the non-firing hand is held within a few inches of the gun during firing, these gases will only be deposited on the back of the firing hand.

- The palm of the firing hand will be protected from the deposition of any GSR particles during firing, as it is wrapped around the grip.

- In a weapon which has been fired, both the muzzle and the breech end of the barrel will be contaminated with GSR. Handling these areas of a fired weapon will deposit GSR particles onto the palms of the hands.

- Immediately after firing a weapon, the GSR distribution pattern on the hands will be fairly predictable. With time, however, there will be some redistribution of particles over the hands. The interpretation of GSR distribution vs. time patterns can be difficult.

Bearing in mind the above, there are four basic GSR distribution patterns which may be encountered. These are as follows:

1. *GSR particles found only on the taping taken from the back of the right (or left if the person is left-handed) hand.* This is highly indicative of the person having fired a weapon in that hand.

2. *GSR particles found only on the tapings taken from the backs of both hands.* This is highly indicative that the person fired the weapon in one hand while supporting the firing hand with the other.

3. *GSR particles found on all four tapings.* This would indicate that the person was standing in front of a weapon when it was fired and was enveloped in the large cloud of gases emanating from the muzzle of the weapon. The person could have been either an innocent bystander or part of, say, a gang carrying out a robbery.

4. *GSR particles only on the tapings taken from the palms of both hands.* This could indicate that the person had merely handled a weapon which had been recently fired.

When considering these interpretations, it must be kept in mind that the longer the elapsed time between the firing incident and taking the tapings, the greater the redistribution of particles. As the elapsed time increases, greater emphasis must be placed on the interpretation of indicative GSR particle distribution and the indicative GSR to confirmed GSR particle ratio (see below). This interpretation is purely a matter of experience.

14.0.7 Interpretation of results

Merely looking for particles on hand tapings which match, in elemental composition, those taken from a control cartridge case is simply not enough. Not all primer residue particles formed during the firing of a weapon will contain all the of elements present in the original primer mix. If a standard primer composition of lead styphnate (or lead peroxide), barium nitrate and antimony sulphide is taken, then only particles which contain lead (Pb), barium (Ba) and antimony (Sb) can be positively identified as being GSR particles. There will, however, be a very much larger number of **indicative GSR particles** formed at the same time. These indicative GSR particles can contain Pb/Sb, Pb/Ba or Ba/Sb.

There will be, depending on the ammunition type and make, a very approximate relationship between the ratios of these confirmed GSR particles and indicative GSR particles.

Other particles of indeterminate origin will also be present which contain only Pb, Ba or Sb. If the bullet is plain lead or has an exposed lead base, there will also be a distinct GSR/Pb ratio from lead volatilised from the base of the bullet.

The ratio of plain lead particles to GSR particles (in ammunition containing a plain lead bullet) will be higher at the muzzle than at the breech end of the barrel. This can be accounted for by:

- the hot gases emerging from the muzzle having had longer to volatilise the lead from the base of the bullet than those emerging from the breech;

- the fact that particles of lead are torn off the sides of the bullet as it passes down the rifling.

This can be extremely useful when determining whether particles found on a suspect's hands were from actually firing a weapon or whether they were from merely being in front of the weapon, possibly as an innocent bystander, when it was fired.

For example, at the breech end of the barrel, Winchester .38″ Special calibre plain lead ammunition the residues have a ratio of approximately 15 plain lead particles to every confirmed GSR particle, but at the muzzle this will be in excess of 35 plain lead particles to every GSR particle.

These ratios are only very approximate and can only be obtained from controlled test firings, not only with different types of ammunition but also barrel lengths. Likewise, they are only of use in ammunition which have plain lead (i.e. non-jacketed) bullets.

The situation with fully jacketed ammunition is similar, but the Pb/GSR ratio is much lower due to the smaller area of lead that is exposed. Some interpretation of the Pb/GSR ratios at the breech can be made, but this is much more difficult. In this situation, it is probably better to search for Cu/Zn particles which may have been stripped from the bullet jacket by the rifling. These particles should only be present in the residues issuing from the muzzle.

For non-toxic ammunition, it is extremely difficult for such an interpretation to be attempted, due to the vast range of primer compositions and bullet alloys

in use. Any such determination will have to be taken on a case-by-case basis, using exactly the same ammunition as that used in the shooting incident.

Minimum requirements for a positive result

One major question when interpreting GSR results concerns the minimum number of GSR particles that constitute a positive result. If the necessity for associated particle identification is taken into consideration, then the answer must be 'one'. However, the fact that the above ratios for confirmed GSR to indicative GSR particles is based on averages when a number of confirmed particles much larger than one are present must not be forgotten. For example, if the ratio were 1 : 5 for breech-emitted particles, where there are 50 positive GSR particles, then the possibility for there being only one positive GSR particle with no associated particles is high.

Several papers (Singer et al., 1996; DeGaetano& Siegel, 1990; ASTM E1588, 1993) have investigated the common laboratory practice for the threshold limit for a positive finding of GSR on hand tapings. The results are varied, with most coming out in the 1–2 region.

In practice, the situation is a little more complex. If, for example, one is an area where the police force is issued with ammunition containing Pb, Ba, Sb, Al and the criminals are using ammunition containing Hg, Sn, K, Cl, the finding of only one Hg, Sn, K, Cl particle on the hands of a suspect would have far more significance than if both the criminals and the police were using the same kind of ammunition.

In the author's previous laboratory, even though the GSR in ammunition issued to the police and that used by the criminals was radically different, the bench mark of a minimum of two confirmed GSR particles, *together with associated particles*, was considered the absolute lowest limit for a positive result.

14.0.8 Identification of type of ammunition and country or origin from GSR composition

Modern centre fire ammunition from western countries (i.e. Europe, North America, Australia, New Zealand, etc.) all contain a very similar priming composition, the basic elements found being Pb, Ba and Sb, with calcium silicide and/or powdered glass giving silicon (Si). With so little variation, it is therefore very difficult to make any differentiation between calibres and origin.

Aluminium (Al), magnesium (Mg) or titanium (Ti) can also often be added to increase the temperature and the burn time of the flame produced. This is usually found in the higher pressure cartridges (e.g. 9 mm PB, .357″ Magnum and + P cartridges). This can, sometimes be useful in identifying the type of ammunition fired.

Centre fire ammunition from what was previously called the Warsaw Pact countries (i.e. Russia, Poland, Czechoslovakia, Hungary, Rumania, etc.), as well as China and Korea, tend to have a completely different primer composition. Generally speaking, these priming compounds are much more corrosive than those found elsewhere in the world.

The basic elements found in these priming compounds are:

- Mercury (Hg);

- Tin (Sn);

- Antimony (Sb);

- Phosphorous (P);

- Potassium (K);

- Sodium (Na);

- Silicon (Si); and

- Calcium (Ca).

Other compounds occasionally encountered include:

- Lead (Pb);

- Barium (Ba);

- Silver (Ag);

- Zinc (Zn);

- Copper (Cu);

- Magnesium (Mg);

- Aluminium (Al); and

- Lanthanum/cerium/Iron (basically lighter flint or Mischmetal).

It is this great diversity of elements which, in some circumstances, enables the identification of calibre, country of origin and sometimes even a factory code from the GSR composition. In rare instances, it is even possible to give an approximate date of manufacture for the ammunition based solely on the GSR composition.

Illustrative Case 2

After robbing a bank of several tens of millions of dollars, a very large and determined gang of heavily armed robbers became involved in a running shoot-out with the police through the streets. At one point, an innocent bystander turned a corner and was shot in the head by one of the culprits. The bullet was a .357″ Magnum, and GSR found on the base of the bullet contained Pb, Ba, Sb, Si and Al. This was the only round of .357″ Magnum fired during the chase, the rest being .38″ Special, none of which contained aluminium in the GSR. Some time later, a number of string gloves were found on a hillside, along with some of the stolen money and guns. It was easy to determine, from GSR found in the weave of the gloves, which one had been used to fire the .357″ Magnum round, and it was easy to determine which of the guns had fired the fatal bullet. Luckily, the glove in question also had some blood from where the wearer had cut his hand on a piece of glass. Eventually, suspects were located, and it was just a matter of blood-grouping them to determine who had been wearing the glove that had been used to fire the fatal shot.

14.0.9 Environmental contaminants

When interpreting GSR/Pb ratios, great care should be exercised to correctly identify particles containing lead and bromine (Br). These particles have been found in the emissions from car exhausts and came from the ethylene dibromide which was used to remove the lead in the petrol anti-knock compound lead tetraethyl. Although petrol containing ethylene dibromide has been unavailable for many years now, there is still so much Pb/Br from this in the general environment that it is still occasionally found on people's hands.

Likewise, barium is also utilised in face powders and as a filler in paper. In these situations, it is nearly always associated with sulphur (S) and should be readily identified.

With modern non-corrosive ammunition of a Western origin, it is very rare to find sulphur in a priming compound. In $7.62 \times 25\,mm$ and $7.62 \times 39\,mm$ ammunition, however, barium and sulphur are often found together in the priming compound, and thus confusion can arise.

Lead is alloyed with antimony in battery plates and type metal. It is also alloyed with tin and/or antimony in solder. This is a common contaminant, especially with anyone working in the printing or car repair trade.

Antimony is also used, as its oxide, as a fire retardant in cotton and polyester blend fibres.

Zirconium and titanium (used in lead free primer compounds) is used as fluoro complexes in the treatment of wool.

Sources of elements commonly found in lead-based gunshot residues

Table 14.0.1 Some of the More Common Lead Alloys

Alloy	Uses
Pb-Sb	Tank linings, coils, pumps, valves, lead-lined pipes, car storage batteries, collapsible tubes, bullets, lead shot, insoluble anodes.
Cu-Pb-Sb	Type metals, bearings, special casting alloys
Ca-Pb	Grids of industrial storage batteries, tape to separate double-glazing panes
Cu-Pb	Car and aircraft bearings and bushings
Ag-Pb	Solders, insoluble anode in electro-winning of Zn, manganese refining
Te-Pb	Pipe and sheet in chemical installations
Sn-Pb	Solders (tin cans, circuit boards), manufacture of car radiators, heat exchangers, car industry (covering welded body sections), corrosive protective coatings on steel and copper, gaskets, metal furniture, gutter piping and fittings, roof flashing, coating on steel and copper electronic components
Sn-Sb-Pb	Sleeve bearings, casting alloys, slush castings, journal bearings (railway freight cars)
Pb-Sn-Bi-Cd	Sprinkler systems, foundry patterns, moulds, died and punches, chucks, cores, mandrills, low-temperature solders

Table 14.0.2 Some of the More Common Lead Compounds

Compound	Use
Lead arsenates	Insecticides
Lead azides	Explosives, priming compounds
Lead borate	Glazes, enamels on pottery, porcelain, china work, drier in paints
Basic lead carbonates	Exterior paints, ceramic glazes and enamels
Lead chromates	Paint pigments
Lead silichromates	Paint pigments
Lead cyanamide	Anti-rust paints
Lead 2-ethylhexoate	Driers, metallic soap
Lead fluorosilicate	Electrolyte in electrolytic refining of lead

(continued)

Table 14.0.2 (*Continued*)

Compound	Use
Lead formate	Manufacture of specialised rubber compounds
Tetrabasic lead fumarate	Heat stabiliser for plastisols, records, electric insulation, vulcanisation reagent
Lead chloride	Laboratory drying agent
Lead lineolate	Driers, metallic soaps
Lead maleate	Vulcanising agent for chlorosulphonated polyethylene
Lead molybdate	Anticorrosive paint pigment
Lead nitrate	Match industry, pyrotechnics
Lead oleates	Metallic soap
Lead monoxide	Litharge – ceramic industry, manufacture of glasses, glazes, vitreous enamels, oil refining, insecticides
Trilead tetroxide	Storage batteries, paints, ceramic industry, lubricants, petroleum, rubber
Lead dioxide	Manufacture of dyes, chemical, matches, pyrotechnics, rubber substitutes, polysulfide polymers
Lead seleride	In IR detectors
Lead silicates	Glass, ceramics, high temp dry lubricant
Lead stannate	Manufacture of ceramic and electronic bodies
Lead sulphate	Paint pigments, stabilisers for vinyl and other plastics, lead storage battery
Lead sulphide	Semiconductors, photoelectric cells, photosensitive resistor circuits
Lead tellate	Driers, metallic soaps
Lead telluride	Semiconductors, IR detection, heat sensing instruments
Lead thiocyanate	Matches, explosives, priming compounds
Lead thiosulphate	Vulcanising rubber, deposition of lead mirrors
Lead tungstate	Pigment
Lead zirconate	Ferroelectric characteristics, memory devices for computers
Tetraalkyllead	Gasoline industry, organomercury fungicides

Table 14.0.3 Some of the More Common Antimony Compounds

Compound	Use
Pure antimony	Ornamental applications
Antimony alloys	Type metal, battery grids, bearing metal, cable covering, sheet and pipe, plumbers solder, pewter, Britannia metal, bullets, shrapnel
Antimony oxide	Flame retardant, glasses, ceramics, vitreous enamels, opacifier
Antimony fluoride	Mordant in dyeing
Antimony chloride	Catalyst and mordant in calico dyeing
Antimony sulphide	Fireworks, matches, priming compounds
Tartar emetic	Medicines, insecticide, mordant in dyeing

Table 14.0.4 Some of the More Common Barium compounds

Compound	Use
Barium carbonate	Ceramic industry, optical glasses, flux, steel carburising, paper industry
Barium sulphate	Paper industry
Barium ferrite	Inexpensive magnetic materials
Barium chloride	Blanc fixe for photographic paper, leather and cloth, case hardening, heat-treating baths
Barium nitrate	Pyrotechnics, green flares, tracer bullets, primers, detonators
Barium sulphate	Barium meal X-rays, anti-diarrhoeal and demulcent powder, manufacture of linoleum, oilcloth, storage battery, rubber, cosmetics face powder, paint and pigments, oil well treatment, paint filler
Barium titanate	Transducer crystal used in sonar equipment, record pick-up cartridge and other electronic equipment

14.0.10 Extending the period over which GSR particles can be recovered

As stated earlier, GSR particles will be lost rapidly from the surface of the hands through everyday activities. Within three hours – four at the absolute most – all GSR particles will have been lost from the hands. It should be noted here that the resolution of the SEM will ultimately determine the time limit for the identification of GSR particles. If the instrument cannot resolve an image smaller than 2 μm, then one is unlikely to identify GSR particles after two hours. If the resolution for GSR particles is 0.25 μm, then four hours might be a possibility. It is, therefore important to establish the exact parameters within which the instrument operates.

In the search for alternative sampling sites where these particles might be retained for longer periods, the face, hair cuffs of jackets and the front of any clothing worn have been examined. Although some of these areas showed promise, they all suffered from the same problem – that is, the GSR vented from the breech end of a pistol is of low velocity and, as such, particles can only be found on the surfaces immediately surrounding the breech of the weapon (i.e. the hands). Therefore, the likelihood of any GSR particles being found on any of these alternative sites, unless a strong wind is blowing towards the firer, is extremely small.

However, it has been found[2] that if the firing hand is put into a trouser pocket, some of the GSR particles are transferred from the back of the hand onto the inside surfaces of the pocket. With time, these particles gravitate to the bottom of the pocket and become trapped within the folds of material and general pocket fluff and debris that accumulate in this area. The particles are protected so well by this debris that they are not affected by repeated washing and dry cleaning of the trousers. GSR particles have been recovered up to 16 months after a shooting incident.

However, recovery of GSR particles from the inside of a pocket is somewhat problematical, as they become associated with large quantities of organic and inorganic material. This debris not only makes efficient recovery difficult, it also interferes with the SEM examination.

Using a vacuuming system has been suggested, but recovery rates have been found by the author to be unacceptably low. This is probably due to the requirement for a filtering medium (usually a paper thimble inside a specialised holder) of sufficiently small pore size to trap GSR particles of 1 μm or less but still able to provide sufficient negative pressure to pick up the debris. With high vacuum pressures, it was found that the small particles are sucked straight through the paper thimble and lost.

Picking up the debris with an adhesive-covered (a high molecular weight polyisobutylene) aluminium disc, then dissolving the adhesive material from the disc in an organic solvent, has been tried with some success[3]. In this system, the debris-covered adhesive is removed from the disc by dissolving it in a suitable solvent. The resulting solution, together with suspended debris, is then passed though a two-stage filter system. The first filter, which is generally of about 100 μm pore size, is to filter out the general debris. The second, of pore size 0.5 μm or 1 μm and of the nucleopore type, collects any GSR particles which are present.

Whilst the vacuum and solvents used in this method tend to result in the GSR particles losing their distinctive morphology, it does leave a fairly clean sample for analysis. Unfortunately, the potential for GSR loss is, once again, quite high. There is also a high risk of contamination, not only due to the number of processes that must be gone through but also to the high vacuum required for the filtration sucking in airborne contamination.

A much better recovery rate can be obtained by lifting the debris from the pocket with a 1.5 × 1.5 cm taping and removing the excess organic debris by treatment in a low temperature oxygen plasma asher. The plasma asher 'burns' off the organic debris by way of a highly reactive form of oxygen at a temperature not much higher than ambient. By careful manipulation of the oxygen plasma, it is possible to remove virtually all of the general organic debris without touching the adhesive material on the strip.

---

[2] Unpublished work by author.

[3] Wallace, *J. Northern Ireland Forensic Science Laboratory Methods Manual.*

Illustrative Case 3

A case which illustrates the use of GSR in the investigation of crime and the recovery of particles from trouser pockets involved a robbery at a jewellers shop in Central District of Hong Kong.

One robber was posted outside of the shop as a lookout, while the rest robbed the shop. A police constable on normal patrol noticed that something was amiss and ran towards the shop. At that stage, the lookout fired a shot at the constable which, luckily, missed. While the officer dived for cover in an adjacent shop doorway, the robbers came out of the shop and threw a hand grenade into the street to deter any would-be pursuers. They made good their escape in a waiting car.

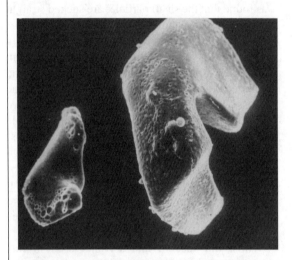

Figure 14.0.5 Propellant particle recovered from sign.

An examination of the scene did not reveal the presence of any bullets or cartridge cases, but there was a bullet ricochet mark on a traffic sign under which the constable had been standing when the shot was fired. The relevant portion of the traffic sign was removed and tapings taken from the impact area for examination under the SEM.

The examination revealed the presence of microscopic fragments of steel with a thin coating of copper, along with a smear of lead and a small fragment of partially burnt propellant (Figure 14.0.5). On the propellant particle were two spheres of GSR (Figure 14.0.6). An EDX analysis of the GSR particles showed them to contain mercury, tin, antimony, potassium, chlorine and phosphorous. This type of GSR composition was typical of that found in 7.62×25 mm Chinese ammunition (Figure 14.0.7), but nothing exactly matching such a composition had ever been encountered before.

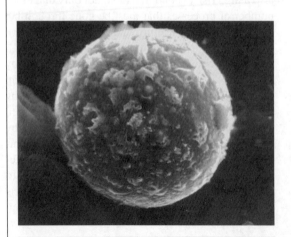

Figure 14.0.6 GSR on propellant particle.

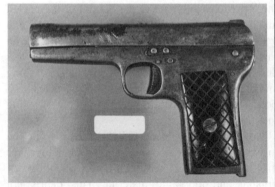

Figure 14.0.7 Home-made 7.62×25 mm pistol.

Steel covered with copper is also typical of 7.62×25 mm ammunition. The presence of a smear of lead with GSR particles would suggest that the bullet was tumbling at the time of impact and probably travelling backwards. This was probably due to the bullet having been fired through a home-made, non-rifled barrel.

Some eight months later, a suspect was arrested, and in his flat was found a home-made 7.62×25 mm pistol with an unrifled barrel. Tapings taken from inside the barrel showed the last round of ammunition to have been fired had exactly the same GSR composition as that found on the traffic sign. This taping also showed that the last round of ammunition to have been fired had a copper-coated steel bullet. A search through the suspect's clothes revealed a pair of trousers fitting the description of those worn by the robber who fired the gun at the constable. Tapings from inside the pockets revealed the presence, in the right-hand pocket only, of particles of GSR with exactly the same composition as those found in the barrel and on the sign.

While these results could not convict alone, they did form very strong supportive evidence.

Illustrative Case 4: The Jill Dando Murder.

In April 1999, Jill Dando, a highly respected TV newsreader, was found dead outside her home. Death had been caused by a single, contact shot to the head from a 9 mm PB pistol. Almost a year later, a suspect, Barry George, was arrested and charged with her murder.

The evidence against Barry George was almost entirely circumstantial and based around his interest in toy replica firearms, a history of stalking and the fact that he was seen in the vicinity on the day of the shooting. This last piece of circumstantial evidence was, however, largely discounted as he lived in a street quite close to where the victim lived.

The only forensic evidence was a single, spherical particle of gunshot residue in the pocket of one of his coats. This particle contained lead, barium, antimony and aluminium, the same as that found around the fatal wound. There has never been mention of any associated/indicative particles being found.

During the trial, the prosecution said that the spherical particle found in Barry George's coat pocket provided 'compelling' evidence of guilt. In July 2001, he was found guilty by a 10–1 majority and sentenced to life imprisonment.

In July 2002, George lost an appeal against an unsafe conviction, and in December 2002, the Final Court of Appeal once again refused an application for appeal. However, in June 2007, the Criminal Cases Review Board granted George the right to appeal on the grounds that conviction on little more than a single particle was unsafe.

It transpired that the coat on which the particle had been recovered had been placed on a dummy at the police photographic section. It was accepted by the photographic section that this dummy could well have been contaminated with GSR from other exhibits. It was also noted that, at the time of the murder, the police were also using ammunition which contained lead, barium, antimony and aluminium in the primer.

Three appeal judges decided that George's murder conviction at the Old Bailey in July 2001 was unsafe, as the jury had been misled about the significance of a single microscopic speck of GSR found on the lining of an inside pocket of his overcoat. Lawyers for George argued in the appeal hearing that the Crown had advanced the speck as significant evidence of his guilt, but now, scientists – including the principal forensic witness for the prosecution – accepted that its evidential value was 'neutral.'

In essence, the experts now agreed the single speck was 'no more likely to have come from a gun fired by George than from any other, non-incriminating source'.

How many particles the Metropolitan Police Forensic Science Services Laboratory now consider relevant, and whether they require the indicative/associated ratios to be correct before a positive result is reported, is unclear.

This case does, however, illustrate the importance of a requirement for a number of GSR particles greater than one to be necessary, and for the indicative/associated particle ratio to be taken into consideration.

In all cases examined by the author[4] involving the transfer of GSR from the hands or from the discharge of a weapon to the clothes, there has always been associated/indicative particles present in approximately the correct ratio.

Illustrative Case 5

A report appeared in the Scotland Herald, on 5 May 2012, that an independent inquiry has been launched into forensic evidence at the trial of a man who was dramatically cleared of murdering a Glasgow gangland figure:

'Ross Monaghan, 30, was acquitted yesterday on the orders of a judge at the High Court in Glasgow, where he had been accused of shooting Kevin "Gerbil" Carroll outside ASDA, in Robroyston, Glasgow. The judge, Lord Brailsford, heavily criticised police after a firearms officer admitted he and his colleagues were wearing the same uniforms they had earlier worn to a gun training exercise during a raid on Mr Monaghan's home. The clothing would have been covered in bullet residue, contaminating the evidence. Lord Brailsford said: "It was absolutely clear that the search of the house and the jacket seizure gave rise to contamination. I was told the search was, in scientific terms, horrendous and that is also my conclusion."'

Lord Brailsford heard two days of submissions by defence QC Derek Ogg, which revealed 'disturbing' issues surrounding forensics. A single particle of firearms discharge residue was found on a jacket seized during a raid of Mr Monaghan's home in July 2010. However, SPSA forensic expert Alison Colley said that a single particle was insufficient to draw any scientific conclusion. Ms Colley had previously prepared a report stating that the residue was of a similar type to that used in cartridges recovered from the crime scene, but she admitted in court that she had formed her conclusion at the request of a detective superintendent involved in the investigation.

Lord Brailsford said: 'Miss Colley displayed great candour and said she had been told to file her report in the way she did by a detective superintendent. I find this evidence to be disturbing.'

14.0.11 General considerations to be made when examining GSR analysis results

Particle composition

The following list of particle compositions would be relevant for standard Pb, Ba, Sb based ammunition:

Sb/Ba: Indicative
Sb/Pb: Indicative
Ba/Pb: Indicative

Sb/Sn: Indicative
Pb: Indicative

The above does not, as a result of the very large number of possible combinations, include ammunition from Eastern Europe, China or Warsaw Pact countries. For such ammunition, each case will have to be taken on its own merit.

If the following elements are found alone, they can be considered as environmental contaminants:

Sb   Environmental
Cu/Zn   Environmental/bullet jacket material
Ni   Environmental

---

[4] Unpublished paper by B. Heard.

Sn	Environmental
Au	Environmental
Ce/La	Environmental
Fe	Environmental
Cu	Environmental

Particle size

No GSR particle above 20 μm should ever be present on the hands. Any particle of a size greater than this will fall off almost immediately. In over 4,000 hand lifts examined by the author, no particle of this size has ever been detected. If a particle of this size is encountered, it should be viewed with great suspicion.

Perfectly spherical particles of GSR

These should also be viewed with suspicion and appropriately 'flagged'. GSR particles are invariably spheroidal, but they are rarely spherical. Cases have been examined where a fired cartridge case has been held over a stub and shaken to produce a positive result. These (fortunately very rare) instances are easily identified by the number of spherical particles associated with very large amorphous, partially burnt propellant particles coated with spherical GSR particles. In one published paper, the imprint of a cartridge case mouth can clearly been seen on the stub of a sample allegedly taken from a suspect. Large numbers of perfectly spherical and amorphous GSR particles were, not unsurprisingly, located on the stub! In another article, the SEM image shown in Figure 14.0.8 appeared.

While the particle in Figure 14.0.8 was not purported to having been recovered from the hands or clothing, in the author's experience, nothing of this extreme size has ever been recovered even a few seconds after test firings. Any such particles reported as being found on the hands or clothing of a suspect should be treated with extreme suspicion.

Particles to be eliminated as having no relevance

- **Particles containing only barium** can be ignored. While there is some possibility of Barium from a standard Pb, Ba, Sb, primer being present alone, it

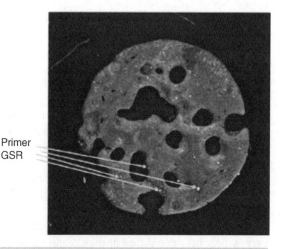

Primer
GSR

Figure 14.0.8 SEM image of GSR on propellant particle.

is far more probable that it will be a contaminant $BaSO_4$ particle from paper, or even from ladies' makeup.

- **Antimony** is, for some unknown reason, very rarely encountered alone. Once again, if a pure antimony particle is located, it is most probably a contaminant.

- **Particles containing Pb and Sn** are invariably from type metal or plumber's solder. The latter is another material that is also available in non-toxic form and nowadays contains tin, copper, silver, and sometimes bismuth, indium, zinc, antimony, and other metals in varying amounts.

Storage of GSR samples

If a GSR Outstanding Crime Index (Unsolved Crime Index) is maintained – something which is entirely possible when dealing with Eastern European, Russian and Chinese ammunition – then stored case GSR samples cannot be relied upon to have the same elemental composition as when first examined. This is due to the high volatility of mercury; over time, the mercury evaporates from the GSR particles, eventually disappearing altogether. This is very dependent on ambient conditions and can be as little as a few months to several years.

Positive/indicative particle ratios

Taking the standard Pb, Ba, Sb primer composition an example, to classify a particle as being positive GSR, it would have to contain all three elements – i.e. Pb, Ba and Sb – in one particle.

As previously explained, indicative particles in a standard Pb, Ba, Sb type primer would include Pb, Pb/Sb, Pb/Ba and Ba/Sb particles.

The ratio of positive to indicative particles can vary widely between different makes and (particularly) types of ammunition. With a plain lead bullet and a Pb, Sb, Ba primer, the positive/indicative ratio would be in the region of 1 : 40 or even more. For a jacketed hollow-point bullet, the positive to indicative particle ratio would be in the region of 1 : 10.

14.0.12   Discussion

GSR testimony can be challenging because of the difficulty in interpreting the results. An expert assumes the role of teacher when describing gunshot residue and its analysis. After instructing the court on the definition, production, collection, preservation, and analysis of GSR, the examiner then must present the results in a simple, truthful and unbiased manner.

The difficulty lies in the fact that while analysts can report that the particles came from a fired weapon, they cannot describe how they were deposited on the item. A distribution pattern of GSR can give an indication as to the circumstances, but only if the tapings were taken shortly after the firing.

Examiners called to testify on GSR results cannot identify the person who discharged a firearm in the commission of a criminal act unless, of course, he has been apprehended and residues were found on his hands with the correct distribution.

A positive GSR finding is of most use where a suspect denies proximity to a discharged firearm because GSR is not common to the average person's daily environment. A negative finding does not imply that the subject was not in the vicinity of a recently discharged firearm; it only indicates that no evidence of primer residue was found on the items tested.

Often, defence lawyers will raise questions at trial as to why GSR was not collected, under the guise that negative results would have been vital to the defence's strategy and would ultimately have exonerated the suspect.

So, the question arises, 'Why analyse for GSR?'

- The technology behind the analysis of gunshot residue is unquestionably scientifically sound. SEM/EDS analysis has existed for a long time and been used in GSR analysis since the 1970s.

- Studies have shown that, generally, people do not have gunshot residue on their hands, but that someone who fires a gun most likely will for a period of time.

- Despite efforts by forensic scientists to disprove the uniqueness of GSR to firearms, research has only strengthened the position of naming spheroid/spheroidal Pb, Ba, and Sb particles as having come from a fired weapon.

- While studies of contamination issues continue, the likelihood of transfer from another source remains small in most cases.

- The reason for analysing for GSR lies in the fact that most trace evidence is not conclusive but supportive.

- GSR found on the hands of a suspected shooter is significant and is worthy of consideration by the jury.

For a court to understand the significance of the findings, experts must discuss all aspects of the sample collection, analysis and interpretation at trial. Sources of contamination, and an explanation as to whether the analyst could account for any anomalies in the findings, also should be included in the testimony. In some cases, the sample collection officer should give testimony first to provide context for the results that an analyst may report. Ideally, the firearms examiner should be the one who collects the samples, but only under the strict anti-contamination procedures outlined earlier.

References

1 Walker, J.T. (1940). Bullet Holes and Chemical Residues in Shooting Cases. *Journal of Crime Law & Criminology* 31, 497.

2 Andrasko, J. (1992). Characterisation of Smokeless Powder Flakes from Fired Cartridge Cases and from Discharge Patterns on Clothing. *Journal of Forensic Sciences* 37, 1030–1047.

3 Harrison, H.C. & Gillroy, R. (1959). Firearms Discharge Residues. *Journal of Forensic Sciences* 4, 184–199.

4 Ruch, R.R., Buchanan, J.D., Guinn, V.P., Bellanca, S. C. & Pinker, R.H. (1964). Neutron Activation Analysis in Scientific Crime Detection. *Journal of Forensic Sciences* 9 (1), 119–33.

5 Green, A.L. & Sauve, J.P. (1972). The Analysis of Gunshot Residue by Atomic Absorption Spectrophotometry. *Atomic Absorption Newsletter* 11 (5), 93–95.

6 Sen, P., Panigrahi, N., Rao, M.S., Varier, K.M., Sen, S. & Mehta, G.K. (1982). Application of proton-induced X-ray emission technique to gunshot residue analyses. *Journal of Forensic Sciences* 27 (2), 330–339.

7 Brihaye, C., Machiroux, R. & Gillain, G. (1982). Gunpowder Residues Detection by Anodic Stripping Voltammetry. *Forensic Science International* 20, 269–276.

8 Hellmiss, G., Lichtenberg, W. & Weiss, M. (1987), Investigation of Gunshot Residues by Means of Auger Electron Spectroscopy. *Journal of Forensic Sciences* 32 (3), 747–760.

9 Matricardi, V.R. & Kilty, J.W. (1977). Detection of gunshot residue particles from the hands of a shooter. *Journal of Forensic Science* 22, 725–738.

10 Wolten, G.M., Nesbitt, R.S., Calloway, A.R., Loper, G.L. & Jones, P.E. (1977). *Final Report on Particle Analysis for Gun Shot Residue Detection.* Report ATR-77 (7915)-3, The Aerospace Corporation, El Segundo, CA, USA.

11 DeGaetano, D. (1992). A Comparison of Three Techniques Developed for the Sampling and Analysis of GSR by SEM/EDX. *Journal of Forensic Sciences* 37, 281.

12 Zeichner, A., Levin, N. & Dvorachek, M. (1992). GSR Particles Formed by Using Ammunition that have Mercury Fulminate Based Primers. *Journal of Forensic Sciences* 37, 1567.

13 Gunaratnam, L. & Himber, K. (1994). The Identification of GSR from Lead-free Sintox Ammunition. *Journal of Forensic Science* 39 (2), 532–536.

14 Zeichner, A., Foner, H.A., Dvorachek, M., Bergman, P. & Levin, N. (1989). Concentration Techniques for the Detection of Gunshot Residues by Scanning Electron Microscopy/Energy- Dispersive X-Ray Analysis (SEM/EDX). *Journal of Forensic Sciences* 34 (2), 312–320.

15 Wallace, J.S. & McQuillan, J. (1984). Discharge Residues from Cartridge-Operated Industrial Tools. *Journal of the Forensic Science Society* 24 (5), 495–508.

16 Singer, R.L., Davis, D. & Houck, M.M. (1996). A Survey of Gunshot Residue Analysis Methods. *Journal of Forensic Sciences* 41 (2), 195–198.

17 DeGaetano, D., and Siegel, J.A. (1990). Survey of Gunshot Residue Analysis in Forensic Science Laboratories. *Journal of Forensic Sciences* 35 (5), 1087–1095.

18 ASTM E1588 (1993). *Standard Guide for the Analysis of Gunshot Residue by Scanning Electron Microscopy/Energy-Dispersive Spectrometry.* Philadelphia, PA, ASTM.

19 Stephen Kiehl, 'Defender Spotlights Faulty Forensics,' *Baltimore Sun,* November 5, 2007.

20 Errors in gunshot residue assessment by scanning electron www.meixatech.com/MISTAKES3.pdf

15.0

Gun Handling Tests

15.0.1　Introduction

In armed robbery incidents where no shot has been fired, it is often necessary to demonstrate a link between the suspect and a recovered weapon. As GSR particles will not be present on the hands, the only way this can be affected is through the detection of any metal traces that may have been transferred from the weapon to the hands.

The quantity of metal traces transferred from the weapon to the hand is extremely small, and probably below the threshold for analytical detection by conventional instrumental methods. Even if the quantity of metal were sufficient to perform an analysis, the only information available would be that there were traces of iron (or aluminium if it was an aluminium-framed weapon) on the palm of the hands. This would be of little or no evidential value whatsoever.

Due to the very characteristic shape of a weapon, the way it is held in the hand and the fact that large portions of it are covered by non-metallic materials in the form of the grip plates, the signature from the metal traces left on the hands should be readily identifiable as that of a firearm. Visualisation of the metallic traces left on the hands using trace metal detection (TMD) sprays is a very easy technique and one that can return dramatic results.

Interpretation of the results is, as in many forensic disciplines, the keyword. It is so easy, especially late at night in a darkened police station, to imagine what should be there from fragmentary patches of magenta colouration. The essence of this test is experience with the interpretation of the results of positive reactions from control tests. Basics should include knowledge of what metals react to the test, at what concentrations, the colours that are produced, how they can be distinguished from that given by iron or steel, and why everyday objects such as kitchen utensils will not normally give a positive result.

Even if the examiner is not a qualified chemist, he or she should be expected to be able to explain:

• what causes the reaction to give the magenta colouration;

• how the pH affects the results;

• the use or otherwise of pH buffers;

• how UV light catalyses the reaction;

• why this is a qualitative and not quantitative test.

Following on from these basics, the examiner should be able to explain what specific patterns are likely with various firearms and how, for example, a self-loading pistol can be differentiated from a revolver.

The examiner should also be able to explain how each and every area of a positive reaction relates to the various parts of the weapon in question, and why some parts, such as an escutcheon, have not produced a result, while others have.

Forensic Ballistics in Court: Interpretation and Presentation of Firearms Evidence, First Edition. Brian J. Heard.
© 2013 John Wiley & Sons, Ltd. Published 2013 by John Wiley & Sons, Ltd.

The interpretation of blind tests should be part of every firearm examiner's training. Ideally, the examiner should be certificated (either internally or externally) via proficiency tests and be able to produce such certificates. In the author's laboratory, an examiner could not attend court unless he or she possessed the correct certificate for the evidence to be presented.

15.0.2 History

Probably the first recorded instance of the use of trace metal detection (TMD) sprays was during the Vietnam War. During this action it was often necessary to differentiate between innocent farmers going to work in the morning and Viet Cong guerrillas who had been out at night with their AK47 assault rifles. A simple spray test[1,2] was developed, which would visualise, under ultraviolet (UV) light, a number of different metals. The reagent used in this spray was a 0.2 per cent solution of 8-hydroxyquinoline in isopropyl alcohol. This reagent reacts with iron to give a bright blue fluorescence under UV light. Many other metals also react with this reagent, including, aluminium, lead, zinc and copper, some of which fluoresce and some of which adsorb the UV light.

While this test is very sensitive and it is quite easy to distinguish between the various metals, the results can be very confusing. The outline of a weapon might be overlaid with that from an aluminium door handle, and the nickel and copper from handling small change. There is also the problem of carrying round a large UV light cabinet to enable the result to be seen, as well as special photographic equipment to record it.

Another reagent is Ferrozine, or 3-(2-pyridyl)-5,6-diphenyl-1,2,4-triazine-p,p'-disulphonic acid, disodium salt trihydrate (also known as PDT – see Goldman & Thornton, 1976). This has been found to be far superior to the 8-hydroxyquinoline and does not require a UV light box for visualisation. The reagent also has no known toxic side effects.

In this test, the reagent is made up as a saturated (0.2 per cent) solution in methanol, which is simply sprayed onto the hands. A positive reaction to iron is visualised as a deep magenta colour. This colour results from the formation of a bidentate ligand with any ferrous (Fe(II)) traces which may be present. The iron that is transferred from a weapon to the hands is, however, predominately in the ferric (Fe(III)) form, which does not give a reaction with ferrozine. It has been found (Lee, 1986) that by adding 1 per cent ascorbic acid to the ferrozine solution, the Fe(III) is effectively reduced to the Fe(II) state, thus increasing the sensitivity by six or seven fold.

It has been suggested that a buffer be used in addition to the ascorbic acid. However, while this can help in the elimination of interfering metal traces, the extra spray has been found to dilute the results rather than enhance them.

Of the other metallic elements which give a colour reaction with ferrozine, only Cu(II) and Al(III) are of note. They are, however, of little significance, as Cu (II) gives only a weak golden brown coloration and Al(III), which does give a similar colour to Fe(III), is so insensitive that a positive reaction can only be obtained in a test tube at untypically high concentrations.

Recent advances[3] in the use of Ferrozine spray include the use of the base chemical rather than the sodium salt. The advantages of this over the sodium salt include a much greater sensitivity and the ability to make solutions in excess of 0.2 per cent strength. The higher strength solutions mean that less of the spray has to be applied, thus reducing the tendency for the result to diffuse by running over the hand. The solution is also made up in ethanol, rather than methanol, which is quite poisonous.

The use of 2-nitroso-1-naphthol[4] has been suggested as an alternative to Ferrozine, but this gives coloured complexes with iron, copper, zinc and silver. As a result, it has gained little support.

[3] Unpublished paper by author & Dr C.M.LAU of the HK Govt Laboratory.
[4] Kokocinski, C.W., Brundage, D.J. & Nicol, J.D. (1980) A Study of he Uses of 2-Nitroso-1-Naphthol as a Trace Metal Detection Reagent. *Journal of Forensic Sciences* 25(4), 810–814.

[1] US Government Printing Office Publication, 1972
[2] Stevens, J.M. & Messler, H. (1974). Ferrous metal detection. *Journal of Forensic Science* 19, 496–503.

15.0.3 Methodology for the use of Ferrozine

Unlike GSR particles, which are merely lying on the surface of the skin, Fe(II) traces transferred to the hands through the holding an iron object appear to be absorbed into the skin. As such, they are not easily removed and are often detectable with Ferrozine spray eight hours or more after an incident.

This is a fairly simple test to apply, but some background knowledge of the influencing factors will assist in obtaining the best from it. Following are a few considerations one should bear in mind.

As the coloured complex formed is soluble in the ethanol used to make up the reagent, the results will run if too much reagent is applied at one time. Far better results will be obtained with several light applications of the spray, allowing each to dry before applying the next.

The reaction between Fe(II) and ferrozine is catalysed by short-wave UV light. In a dark office at night, with only strip lighting or with very weak transfers, the result can take an hour or more to develop. A simple hand-held short-wave UV source will be sufficient to speed up and enhance the development of the reaction.

Weak reactions, even when using the UV light source as a catalyst, can take anything up to an hour to develop. Additional light sprays of the reagent, exposure to UV light and some patience will be required for light transfers or when the elapsed time approaches eight hours.

This test is mutually compatible with the taping of hands for GSR. The taping must be completed before the Ferrozine spray is started. However, if the weapon has a slightly rusty surface, it is possible to obtain a positive reaction from cotton gloves.

Painted or plated weapons will not give a positive reaction to the test. Neither will aluminium- or stainless steel-framed weapons.

A conventional blue or 'Parkerised' (phosphated) finish to the weapon will not affect the test. In fact, some of the best results obtained by the author concerned 'Parkerised' weapons.

Black and white film does not appear to be very sensitive to the magenta part of the spectrum. Photography of the results should be carried out with colour film, preferably with a green background for added contrast.

If it was raining during the holding of the weapon, the test will always return a negative result. The reason for this is unknown.

If the hands are damp due to nervous sweat, a light application of a hot air blower will assist. The hot air blower should also be applied between applications of the spray. This will not only speed up the reaction, it will also stop the reagent running over the hand and spoiling the result.

Washing the hands with soap and water will only remove about 50 per cent of the transfer. It appears that, once the transfer has been made, the skin has a greater affinity for the metal traces than does water.

The hands must never be placed in plastic bags to conserve any transfer. As soon as the hands start to sweat, the results spread over the entire hand and the result will be meaningless.

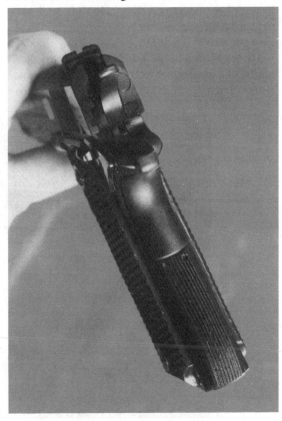

Figure 15.0.1 Colt 1911A1 pistol showing grooved back strap.

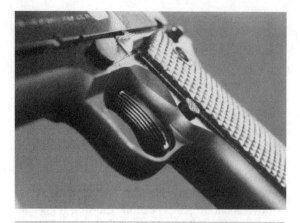

Figure 15.0.2 Colt 1911A1 pistol showing grooved trigger.

Protect the hands with paper bags and do not restrain the hands with steel handcuffs. Likewise, do not place the suspect in a cell with steel bars. Neither should the suspect be allowed to urinate on his/her hands. While this does not remove all of the Fe(III) traces from the hands, it does place the hand in an acidic state, which interferes with the bidentate ligand formation.

If the hands of a deceased person have to be tested, *never* allow the body to be placed into the refrigerator before carrying out the test. Once the body has cooled down below ambient temperature, it is impossible to obtain a positive result, even if the hands are reheated. The reason for this is unknown.

It should be emphasised here that, used in the above way and for the above reason, the reagent Ferrozine is being used as a qualitative (what is there) rather than a quantitative (how much is there) test.

It should be remembered that Ferrozine is, however, a recognised quantitative reagent for the analysis of the iron content in, for example, water in boiler systems. Here, the test is being used to estimate the breakdown of the boiler via the amount of iron that is being dissolved in the water.

Case notes

It is interesting to note that in all cases of suicide with a revolver which have been examined by the author, there has been a very distinctive positive reaction on the pad of the right thumb. It is assumed that there is

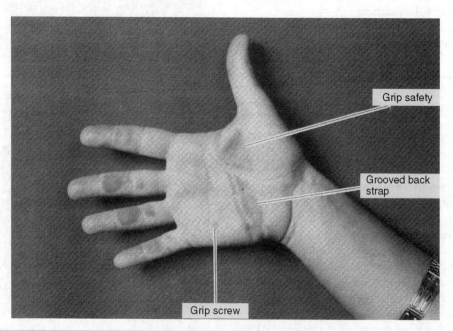

Figure 15.0.3 Hand after spraying with Ferrozine.

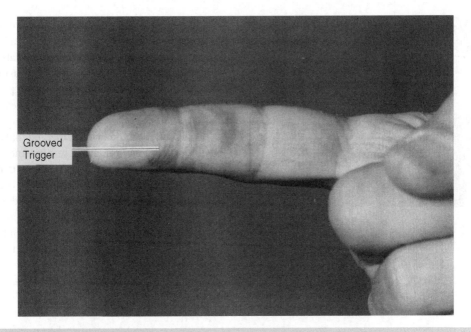

Grooved
Trigger

Figure 15.0.4 Trigger finger after spraying, showing grooves on trigger.

some trepidation over committing the act, and that the hammer has been cocked and uncocked several times.

The Ferrozine test is not exclusive to firearms and will give a positive with any iron object. Spanners, car jacks, crowbars, etc. can all give a positive reaction.

Discussion

This test is a useful adjunct to an investigation of those crimes where a firearm has been held but not fired. It can be carried out in the field by a scene of crime officer or a technician, but only with extensive training. The results from this test can only be interpreted by an experienced forensic firearms expert who has had extensive experience in the application of this reagent.

It is extremely easy to imagine what might be there and to make an incorrect assessment. In addition, it is often the case that what can be seen on the hands is not faithfully reproduced on film. As mentioned earlier, black and white photography is not particularly sensitive in the magenta region of the spectrum, so any photographic work should be made in colour with a green background. With modern photo-manipulation

---

Illustrative Case 1

A well-known blood grouping forensic scientist was attempting to make a name for herself as a forensic firearms defence expert. She went to great lengths trying to persuade the jury in a case which involved the holding, but not firing of a firearm, that the police examiner did not know what he was talking about. Her argument was that he did not know the exact quantity of Ferrozine and ascorbic acid that was being sprayed onto the hands and, therefore, the results were meaningless. After it was patiently explained to her that this was not a quantitative test, but rather a qualitative test, and after being shown the relevant papers on the subject, her evidence was discredited by the judge. She never attempted to give evidence in a firearms case again.

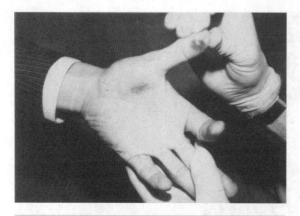

Figure 15.0.5   Results of Ferrozine test on suicide case, showing mark on thumb as well as the back strap.

programs (e.g. *Paint Shop Pro*), the photographically recorded results can be significantly enhanced by the use of various filters and the manipulation of the colour temperature. This, however, can easily be taken too far, and copies of the unenhanced photographs must also be made available. Ideally, the results should also be captured on video.

Above all, it should be remembered that a negative result is not an eliminating result, since so many factors can affect a positive outcome from this spray.

Several precautions are necessary when one is utilising the developed pattern on the hand of a suspect to provide evidence. The Ferrozine method of developing patterns of iron residues on the hands from the handling of a weapon – or, for that matter, tools – has

---

Illustrative Case 2

An example of how useful this can be in non-firearms related cases involved a breaking and entering case, where a row of shops had their front door locks drilled out. A suspect was spotted in the act of drilling a door lock and, when approached, he fled, leaving his equipment behind. This equipment consisted of a motorcycle starter motor with a drill chuck attached to the spindle. This was driven by a battery held in a shoulder bag. A suspect was eventually located some four hours later and, when his hands were sprayed with the Ferrozine reagent, a perfect imprint of the castellated chuck was observed. He denied all knowledge of the burglary incidents, passing the chuck mark off as from a drill at his home. Fortunately, the chuck on the starter motor had half of one of the castellations missing, which matched perfectly with that on his hand.

Illustrative Case 3

This involved a stolen police weapon being used in an armed robbery. The weapon had been abandoned at the scene of the crime. A suspect was arrested, but he denied all knowledge of the incident until his hands were sprayed with Ferrozine. This not only revealed a positive result that was typical of a revolver being held, but also the weapon's serial number, which had been stamped on the back strap, was clearly visible.

Illustrative Case 4

Another very positive case concerned the use of a military rifle by three very drunk soldiers in a very amateur attempt to hijack an airliner at an international airport. The weapon was fired several times at various objects in the airport and, due to the fact that they were all soldiers on active duty, they were all covered in GSR. The Ferrozine test was likewise somewhat compromised, due to the fact that all three had been carrying rifles earlier in the day. As a rifle is held up to the cheek during aiming and firing, it was decided to spray the soldiers' faces as well. This clearly revealed the serial number, which was stamped on the side of the rifle's receiver, on the right cheek of one soldier.

inherent limitations that must recognised and understood. First, the object held must have a distinctive or characteristic morphology, and the pattern produced on the skin must reflect this if it is to be used as associative evidence. Several factors, as given above, can affect the fidelity of the pattern. In the more commonly encountered situation, where there is a reaction, but where the pattern is less distinct, the results may be useful, but only as an investigative aid.

In the end, however, it all comes down to interpretation by the examiner. Such questions as: 'How does this result differ from the holding of a spoon?'; 'Will a knife give a similar result? Or a spanner?', etc. will distinguish between a witness who has the necessary experience to give evidence and one who has not.

Further reading

1 Goldman, G. & Thornton, J. (1976). A New Trace Ferrous Metal Detection Reagent. *Journal of Forensic Science* 21 (3), 625–628.

2 Leifer, A., Wax, H. & Almog, J. (2001). Who held the gun? Decipherment of suicide homicide cases using the PDT reagent. *Journal of Forensic Identification* 51, 346–360.

3 Glattstein, B., Nedivi, L. & Almog, J. (1998). Detection of firearms on hands by Ferrotrace spray: profiles of some common weapons. *Journal of Forensic Identification* 48 (3), 257–272.

4 Almog, J. & Glattstein, B. (1997). Detection of firearms imprints on hands of suspects: study of the PDT-based field test. *Journal of Forensic Science* 42 (6), 993–996.

5 Lee, C-W. (1986). The Detection of Iron Traces on Hands by Ferrozine Sprays: A Report on the Sensitivity and Interference of the Method and Recommended Procedure in Forensic Science Investigation. *Journal of Forensic Sciences* 31 (3), 920–930.

6 Pearson, J. & Lennard, C. (2000). A forensic evaluation of PDT reagents for the detection of latent residues on the hands. http:\\www.bit.net.au/'qpolfsb/abst-PQ.htm.

7 Almog, J., Hirshfeld, A., Glattstein, B., Sterling, J. & Goren, Z. (1996). Chromogenic reagents for iron (II): studies in the 1,2,4-triazine series. *Analytica Chimica Acta* 322, 203–208.

16.0

Laser-etched Serial Numbers and Bar Codes

16.0.1 Introduction

On the face of it, laser etching the serial number of a firearm on the firing pin or inside the barrel in the form of a bar code is an excellent idea. It would do away with the lengthy process of matching fired bullets via stria and the difficult process of comparing stria on deeply impressed firing impressions. The serial number would be imprinted directly on primer of any ammunition fired in that weapon. Likewise, a bar code transferred from the inside surface of the barrel would be imprinted on a fired bullet. All that would be needed is a bar code reader, and not only would be weapon be identified, but also the owner.

Unfortunately, it is not that simple.

16.0.2 Laser-etched serial numbers

By the late 1990s, H&K, at their Nottingham-based factory, were laser-etching serial numbers onto their HK MP5 weapons. Marlin rifles, S&W Sigma pistols, Dan Wesson revolvers, Colt AR15 rifles, Thompson, Centre Arms Company and many other manufacturers also laser-etch their serial numbers either numerically or via a bar code system.

Laser-etched bar codes are also under consideration in the UK, Europe, Australia and New Zealand, and will become far more prevalent in the future.

Laser-etching of serial numbers onto the firing pin (Figure 16.0.1)

Laser-etching serial numbers onto the firing pin and/or the breech face is a much more recent addition to this technique, which has now reached the point of being mandatory in parts of the USA. California was the first state to pass the micro-stamping legislation. Massachusetts and Rhode Island have introduced similar legislation, and the Maryland Police Department is promoting consideration as well. It is intended that legislation be introduced to require micro stamping on a Federal level throughout the US. The UK, Europe and Australasia are also looking into this technique.

It remains to be seen how long the laser etched marks remain on the firing pin, although Neuman Micro Technologies Inc. of New Hampshire do report that the serial number is still present after 30,000 cycles.

In a study, George G. Krivosta (2006), referring to these laser etched markings as 'NanoTags', asked:

- Would the NanoTag markings be reproducible and readily decipherable?

- How resistant to wear would the NanoTag engraved firing pin be under normal use?

- How susceptible would the NanoTag engraved firing pin be to intentional defacement?

Forensic Ballistics in Court: Interpretation and Presentation of Firearms Evidence, First Edition. Brian J. Heard.
© 2013 John Wiley & Sons, Ltd. Published 2013 by John Wiley & Sons, Ltd.

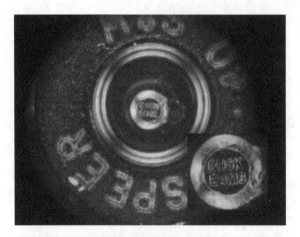

Figure 16.0.1   Firing pin impression from laser-etched serial number on firing pin.

He stated that in reviewing cartridge cases previously expended in firearms with NanoTag micro-laser engraved firing pins, the NanoTag markings were illegible and non-reproducible due to the fact that the firing pin usually strikes the cartridge multiple times, and that the additional impacts overlap. Furthermore, the vast majority of the micro-laser-engraved serial numbers never showed up on any of the cartridge cases fired, and those that did were very difficult to decipher. In addition, after test firing only 1,000 rounds, he found that the micro-laser-engraved markings were softening in their sharpness as a result of the metal peening. The study also revealed that the markings could be removed in seconds using common household tools. Subsequent test firing established that removing the markings did not render the firearm inoperable.

The *AFTE Journal* opines that: 'implementing this technology will be much more complicated than burning a serial number on a few parts and dropping them into firearms being manufactured'.

16.0.3   Bar codes

Bar codes laser-etched inside the barrel

Laser-etched bar codes inside the muzzle of the weapon (United States Patent 6462302 and many others), which are transferred onto a fired bullet, are also under consideration.

The bar code would be transferred to the bullet on firing and could be read with a specialised peripheral bar code scanner. The bar code would include the serial number of the weapon, its make and model as well as the owner's name and address.[1,2]

Once again, the life expectancy of such a bar code in a very hostile environment would be the biggest drawback to the implementation of such technology. In addition, most bullets recovered from crime scenes tend to be damaged to some extent. The likelihood of recovering an intact bar code from such would appear to be problematical.

Removing such a bar code would not be very difficult, and restoring it would be even more difficult, if not impossible.

Bar-coded ammunition

Ammunition Accountability is a company that states they have the solution to gun crime by laser micro-etching a serial number on the base of the projectile (Figure 16.0.2) that matches with the serial number on the inside of its cartridge case. The plan is to sell

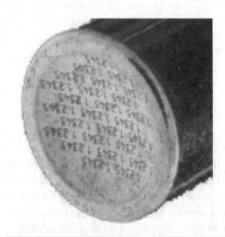

Figure 16.0.2   Laser-etched serial number on bullet.

[1] Valerie Coffey, *Laser Focus World*, 01-12-2002
[2] Rifled Weapon Barrel Engraver and Scanner Intellectual Property Organisation, WO/2002/

ammunition in boxes with unique codes that can be tracked and recorded by law enforcement. They admit that they will not be able to identify 'who pulled the trigger', but it 'will provide law enforcement with a valuable lead and a starting point to quickly begin their investigations'.

Ammunition Accountability is also pressing for legislation which would require an ammunition code database. The database would hold the bar code of each box of ammunition sold, along with the state-issued ID of the person who purchased it.

The logistics of such a move, especially when considering that the company is the sole provider of such technology, the cost involved and the fact that every single round of non-stamped ammunition would have to be recalled, would make this a non-viable consideration. As of 2009, 33 Bills had been presented in Congress, all of which had failed.

16.0.4   Conclusion

It is doubtful whether micro- (or nano-) laser-etching of serial numbers on firing pins and barrels will ever be a successful technique. As for laser etching serial numbers onto bullets and cartridge cases, this is even less likely to be successful, let alone be put into law.

Further reading

1 Page, D. (2008). *Microstamping calls the shot: A revolutionary gun identification technology finds favor and foes*. In Studies/research reports (p. 5). Fort Atkinson, WI: Cygnus Business Media.
2 'Cracking the Case: The Crime Solving Promise of Ballistics Identification'. Educational Fund to Stop Gun Violence Report on Micro stamping, 2004.
3 Krivosta, G.G. (2006). NanoTag Markings from Another Perspective, *AFTE Journal* 38 (1), 41–47.

17.0

Classification of Firearms-related Death

17.0.1 Introduction

Much of the research on firearms focuses on injuries and deaths that occur when people misuse firearms, and the role that firearms play in the rising violence of some societies.

Injuries caused by firearms are classified as either 'fatal' or 'non-fatal'. Homicide, suicide and accidental death are the three types of fatal injuries caused by firearms. Non-fatal injuries are called 'assaultive', 'self-inflicted' and 'accidental'.

This chapter presents an overview of the role of firearms in deaths and injuries, how they may be classified and the frequency for various countries, compared with the number of legally held weapons.

17.0.2 Basics

Unfortunately, there is no single characteristic appearance, position or type of gunshot wound that defines the exact manner of death. Such a determination requires analysis of multiple pieces of evidence, including;

- the scene investigation;

- the examination of the body;

- ballistics evidence;

- trace metal detection on the hands;

- analysis for gunshot residue; and

- interviews of persons involved with the decedent and the scene of death.

The presence of multiple entrance wounds may not exclude suicide. Kohlmeier *et al.* (2001) have analysed 1704 suicidal firearms deaths and determined characteristics of those injuries.

The type of weapon used was:

- A revolver in 49.8 per cent of cases;

- A self-loading pistol in 19.5 per cent of cases;

- A rifle in 30.0 per cent of cases; and

- Some other firearm in 0.7 per cent of cases.

The site of the entrance wound involved:

- The head in 83.7 per cent of cases;

- The chest in 14.0 per cent;

- The abdomen in 1.9 per cent; and

- A combination of sites in 0.4 per cent.

Table 17.0.1 identifies the site of the entrance wound by type of weapon used in suicidal firearms deaths.

Forensic Ballistics in Court: Interpretation and Presentation of Firearms Evidence, First Edition. Brian J. Heard.
© 2013 John Wiley & Sons, Ltd. Published 2013 by John Wiley & Sons, Ltd.

Table 17.0.1   Suicidal Firearms Deaths

Site	Handgun (%)	Rifle (%)	Shotgun (%)
Right temple	50.0	22.9	9.3
Left temple	5.8	3.3	3.7
Mouth	14.5	24.3	31.7
Forehead	5.9	15.7	8.1
Under chin	2.4	9.1	10.6
Back of head	3.6	3.8	1.2
Chest	13.2	15.7	19.9
Abdomen	1.4	1.9	5.6
Other	3.2	3.3	9.9

In the above series, contact wounds were found in 97.9 per cent, near contact in 2.0 per cent, and a combination of these or an unknown range in the remainder.

Gunshot residue deposition (see Chapter 14) will, in many cases, be only indicative in determining the exact cause of death. Deposition of residues only on the palms of the hands are indicative of them being held up in self-preservation, but in those cases where it is located on the back of either one or both hands, it is indicative of that person having fired the weapon.

GSR deposition is extremely difficult to fake convincingly, and any competent electron microscopist specialising in GSR interpretation should easily be able to spot any such attempt. In the few cases that the author has dealt with where such an attempt has been made, it has been easily identifiable by:

• the size of the GSR particles (where they have been shaken out of a fired cartridge case);

• their morphology (predominantly spherical, with large, amorphous, partially burnt propellant particles covered in GSR particles);

• incorrect positive/indicative GSR ratios;

• the presence of large quantities of semi-burnt propellant particles, once again shaken out of a fired cartridge case.

The deciding factor, when taken in the light of GSR deposition, can often be via trace metal detection,

using either PDT or Ferrozine (Chapter 15). With TMD results being even more difficult to fake than GSR deposition, this is crucial in deciding the true nature of the crime.

The following are problems with attempting to fake a TMD result.

• Sweat is crucial in the transfer of iron in its ferric (Fe^{3+}) form.

• Dead bodies do not sweat and, as any sweat that may be present at the time of death soon evaporates, it is therefore extremely difficult to affect any substantial transfer. This is especially so once the body starts to cool down.

• The transfer requires a conscious and sustained pressure upon the weapon, which is all but impossible to recreate convincingly with a dead body – especially one with rigor mortis.

In addition to the above, in every case of suicide involving a revolver that I have dealt with, there has always been a very positive result on the thumb of the deceased. This, I can only conclude, results from some trepidation over committing the act, and the hammer has been cocked and un-cocked several times before the weapon is eventually fired.

In the realm of accidental death, there are too many variables to list here. Personally, however, the author has never encountered a case in which accidental death was caused during the cleaning of a firearm. Naturally, this does not exclude the possibility of such an event.

While it is of little more than academic interest, the following Table 17.0.2 shows the ratio of violent deaths vs. suicides for various countries.

17.0.3   Multiple shot suicides

Multiple shot suicides engender controversy, due to the misconception that it is impossible to inflict more than one gunshot upon oneself. Tied in with this mistaken belief of instant incapacity are fallacies such as 'the impact of the bullet would send you reeling backwards', 'the gun would fly out of your hand' and so on.

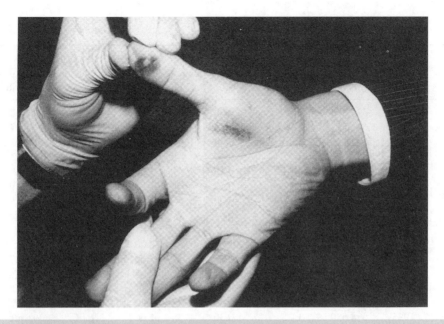

Figure 17.0.1 Positive Ferrozine reaction on pad of thumb in suicide case.

Table 17.0.2 International Violent Death Rate Table (Death Rates are per 100,000)

Country	Year	Population	Total Homicide	Firearm Homicide	Total Suicide	Firearm Suicide	Percentage Households with Guns
Estonia	1994	1,499,257	28.21	8.07	40.95	3.13	n/a
Hungary	1994	10,245,677	3.53	0.23	35.38	0.88	n/a
Slovenia	1994	1,989,477	2.01	0.35	31.16	2.51	n/a
Finland[1]	1994	5,088,333	3.24	0.86	27.26	5.78	23.2
Brazil	1993	160,737,000	19.04	10.58	3.46	0.73	n/a
Denmark	1993	5,189,378	1.21	0.23	22.13	2.25	n/a
Austria	1994	8,029,717	1.17	0.42	22.12	4.06	n/a
Switzerland[2]	1994	7,021,000	1.32	0.58	21.28	5.61	27.2
France	1994	57,915,450	1.12	0.44	20.79	5.14	22.6
Mexico	1994	90,011,259	17.58	9.88	2.89	0.91	n/a
Belgium	1990	9,967,387	1.41	0.60	19.04	2.56	16.6
Portugal	1994	5,138,600	2.98	1.28	14.83	1.28	n/a
United States[3]	1993	257,783,004	5.70	3.72	12.06	7.35	39.0
Japan	1994	124,069,000	0.62	0.02	16.72	0.04	n/a
Sweden	1993	8,718,571	1.30	0.18	15.75	2.09	15.1
Germany	1994	81,338,093	1.17	0.22	15.64	1.17	8.9
Taiwan	1996	21,979,444	8.12	0.97	6.88	0.12	n/a
Singapore	1994	2,930,200	1.71	0.07	14.06	0.17	n/a
Canada	1992	28,120,065	2.16	0.76	13.19	3.72	29.1
Mauritius	1993	1,062,810	2.35	0	12.98	0.09	n/a
Argentina	1994	34,179,000	4.51	2.11	6.71	3.05	n/a

(continued)

Table 17.0.2 (*Continued*)

Country	Year	Population	Total Homicide	Firearm Homicide	Total Suicide	Firearm Suicide	Percentage Households with Guns
Norway	1993	4,324,815	0.97	0.30	13.64	3.95	32.0
N. Ireland	1994	1,641,711	6.09	5.24	8.41	1.34	8.4
Australia	1994	17,838,401	1.86	0.44	12.65	2.35	19.4
New Zealand	1993	3,458,850	1.47	0.17	12.81	2.14	22.3
Scotland	1994	5,132,400	2.24	0.19	12.16	0.31	4.7
Hong Kong	1993	5,919,000	1.23	0.12	10.29	0.07	Nil
Netherlands	1994	15,382,830	1.11	0.36	10.10	0.31	1.9
South Korea	1994	44,453,179	1.62	0.04	9.48	0.02	n/a
Ireland	1991	3,525,719	0.62	0.03	9.81	0.94	n/a
Italy	1992	56,764,854	2.25	1.66	8.00	1.11	16.0
England/Wales	1992	51,429,000	1.41	0.11	7.68	0.33	4.7
Israel	1993	5,261,700	2.32	0.72	7.05	1.84	n/a
Spain	1993	39,086,079	0.95	0.21	7.77	0.43	13.1
Greece	1994	10,426,289	1.14	0.59	3.40	0.84	n/a
Kuwait	1995	1,684,529	1.01	0.36	1.66	0.06	n/a

Notes:

1. The United Nations International Study on Firearm Regulation reports Finland's gun ownership rate at 50 per cent of households.
2. Percentage of households with guns includes all army personnel.
3. Total homicide rate and firearm homicide rates are for 1999 (FBI Uniform Crime Report, 1999).

Incapacitation can be divided into three major groups:

- **Instant incapacitation** this can only result from a cessation in the functioning of the central nervous system via direct disruption of brain stem tissue.

- **Rapid incapacitation** can be achieved via massive bleeding from the heart, the thoracic aorta, the pulmonary artery or other major vein or artery. This can take five minutes or more.

- **Delayed incapacitation** from damage to other major organs, e.g. the lungs, kidney, liver. With such damage to the internal organs, total incapacitation can take a considerable period of time.

Although multiple shot suicides are uncommon, they are by no means rare. Of the cases the author has dealt with, the following are of note:

- An Australian who shot himself in the back seven times with a .22″ calibre rifle,

- A police officer who shot himself twice with a .410″ shotgun. The first shot was with the muzzle in the mouth. The shot shredded the tongue, then went through the back of the neck, missing the spine. The second shot was also in the mouth, but angled upwards through the roof of the mouth and into the brain.

- Another police officer shot himself five times in the chest with a .38″ S&W calibre revolver.

All of these cases were conclusively shown to be suicide, with no external influences.

Betzt *et al.* (1994) states that of 117 gunshot suicides examined in a study, seven showed more than one gunshot wound. Two of these were unusual, in that the second shot was fired directly into the first wound.

Hudson (1981) reports that from 7,895 gunshot deaths, 3,522 were suicides. Of these, 58 (0.7 per cent) were multi-shot suicides.

Introna & Smialek (1989) reports than in six years at the Office of the Chief Medical Examiner, nine cases of multiple-shot suicides were examined, with each victim suffering 3–5 gunshot wounds. No preferential sites for the wounds were of significance.

In conclusion, one must approach any such case with severe scepticism, and every avenue of investigation must be thoroughly examined before reaching a decision as to the exact circumstances leading up to the death.

References and further reading

1 Kohlmeier, R.E., McMahan, C.A. & DiMaio, V.J.M. (2001). Suicide by firearms. *American Journal of Forensic Medicine and Pathology* 22, 337–340.

2 Betz, P., Peschel, O. & Eisenmenger, W. (1994). Suicidal Gunshot Wounds – Site and Characteristics. *Archiv Fur Kriminologie* 193 (3–4) 65–71.

3 Hudson, P. (1981) Multishot Firearms Suicide. Examination of 58 Cases. *American Journal of Forensic Medicine and Pathology* 2 (3), 239–242.

4 Introna, F. & Smialek, J.E. (1989). Suicide from Multiple Gunshot Wounds. *American Journal of Forensic Medicine and Pathology* 10 (4), 275–84.

5 Miller, M., Azrael, D. & Hemenway, D. (2001). Firearm Availability and Unintentional Firearm Deaths. *Accident Analysis and Prevention* 33 (4), 477–484.

6 Miller, M. & Hemenway, D. (2008). Guns and suicide in the United States. *The New England Journal of Medicine* 359 (10), 989–991.

7 Barber, C.W., Azrael, D., Hemenway, D., Olson, L.M., Nie, C., Schaechter, J. & Walsh, S. (2008). Suicides and suicide attempts following homicide: Victim-suspect relationship, weapon type, and presence of antidepressants. *Homicide Studies* 12, 285–297.

8 Miller, M., Hemenway, D. & Azrael, D. (2004). Firearms and Suicide in the Northeast. *Journal of Trauma* 57, 626–632.

9 Miller, M., Azrael, D., Hepburn, L., Hemenway, D. & Lippman, S. (2006). The Association between Changes in Household Firearm Ownership and Rates of Suicide in the United States, 1981–2002. *Injury Prevention* 12, 178–82.

10 North, M. (2000). *Dunblane: Never Forget*. Mainstream Publishing.

11 Cukier, W. & Sidel, V.W. (2006). *The Global Gun Epidemic. From Saturday Night Specials to AK-47s.* Praeger Security International.

18.0

Practical Considerations in a Firearms Case from a Legal Point of View

18.0.1 Introduction

Safety is a key concern whenever a firearm is introduced into evidence. No weapon will ever leave the forensic science laboratory loaded, but one never knows what happens between there and the court, as some of the previous illustrative cases have shown. Normally, police will have ensured that the firearm is not loaded when it is withdrawn from the exhibit store for submission to the trial court. However, a lawyer should still check the firearm before handling it, and do this in the judge and jury's presence when the firearm is marked as an exhibit.

If the lawyer does not know how to check a specific firearm, it should be researched ahead of time by talking with a firearms dealer, the manufacturer, or an expert. Showing knowledge of the subject firearm will always create a positive image with the court.

Although no one has yet been shot in a courtroom by an exhibit assumed to be unloaded, a moment's precaution will maintain that safety record. In addition, checking the firearm in the correct way in front of the jurors or judge will reassure them that the firearm is safe and that the lawyer is familiar with safe gun-handling.

Firearms instructors teach students that it is unsafe to point the muzzle of even an unloaded firearm at any person or to put a finger inside the trigger guard while handling it.

Always resist the temptation to point the firearm at anyone or to put your finger on the trigger (rest it on or along the frame instead). If it is necessary to demonstrate how a weapon was held, for example, against a victim's head, then use your own head, not someone else's.

If someone has a specific reason to manipulate the trigger, make certain that the muzzle is pointed in a safe direction away from any person, and preferably at some solid object such as a wall. Resist the temptation to 'dry fire' the weapon, as this can damage the firing pin. If the trigger has to be pulled, obtain a 'snap cap' from the firearms examiner or a dealer.

If the judge or jury requires access to a weapon during a trial, always show them, no matter how many times this happens, that the weapon is not loaded, either by working the action in a self-loading pistol or by opening the cylinder in a revolver.

When demonstrating the workings of a self-loading pistol or showing that it is not loaded, **always, always** take the magazine out first. The magazine could have a round in it, and working the action will simply load this round into the chamber, cocking the action in the process. This places the weapon into a state where it is ready to fire.

If both firearms and ammunition are exhibits are requested by the jury, think carefully about the pros and cons of sending both into the jury room at the same time. Likewise, unless the ammunition is in a

Forensic Ballistics in Court: Interpretation and Presentation of Firearms Evidence, First Edition. Brian J. Heard.
© 2013 John Wiley & Sons, Ltd. Published 2013 by John Wiley & Sons, Ltd.

safely sealed bag, never give both the weapon and ammunition to anyone.

In general, look at the physical evidence:

- Is the firearm in good repair?

- Are the recovered cartridge cases, bullets, and fragments in good condition?

- How might their condition affect the examiner's results?

- Is the condition consistent with the prosecution's theory of the case?

- What happened at the crime scene between the crime and the police arrival? Could evidence have been removed, moved, or damaged by the victims or bystanders?

What did the police do at the crime scene? Look at the crime scene photographs and sketches to see where evidence was found. Look specifically at the chain of custody documentation for any indication of fabrication or fraud. Over-zealous investigators have been known to have falsified evidence in fingerprint cases; it could happen in other cases as well.

Look carefully at any GSR images, bearing in mind that spherical particles and particles over 2 μm are almost never found on the hands.

What did the examiner know when the evidence was submitted to him or her?

- Was this a high-profile case?

- Was the examiner rushed?

- Did the examiner have any expectation about the results of his or her tests before making them?

Ideally, the examiner should be given the absolute minimum amount of information about the circumstances surrounding the case, to prevent any chance of a predisposition towards one outcome. This can have its drawbacks, however, as can be seen from Illustrative Case 3.

18.0.2   Key questions

- What methods were used to determine the examiner's opinion? Are they the methods recommended in the examiner's training materials and/or laboratory procedures?

Illustrative Case 1

When working in the Far East, the author was surprised at the number of times, after a large exchange of fire had taken place, how few — if any — fired cartridge cases and bullets were found at the scene. It transpired that there was a large market in such items, especially if the case was a high-profile one.

Illustrative Case 2

A paper was published, illustrating how gunshot residues solved a particularly difficult murder case. Photographs of particles supposedly found on the hands of the suspects not only showed very large spherical GSR particles and partially burnt propellant particles, but also the circular indentation where a cartridge case had been upended and tapped on the taping to shake out some residues! This could, of course, have simply been a mix-up with the photographs, and the one in the article was simply a control sample of GSR. However, in court, such a mix up would have severe consequences as to the reliability of the evidence.

Illustrative Case 3

This case involved a bank robbery using a double-barrelled sawn-off 12-bore shotgun which was used to kill a bank teller. When the exhibits were submitted, the police submission simply stated that a number of people had been arrested, and the police had also taken a sawn-off shotgun and several gloves. The gun went through the normal examination, which showed that both barrels had been recently fired and that it was in good condition, good working order, had acceptable trigger pressures and was not at all prone to accidental discharge. Tapings from the gloves showed that only one had gunshot residues on its outside surface. The results of the DNA analysis revealed that one of the defendants had been wearing the gloves.

During the trial, I was asked some searching questions about the presence of the GSR on the gloves and whether it could be contamination. I was then asked, 'If the gun was fired in the getaway car, would you expect to see gunshot residues on the hands of the person holding the gun?' The defence barrister then proceeded to produce a series of police photographs showing the inside of the car with a neat 12-bore-sized hole in the floor of the passenger side. This was completely unexpected, and the prosecution asked for a recess. Nobody had told me about this and, of course, it completely destroyed the GSR aspect of the case. If, however, I had known about the shot, I could have determined whether the muzzle was in tight contact with the floor at the time of firing. If it had been it would have placed a completely different aspect on the case.

- Are those methods supported by published, peer-reviewed research?

- Does that research use statistically valid sample sizes and blind testing?

Ask specifically for interim reports, bench notes and photomicrographs showing any match. These can often reveal far more that the witness statement. Ask also for interim reports, notes, and photographs of any distance determination. Make sure the examiner matched the ammunition type as closely as possible in making these tests. Ask specifically for notes and reports on gunshot residue testing.

Check to make sure that proper control samples were taken to identify contamination in the laboratory environment, at the scene of the crime and in the area where any GSR tapings were taken. Check also to make sure that the officers who arrested and handled the suspect before and during testing had not recently fired a gun or handled a fired gun.

How many comparison bullets did the examiner create? Were they of exactly the same type and make as those used in the crime? How many bullets had to be compared to find a match between the test fired bullets and the crime bullets? Are photomicrographs of these comparisons available, and if not, why not?

What are the examiner's criteria for identification? How did he or she reach that conclusion? Is it possible that the breech face marks used for the identification are pre-existing marks on the ammunition made during its manufacture, and not those made by the firearm?

If there is a photomicrograph, is it of the entire circumference or just the part that matches most closely? Was a video showing complete match of all the grooves taken and if not why not?

What kind of training does the examiner have? How does that compare with national law enforcement agencies and similar experts in large departments and in other countries? Due to the costs involved, independent forensic laboratories may not have the same certification and accreditation as a state laboratory. So, is the laboratory accredited? This can be very important because, if it is not, then how can one assess their criteria for stria, firearms examinations and GSR/EDX analysis?

Has the examiner taken proficiency or certification tests? How often are these tests taken (a minimum of one every year would be the normal frequency)? How difficult are the tests in comparison with typical crime scene evidence? Can the court be shown the results of these proficiency tests?

Are there any articles in the forensic identification trade journals discussing this specific firearm or ammunition in the case? Do the articles mention difficulties in making accurate identifications or factors that might produce a false positive result?

18.0.3   Legal challenges to forensic firearms evidence in the USA

Although the following might not be applicable in other jurisdictions, it does provide a starting point for further enquiry.

Firearms identification testimony has been accepted by courts since the early 20th century. Often, a prosecutor or defence counsel may feel there is not much that can achieved other than accept the examiner's opinion. However, in the past few years, there have been challenges to a variety of longstanding scientific disciplines.

In Daubert v. Merrell Dow Pharmaceuticals, Inc. (1993), the US Supreme Court set new standards for scientific evidence. Since then, defence attorneys have used Daubert to challenge a number of long-accepted forensic techniques, including firearms identification.

Both prosecutors and defence counsel should be aware of the concerns raised by the challengers, even though Daubert may not be relevant in their domain. A legal challenge to a firearms expert's methodology and opinion may be based on the following points.

1. Have firearms identification methods been adequately tested, are the published studies statistically valid and do they use sufficient blind and double-blind methods? Has there been sufficient testing to determine the error rate in identifications? Is there sufficient study of the statistical likelihood of coincidental matches?

2. Is the standard used by examiners too subjective? The examiners determine whether the comparison exceeds the best known non-match agreement from experience alone. This standard is built up in the examiner's 'mind's eye' and therefore it can be difficult to explain.

3. Is the standard used by examiners prone to potential problems of confirmation bias, tunnel vision, or pressures in high profile cases?

4. Has the field been given sufficient scrutiny by scientists outside the criminal justice community? DNA matching, for example, is used in medical care and research. Fingerprinting is used by some security systems and in identifying disaster victims. Most firearms tests are only used by forensic laboratories, usually funded by law enforcement agencies.

5. Are training, proficiency, and certification tests sufficiently rigorous, and do they reflect adequately the difficulties encountered with typical crime scene evidence?

6. Has the examiner provided sufficient information (generally photomicrographs of the purported match) to allow the judge or jury to understand the basis for the expert's opinion? If photographs are not introduced, then counsel, judge and jury have to take the examiner's word for his or her results, without seeing the underlying data. This should never happen.

7. Essentially, people are very good at recognising patterns, but sometimes one sees what one expects to see, or wants to see instead of what is really there. If, for example, an examiner tests two bullets known to be fired from consecutively manufactured handguns, he or she expects that the stria will be sufficiently different to show a non-match. Thus, if the examiner's results, published in a trade journal, match that preconception, it is hard to tell whether the examiner truly tested the hypothesis. A scientist in another field would generally perform a blind test, so that the examiner deciding whether the bullet matched or not would not know where it had come from. Preferably, the test would be double-blind, which is where neither the examiner nor the person who provided the samples would know where they came from. Double-blind testing avoids any subconscious cues passed between the person administering the test and the person taking the test. A scientist should also test a large number of bullets from the same and from different firearms, to create a statistically valid sample and eliminate random chance affecting the results.

The same basic principle applies to the individual examiner. If he or she is given information about the case that causes the examiner to expect the recovered firearm to match the crime scene evidence, then he or she may see a match that does not exist. That error occurred in the article quoted at the beginning of this section. The examiner was given information from the detectives suggesting a match was certain, was pressured to have a result quickly, and thus found the expected match. On later review, the examiner's conclusion proved to be wrong in that the evidence did not match the recovered firearm. Expectations, time pressure, and pressure to support a case can all cause mistakes.

A different challenge was raised in United States v. Kain, a Pennsylvania federal district court case in 2004 (the case resulted in a plea bargain before the trial court ruled on the defendant's challenge). The Kain challenge focused on statistical issues, specifically the percentage of coincidental matching and non-matching striations found on firearms evidence. It focused on Biasotti (1959 – a study still regarded as one of the most exhaustive statistical studies in the field) and Masson (1997 – a study discussing similarities between suspect ammunition found in the IBIS database and false negative results on manual examinations of ammunition known to be fired from the same gun).

A lawyer considering a challenge to the statistical likelihood of a random firearm with the same class characteristics as the recovered evidence having sufficiently similar individual characteristics to create a misidentification should look at the Kain pleadings.

So far, only three courts in the USA have limited or excluded a firearms examiner's testimony based on a Daubert challenge.

- In Sexton v. State (2002), the Texas Appellate Court excluded testimony purporting to match marks on recovered cartridges caused by the lips of the magazine; no magazine was recovered. The Sexton holding has not been generalised to other areas of firearms identification.

- In United States v. Green (2005), the Federal District Court of Massachusetts limited the testimony of a Boston Police Department firearms examiner to describing his observations. He could not testify that the recovered evidence matched the recovered firearm to the exclusion of all others. The trial court was critical of the examiner's training, the lack of certification for the examiner or laboratory and the lack of proficiency testing of the examiner by a neutral testing body. The examiner did not follow the AFTE protocol and had provided no notes, recorded observations or photographs. It also held that there were no peer-reviewed publications, as Daubert defined that term, in the firearms identification field. The opinion was also critical of the manner in which firearms evidence is compared, comparing it to a show-up (presumptively suggestive in the eyewitness identification field) rather than a line-up, which would reduce the problems of suggestion and confirmation bias.

- In United States v. Montiero (2006), another decision by the Federal District Court of Massachusetts, the trial court criticised a conclusion by a Massachusetts State Police firearms examiner. It also criticised the examiner's training and lack of neutral proficiency testing, although it noted that the examiner had taken and passed a proficiency test after making the identification in question. It also criticised the examiner's documentation and adherence to the AFTE procedures, and the lack of verification by another examiner. The examiner was precluded from testifying about his opinion until he had met the AFTE standards.

Typically, judges are reluctant to reject evidence that has been accepted without question for decades, even if the lawyer presents compelling evidence that the technique may have problems under the Daubert test. Even if the challenge is rejected, it may give the defence lawyer material to impeach the expert at trial or lead to a favourable settlement. The Kain case resulted in a favourable plea agreement. The Prochilo case in 2002 resulted in the defendant's acquittal; a vigorous challenge can cause a jury to reject the examiner's opinion if it is not adequately supported. Green and Monteiro both resulted in limitations on examiners' testimony, which should prove beneficial at trial.

18.0.4   Conclusion

Ballistics, or firearms identification, includes many aspects of firearms and ammunition. When a firearms expert is expected to testify, take the time to learn about the firearm and ammunition involved. Know the relevant laws and terms of the subject. Investigate the examiner's credentials, methods, and conclusions. Ensure that all the protocols involved with the examination, whether it simply be the identification of a firearm, stria matching or GSR analysis, have been strictly adhered to.

Further reading and references

1 Biasotti, A. (1959). A Statistical Study of the Individual Characteristics of Fired Bullets. *Journal of Forensic Sciences* 4 (1), 34–50.

2 AFTE, Criteria for Identification Committee (1992). Theory of Identification, Range of Striae Comparison Reports and Modified Glossary Definitions – an AFTE Criteria for Identification Committee Report. *AFTE Journal* 24 (2), 336–340.

3 Daubert v. Merrell Dow Pharmaceuticals, Inc., 509 U.S. 579 (1993).

4 Hodge, E.E. (1988). Guarding Against Error. *AFTE Journal* 20 (3), 290–293.

5 Masson, J.J. (1997). Confidence Level Variations in Firearms Identification Through Computerized Technology, *AFTE Journal* 29 (1), 42.

6 Molnar, S. (1970). What Is a Firearms Examiner? *AFTE Newsletter* 8, 36.

7 Schwartz, A. (2005). A Systemic Challenge to the Reliability and Admissibility of Firearms and Toolmark Identification. *The Columbia Science and Technology Law Review* 66, 1–42.

8 Sexton v. State, 93 S.W.3d 96 (Tex. Crim. App. 2002).

9 State v. Moua, No. K5-05-7335 (Anoka County, Minn, 10th Judicial District, July 7, 2006).

10 United States v. Green, 405 F. Supp. 2d 104 (D. Mass. 2005).

11 United States v. Kain, Criminal No. 03-573-1 (E.D. Pa. 2004).

12 United States v. Monteiro, 407 F. Supp. 2d 351 (D. Mass. 2006).

13 United States v. Moses, Criminal No. CCB-02-0410 (D. Md. 2003).

14 United States v. Plaza, 188 F. Supp. 2d 549, 58 Fed. R. Evid. Serv. 1 (2002).

15 United States v. Prochilo, Criminal. No. 96-10321-DPW (D. Mass 2002).

16 Stout, W.S. (1925). Fingerprinting Bullets. *Saturday Evening Post*, June 13, 1925, p. 6.

17 Watson v. Stone, 148 Fla. 516, 524, 4 So. 2d 700 (1941).

19.0

Qualifying the Expert and Cross-examination Questions

19.0.1 Definition

An expert witness is a person who is a specialist in a subject, often technical, who may present his/her expert opinion without having been a witness to any occurrence relating to the lawsuit or criminal case. It is an exception to the rule against giving an opinion in trial, provided that the expert is qualified by evidence of his/her expertise, training and special knowledge. If the expertise is challenged, the legal representative of the party calling the 'expert' must make a showing of the necessary background through questions in court, and the trial judge has discretion to qualify the witness or rule that either he/she is not an expert, or is an expert on limited subjects. In most jurisdictions, both sides must exchange the names and addresses of proposed experts to allow pre-trial depositions.

19.0.2 Introduction

As a consequence of advances in analytical technology and limitations on the way in which suspect interrogation is carried out, there has been an increasing necessity for courts of law to rely on expert testimony. Scientific proof has therefore become a necessity in reconstructing the sequence of events at a crime scene. Such 'scientific proof'

covers a large range of disciplines, varying in value from the indisputable to that of very dubious value.

Data obtained in a forensic laboratory has no meaning or worth until presented to a court of law. It is the expert witness who must serve as the vehicle to present this scientific data effectively to the court in a manner understandable to the layman.

Unfortunately, it is often the interface between the lawyer and the expert that breaks down, leaving the court with a somewhat myopic view of the evidence available. This lack of intelligible dialogue with the expert will often result in both the defence and prosecution failing to utilise fully the testimony of the expert to their best advantage. At times, it is the lawyer's lack of scientific knowledge which is at fault, while at others it is the expert's inability to present his testimony in a clear and precise manner.

It must be stated that it is not the role of the defence – or, for that matter, the prosecution – to verbally batter the expert into submission. This could easily destroy a perfectly well-qualified expert's career and alienate the court towards the lawyer concerned. What is required is for the lawyer to qualify the expert, seek out the relevancy of his experience and qualifications to the matter in question and then delve into the probative value of the evidence tendered.

The questions listed in this chapter are suggested as a starting point for the lawyer. The list is directed towards the forensic firearms examiner but, with

Forensic Ballistics in Court: Interpretation and Presentation of Firearms Evidence, First Edition. Brian J. Heard.
© 2013 John Wiley & Sons, Ltd. Published 2013 by John Wiley & Sons, Ltd.

modification, many of the topics are equally well suited to other disciplines.

It should be taken as nothing other than a series of questions which could arise, along with a possible response. Apart from the opening few questions regarding a witness' background and qualifications, there is no case thread to follow.

19.0.3   Qualifying the expert

Qualifying the expert is becoming increasingly important as there are, unfortunately, growing numbers of so-called defence 'experts' who have little or no knowledge of the scientific disciplines in which they are giving evidence.

To counter this, there is an increasing number of professional associations offering 'accreditation' in various forensic fields. This is a very good starting-point as far as the forensic profession is concerned, and some of the qualifications are very highly regarded. There are, however, less reputable bodies that offer accreditation for a fee or, at best, on the basis of an extremely simple written examination. Academic and professional qualifications should, therefore, be carefully examined.

Possible lines to follow and probable answers

Q1. What are your academic qualifications and how do they relate to your profession as a firearms and toolmark examiner?

A1. In reply, it should be stated that in the past, because it was considered that firearms and toolmark examinations tended to be more technically than academically orientated, experience plus a good secondary education was thus often acceptable. Nowadays, however, a good university degree is a basic requirement. Specialised post-degree qualification in firearms and toolmark examination from an accredited university, the Association of Firearms and Toolmark Examiners or the British Forensic Science Society should also be held.

Q2. What are your professional qualifications?

A2. This should include information on training periods, subject matter covered, attachments to other forensic organisations, papers written for professional organisations, etc.

Q3. Do you hold accreditation from any professional forensic body? If not, why?

A3. In the reply, it should be stated that many of the professional forensic associations now offer accreditation, some of which carry post-degree status. One should, however, be aware of those offered by small colleges and available through mail order or correspondence courses. These are often very elementary, and any competent examiner will look upon their value as dubious.

Two of the best professional qualifications are the British Forensic Science Society's (FSS) Qualification in Forensic Firearms and Toolmark examination, and AFTE's Certification in Firearms, Toolmark and GSR.

Illustrative Case 1

During a highly controversial case to determine whether a victim was murdered or had committed suicide, the layers for the family hired a so-called 'expert witness'. His examination of the exhibits bore no relation to what he should have been doing and his report was farcical, to say the least. During examination, it turned out that he had, before being sacked for dubious practices, worked on the exhibits reception desk for a forensic laboratory. He was also found to have had no knowledge of forensic firearms examination, no experience whatsoever with firearms and he had a long criminal record. His evidence was, not unsurprisingly, discredited.

19.0.4 General background questions

Q4. What is ballistics?

A4. This should not include any reference to forensic firearms examination unless it is to note that it is often misrepresented as 'forensic ballistics'.

Ballistics includes **internal ballistics,** which is the behaviour of a missile within the barrel, **external ballistics**, i.e. what course the missile takes from the muzzle to the target, and **terminal ballistics**, i.e. the bullet's effect on the target. With the exception of the latter, these matters seldom have any relevance to forensic firearms examinations.

Q5. What is the make, model and calibre of the evidence weapon?

A5. One must be equipped with sufficient background information to answer general questions on the evidence weapon, e.g. weight of weapon, magazine capacity, materials it is made from, introduction dates and model variations. If the questioning strays outside of that which the examiner feels comfortable, then the stock answer, 'I can look up the reference for that particular question should you so deem it necessary' should be utilised.

Q6. When you say that this gun is . . . calibre, what do you mean?

A6. A good knowledge of the fact that the calibre is often only indicative of the bore diameter is a prerequisite for court testimony. See Chapter 4.2.

Q7. By examining a fired bullet, can you tell the exact manufacturer of the weapon and its model?

A7. Possibly, but this is of little significance.

The CLIS file on General Rifling Characteristics gives thousands of land/groove widths, and it is possible, though time-consuming, to determine the make and model of a weapon from these measurements. It is, however, of little real value in the investigation of a crime.

J. Howard Mathews's 'Firearms Identification' Vol. I also has quite an extensive (although nowadays outdated) list of rifling characteristics.

Q8. Have you measured the pitch of the rifling on this bullet/in the bore of the weapon concerned?

A8. Possible, but of absolutely no use in the investigation of a crime. It would also be worth explaining what exactly 'pitch' means, i.e. the rifling rate of twist and how it is measured. See Chapter 2.3.

Q9. Did you measure the width of the lands and grooves on this bullet?

A9. With a graticule in the eyepiece of a microscope it is quite easy to obtain these measurements but, once again, these measurements are of little or no importance. It is the microscopic comparison which determines whether a bullet was fired from a particular weapon, not the physical dimensions of the lands and grooves.

19.0.5 Comparison microscopy

Q10. What is a photomicrograph, and did you take one in respect to this case?

A10. A photomicrograph is simply a photograph taken under the magnification of a microscope. This could be a simple photomicrograph, or a comparison photomicrograph. The answer should be 'Yes, I took a/several representative photograph(s) for my own reference, but not specifically for court purposes'.

Q11. If not then why not? Was this an attempt to deny some important knowledge to the court?

A11. Simply put, it takes years of experience to become a competent comparison microscopist. It is thus totally unrealistic to expect members of the court to become instant experts and to be able to interpret the significance of a comparison photomicrograph from a single print. At best, a photograph of a match will be illustrative, and at worst totally misleading.

In addition, a photomicrograph only shows a small portion of any match obtained. To produce a photographic representation of the whole circumference of a bullet, thus illustrating the concordance between the two, would require hundreds of photographs. Despite this, some jurisdictions do require the production of photomicrographs. In these instances, the examiner should make clear to the court the limitations of this type of evidence.

Most, if not all, comparison microscopes are now fitted with a video camera and video recorder, which can simplify the matter considerably. If the court demands this type of photographic evidence, a video recording of the match is the only real way of demonstrating how the positive comparison was made.

As an alternative, the examiner could offer the court access to a comparison microscope. In this way, it will be possible for the judge and jury to see the match at first hand and to have a clearer idea as to the problems involved.

Q12. A question as to the expert's experience with either a pantoscopic camera or a peripheral camera could follow this.

A12. These merely take low magnification photographs of the circumference of a bullet and are totally unsuitable for comparing the microstria. It is also unlikely that a modern laboratory would have one of these cameras.

Q13. Can you see the marks that you are using to prove that the bullet came from the gun in question?

A13. Only gross marks will be visible to the naked eye and it would be impossible even to contemplate making a comparison from these. Having said that, I have observed 'expert witnesses' demonstrating to a court how a comparison was made using a simple hand lens.

Q14. How much magnification do you require?

A14. Between 25 and 80 times as a general rule.

Q15. If you don't use enough magnification, you cannot see all the detail – is that correct?

A15. Yes, but further qualification is required in this answer, as per the following question.

Q16. But if you use too much, you lose sight of the small details?

A16. A nonsense question, but one that can easily trip the unwary. Basically, you require enough magnification to see the fine detail produced on the bullet by manufacturing defects in the barrel. This is generally accepted as being about $40\times$ magnification. Once the magnification rises above $100\times$, stria made by dirt, dust and general debris in the bore becomes visible. This is obviously of no significance but, at this magnification, such very fine stria becomes readily visible and interferes with the overall picture.

Q17. Is it not true that even on a positive match, there are many non-matching stria?

A17. This is true, and it is by experience alone that the examiner is able to determine which are relevant and which are non-relevant stria (see A16). Non-relevant stria would include those made by debris in the bore, microscopic traces of corrosion and fragments of the bullet being torn off by the rifling and becoming trapped between the barrel and the bore of the weapon. The variation in these microstria could be illustrated by taking photographs of consecutively fired bullets. This could help to de-mystify the concepts of comparison microscopy by reducing the subjectivity of the process and increasing the objectivity (i.e. scientific aspects) as much as possible. Reference should be made to the PhD thesis by Dr J. Hamby on matching and non-matching stria.

Q18. When you are comparing the rifling on a bullet, how much agreement do you require before you can identify a bullet as having come from a particular weapon?

A18. An amount that exceeds the best known non-match. See Chapter 7.0.

Q19. How much agreement is required?

A19. A non-quantifiable amount, and one that must be determined by the individual examiner, based on his experience. This is not to say, 'I am the expert, so believe me'; qualification (Chapter 7.0 and A20 below) is required.

Q20. What is the standard amount of agreement required by other firearms examiners?

A20. There is no real standard, but experience of other firearms examiners' work has shown that the 'mind's eye' criteria used is fairly consistent. Every forensic firearms laboratory should be part of an external proficiency review program (ASCLD LAB or similar) for stria matching. There should also be an internal proficiency program. The results of these should be readily available, should they be required by the court.

Q21. Would you expect to find some matching stria between bullets known to have been made by different weapons?

A21. The answer is yes, but with the proviso that with the thousands of stria in any bullet comparison, there are bound to be a number of accidentally matching stria. It is the experience of the examiner that enables him or her to determine which matching stria are relevant and which are accidental.

Q22. Have you ever deliberately compared bullets from different weapons to determine the best known non-match?

A22. The answer here must be a resounding 'Yes', otherwise it would not have been possible for the examiner to formulate criteria for a 'best known non-match'.

Q23. If a barrel is rusty, doesn't each bullet fired through it change its characteristics?

A23. It depends upon the degree of rusting. Light rusting will have little effect on the characteristic stria, while heavy rusting could make it impossible to match successive bullets.

Q24. Could you compare and match the first and the one hundredth bullet fired through the same barrel?

A24. As long as the barrel had not been damaged by rusting or some other external influence (e.g. cleaning with a steel rod, or heavy use of steel wool), the answer to this must be 'most definitely, yes'. This type of comparison should form part of every firearms examiner's training.

Q25. Is it not true that two guns of the same make and model will impart the same characteristics on bullets fired through them?

A25. Class characteristics will be the same, i.e. calibre, number, direction and angle of twist, groove profile, groove depth will be the same. The individual characteristics will not. See Chapter 7.0.

Q26. Would you agree that the matching of bullets is not an 'exact science', such as fingerprint examination, which requires 16 points of similarity?

A26. This should be answered along the lines of:
'I do not understand the term "exact science" – possibly you could elaborate. If you are inferring that 16 points of similarity constitutes an 'exactness', then why not 15, 17 or 63? There being no logical, rational or statistical justification to the selection of the number 16, it cannot, therefore, be inferred as endowing some magic quality of an "exact science" to the subject.

'With striation matches, there are often hundreds, if not thousands, of concording points that constitute a positive identification. That these matching lines are not counted or assigned an arbitrary number makes this type of examination no less of an exact science than fingerprinting.'

19.0.6   Gunshot residue

Q27. Who took the GSR samples in this case?

A27. Ideally they should have been taken by the officer on the stand, who should be able to account for any possibility of contamination. If not, then it will necessary to call to the stand the scene of crime officer who did take the samples.

Q28. What precautions did you take to prevent and contamination of the exhibits?

A28. Preferably, the expert giving evidence has no day-to-day contact with firearms. If not, s/he would have to demonstrate that every precaution had been taken to prevent any contamination from him/herself. This would, at the very least, involve using disposable gloves and disposable coveralls with hair cover. Ideally, it would also include washing their hair and changing into new clothes. Control tapings would have to be taken from the disposable gloves before the suspect's hands were taped. Gloves and, preferably, coveralls, *must* be changed for each subject taped.

Q29. How do you know that the tapings were not tampered with before being examined via the scanning electron microscope (SEM)?

A29. It should be standard procedure to examine the tapings under low power in the SEM before they are scanned. If any tampering has taken place, then the added residues will be visible as particles lying on the top of the tape. Anything picked up from the hands will be impressed into the tape's surface. Once again, this is only learned by experience and by deliberately making control false positive samples.

Q30. What steps have been taken, at the collection point and within the laboratory, to ensure that any chance of contamination has been eliminated?

A30. Disposable gloves and coveralls with hair cover must be used when taking samples from a suspect or dead body. The bags in which these items were stored must be kept in a sealed bag for future examination, should questionable results occur or defence counsel requests it. It should also be laboratory practice to randomly examine used gloves and coveralls as part of contamination review procedures.

Q31. Laboratory procedure should be questioned as to the possibility for environmental contamination.

A31. Ideally, no-one working with weapons should have access to the SEM preparation and examination room. The room should also be positively pressurised to minimise ingress of contamination. There should also be a vestibule in which one dons the anti-contamination suits and shoes prior to entering the SEM room. This should be at a lower pressure than the SEM room, but higher than outside.

Q32. Is there a firing range within half a mile?

A32. An irrelevant question if all of the above precautions have been taken. Having said that, the answer must be available.

Q33. Does anybody in the immediate vicinity of where the samples are examined have any connection with firearms?

A33. A very valid question. Ideally, the SEM operator should be a qualified and practising firearms examiner as s/he will have the necessary experience and background knowledge, as well as up-to-date information on ammunition developments, to recognise the relevance of any ambiguous or questionable results. S/he will also be able to interpret those results and, via his/her knowledge, be able to explain their relevance to the court. There is, however, every possibility of such an operator bringing contamination to the SEM room. If this is the case, the operator will have to demonstrate that every possible precaution has been taken to ensure that contamination has been eliminated.

As part of this daily control, samples from the SEM bench and preparation areas must be taken and scanned for contamination as a prerequisite. In addition, the following should be considered as an absolute minimum:

1. Ensure that any SEM work is carried out before entering any other part of the laboratory.

2. Ensure that the hair is washed prior to entering SEM room.

3. Prior to entering the SEM room, strip off all clothes and put on disposable anti-contamination suit with hair cover, gloves and shoe covers.

4. Complete all tasks in the SEM room in one sitting in order to reduce the number of exits and entries to an absolute minimum. If it is necessary to leave the SEM room, dispose of the anti-contamination kit and put on a new set prior to entering the SEM room again.

Q34. Where were the bags obtained that were used to protect the hands of the suspect?

A34. Often, these are merely envelopes taken from police station supplies or, even worse, plastic bags, and are thus very susceptible to contamination. This contamination could come from either a range within the station, or from officers who carry or use weapons.

The inside and outside of these bags or envelopes should be control taped before use to determine whether they have been contaminated.

Ideally, they should be paper bags obtained from an outside source. These should be randomly taped and examined in the SEM for any possible

signs of contamination. The results of these examinations must be retained for court purposes.

GSR sample kits should be made up by an outside contractor. These should contain surgical gloves, plastic restraints, disposable coveralls, disposable shoe covers, five sampling tubes and an instruction leaflet.

Q35. How were the suspect's hands secured while awaiting the taking of the tapings?

A35. If they were handcuffed, there is a very real possibility of GSR particles being transferred from the cuffs to the hands of the suspect. Research has shown[1] that, during range courses, an officer's clothes, baton, handcuffs and holster will become heavily contaminated with GSR particles. The GSR particles remain in the handcuff pouch and, when the handcuffs are used, these particles will be transferred to the hands of an arrested person. Only plastic cable ties (see A35) should be used as restraints. These can be supplied to police stations in sealed plastic bags.

Q36. How can you be sure that the particles found were, in fact, from the firing of a weapon and not environmental or other contamination?

A36. Knowledge will have to be shown of GSR/indicative GSR particle ratios, as well as GSR particle/lead particle ratios, and how they relate to the case statistics.

Q37. What do you consider to be a minimum number of GSR particles for a positive result and how did you decide on that number?

A37. One is the minimum number, but this would have to be backed up with the relevant GSR particle/lead particle and GSR/indicative particle ratios. As a general rule, two particles, with the aforementioned ratios, is generally considered the absolute minimum requirement for a positive finding.

---

[1] Unpublished paper by author.

19.0.7 Ferrozine test

Q38. How do you know that the results obtained from this test were not caused by a kitchen knife, or a knife, fork and spoon?

A38. Firstly, most kitchen utensils are made from stainless steel or are plated with nickel or chromium, neither of which gives a positive result to this test. In addition, this whole test relies on the interpretation of the visualised marks on the hands. The examiner will, therefore, have to prove beyond reasonable doubt that the marks observed were those from a weapon and not something accidental, such as a pry bar or car jack.

Personally, I always carry a spray can of Ferrozine with me when giving such evidence. A member of the court, jury or even the judge himself can then be asked to hold the object in question and then have his or her hands sprayed. A highly effective technique.

Q39. What other metals give a positive reaction to this test?

A39. The examiner should have knowledge of the interfering metals in this test and how to differentiate between copper and iron. S/he should also be aware, as any forensic chemist should, of the chemical processes involved, i.e. bidentate ligand formation with ferrous ions.

Q40. How many times did you spray the suspect's hands?

A40. A stock question designed to catch out the unwary. This is a qualitative test, not quantitative, and the number of times the hand is sprayed or the quantity of reagent applied to the hands has no bearing on the result.

Further reading

1 Moss, R. (1970). Scientific Proof in Criminal cases, a Texas Lawyer's Guide. *AFTE Newsletter* 10
2 Hodge, E. & Blackburn, B. (1979). The Firearms/Toolmark Examiner in Court. *AFTE Journal* 11 (4), 70–96.
3 Moenssens, A.A., Moses, R.E. & Inbau, F.E. (1965). *Scientific Evidence in Criminal Cases*. Foundation Press, Evanston, IL, USA.
4 Murdock, J.E. (1992). Some Suggested Court Questions to Test Criteria for Identification Qualifications. *AFTE Journal* 24 (1), 69–75.
5 Mathews, J. (1962). *Firearms Identification*, Vol. 1 The University of Wisconsin Press.

20.0
Chain of Custody

20.0.1 Introduction

At its simplest, 'chain of custody' is a legal phrase that describes the provable knowledge of everyone who has handled the evidence and a provability that the evidence is the same as that which was present and collected from the crime scene.

The question that the chain of custody attempts to answer is: 'Is this evidence the same, and unaltered, as the one that was collected at the crime scene?'

Lawyers often believe that proving the chain of evidence is peripheral to the facts of the case. However, hard evidence, i.e. physical exhibits, can have a considerable and vital impact on the outcome of many trials. The regular use of hard evidence in courts today – especially the escalated application of forensic sciences in the process of establishing guilt or innocence – emphasises the increasing importance for lawyers to focus on this area of evidence.

Real evidence is physical evidence, such as a firearm, ammunition or bloodstained clothing that is directly connected with a crime scene.

20.0.2 Basics

From crime scene to forensic laboratory to courtroom, all evidence must be inventoried and secured to preserve its integrity. Evidence admissibility in court is predicated upon an unbroken chain of

---

Illustrative Case 1

At one stage in his career, the author was employed by a police force to upgrade its forensic firearms laboratory. The laboratory was very poorly run and possessed absolutely no exhibit management or case file system. The firearms examiner would simply collect the items he required directly from the crime scene, with no record being kept as to what was recovered by the police exhibits officer. The examiner would assign a single laboratory case number to cover all the exhibits he collected. This number was sequential from the day the laboratory first opened, and it did not even include a date or year qualifier. There were no details on the exhibit as to who had collected it, from where or when. These unsealed exhibits were simply thrown into a heap on the floor. No case file was ever created, and the examiner's notes on his collection and examination were simply handwritten on a stenographer's pad.

The chance of exhibits becoming mislaid, fired ammunition from different cases becoming intermixed and cross contamination was extremely high. As a result, many cases fell at the first hurdle, due to the lack of any credible exhibit handling system. In fact, in many instances, the police officer in charge of the case did not wait for or even (when and if ever it finally arrived) present the examiner's report to the court.

Forensic Ballistics in Court: Interpretation and Presentation of Firearms Evidence, First Edition. Brian J. Heard.
© 2013 John Wiley & Sons, Ltd. Published 2013 by John Wiley & Sons, Ltd.

custody, so it is vital to be able to demonstrate that the evidence introduced at trial is the same evidence that was collected at the crime scene, and that access was controlled and documented.

An understanding of the rules governing chain of custody is vital for any lawyer either prosecuting or defending a case.

20.0.3 Process

After collection at the crime scene by the scene of crime officer or the firearms examiner him/herself, the evidence is turned over to the investigator, who submits it to the laboratory's property and evidence section and obtains a receipt documenting the transfer.

Generally, submissions to the forensic laboratory are done on a 'request for analysis' form, which lists the evidence items and a documented chain of custody.

Each individual who assumes custody of the evidence, from collection through analysis, signs the chain of custody document. Many departments have automated this process via a computerised system, called a Laboratory Information Management System (LIMS), whereby all transfers are securely done using bar codes. The chain of custody report will identify each individual contributing to the analysis of the evidentiary materials.

Once the analysis is complete, the evidence is either returned to the submitting agency or is stored by the laboratory, and the chain of custody will document this disposition. All law enforcement reports, photographs, lab analysis reports and chain of custody documents are kept in the case file, which will be made available to the prosecution and is subject to discovery by defence counsel.

In order to preserve the evidence with credibility, this chain of custody must be maintained and preserved at all costs.

20.0.4 In court

Evidence found at the scene of a crime must eventually be presented and questioned in the courtroom. For the evidence to be of use in a trial, it must make

the journey from crime scene to laboratory and on to court in a validated and secure manner, so that all involved can be assured that it has not been contaminated and that the evidence is relevant to the crime investigation. In order to insure validity, investigators must follow the precept of chain of custody when it comes to collecting and handling evidence.

The first identifiable person to collect an item of evidence – be it a firearm, bullet or piece of bloodstained clothing – will sign their initials and date on its secure packaging. Some jurisdictions advocate marking the actual exhibit itself, either with an engraving tool or a permanent marker. However, this is generally inadvisable as, in the case of expended ammunition components, it could easily damage micro-stria or, in the case of GSR, introduce contamination. It also permanently damages an exhibit, which could be a cause for contention.

An identifiable person must always have the physical custody of a piece of evidence. In practice, this means that a police officer or detective will take charge of a piece of evidence, document its collection and hand it over to an evidence clerk for storage in a secure place. If there is a break during the examination in the laboratory, the exhibit must be stored in a secure area to which only the examiner has access, and this access must be demonstrable.

These transactions, and every succeeding transaction between the collection of the evidence and its appearance in court, should be completely documented chronologically in order to withstand legal challenges as to the authenticity of the evidence. Documentation should include:

- the conditions under which the evidence is gathered;

- the identity of all evidence handlers;

- the duration of evidence custody;

- the security conditions while handling or storing the evidence;

- the manner in which evidence is transferred to subsequent custodians each time such a transfer occurs, together with the signatures of persons involved at each step.

It should be noted at this juncture that it is desirable for the forensic laboratory to have its own laboratory chain of custody system in place. Generally, this will be laboratory-wide and not just in the firearms section, as other sections may well require access to the exhibit for collection of blood, fibres, etc.

These systems are virtually all computer-based, with each person who is likely to handle an exhibit from the reception clerk to the examiner having his/her own bar coded signature. In addition, each exhibit will have its own bar coded exhibit bag to prevent tampering with the exhibit and re-bagging. Such systems can be designed to cover the requirements of the police force as a whole.

When the case is presented in court, the prosecuting lawyer takes over custody of the evidence and signs the chain of custody label to that effect. If the chain of custody procedure is handled correctly, the case can then proceed with all involved being aware of the precise journey that the evidence has taken from crime scene to the court. This allows evidence to be admitted in court, and for witnesses to have the assurance that the item of evidence was indeed present at the scene of the crime, was examined by the forensic laboratory, and to testify accordingly. The judge and jury are then able to use the evidence, along with witness statements and other information, to guide their decision-making process.

Further reading

1 Keatley, K.L. (1999). A review of US EPA and FDA requirements for electronic records, electronic signatures, and electronic submissions. *Quality Assurance* 7 (2), 77–89.

2 Venkatesan, M. & Grauer, Z. (2004). Leveraging Radio Frequency Identification (RFID) technology to improve laboratory information management. *American Laboratory* 36 (18), 11–14.

3 Vermont Department of Environmental Conservation's Environmental Laboratory, 'Section 7: Sample Management and Chain of Custody Procedures'. http://www.anr.state.vt.us/dec/lab/htm/qualitycontrol.htm

4 Tomlinson, J. J. Elliott-Smith, W. & Radosta, T. (2006). Laboratory Information Management System Chain of Custody: Reliability and Security. *Journal of Automated Methods and Management in Chemistry* 2006 (1), 21.

Appendix 1

Standard of Review: 'Daubert Trilogy'

The Daubert standard is a legal precedent set in 1993 by the Supreme Court of the United States regarding the admissibility of expert witnesses' testimony during legal proceedings. The citation is Daubert v. Merrell Dow Pharmaceuticals, 509 U.S. 579 (1993).

A Daubert motion is a motion, raised before or during trial, to exclude the presentation of unqualified evidence to the jury. This is usually used to exclude the testimony of an expert witness who has no such expertise or who has used questionable methods to obtain the information.

In Daubert, the Supreme Court held that federal trial judges are the 'gatekeepers' of scientific evidence. Under the Daubert standard, the trial judges must evaluate proffered expert witnesses to determine whether their testimony is both 'relevant' and 'reliable' – a two-pronged test of admissibility:

- **The Relevancy Prong** the relevancy of a testimony refers to whether or not the expert's evidence 'fits' the facts of the case. For example, you may invite an astronomer to tell the jury if it had been a full moon on the night of a crime. However, the astronomer would not be allowed to testify if the fact that the moon was full was not relevant to the issue at hand in the trial.

- **The Reliability Prong** the Supreme Court explained that in order for expert testimony to be considered reliable, the expert must have

derived his or her conclusions from the scientific method (Daubert v. Merrell Dow Pharmaceuticals, Inc. (1993) 509 U.S. 579, 589.) The court offered 'general observations' of whether proffered evidence was based on the scientific method, although the list was not intended to be used as an exacting checklist.

A third prong, **Empirical Testing**, is also taken into account, i.e.:

- The theory or technique must be falsifiable, refutable, and testable.

- It must be subjected to peer review and publication.

- There must be a known or potential error rate and maintenance of standards concerning its operation must be in existence.

- The theory and technique must be generally accepted by a relevant scientific community.

Trial judges have always had the authority to exclude inappropriate testimony but, previous to Daubert, trial courts often preferred to let juries hear evidence proffered by both sides.

Once certain evidence has been excluded by a Daubert motion because it fails to meet the relevancy and reliability standard, it will likely be challenged

Forensic Ballistics in Court: Interpretation and Presentation of Firearms Evidence, First Edition. Brian J. Heard.
© 2013 John Wiley & Sons, Ltd. Published 2013 by John Wiley & Sons, Ltd.

when introduced again in another trial. Even though a Daubert motion is not binding to other courts of law, if something has been found not trustworthy, other judges may choose to follow that precedent.

The Daubert decision was heralded by many observers as one of the most important Supreme Court decisions of the last century, imparting crucial legal reforms to reduce the volume of what has disparagingly been labelled 'junk science' in the courtroom.

Many of these individuals were convinced by Peter Huber's 1991 book, *Galileo's Revenge: Junk Science in the Courtroom*, which argued that numerous product liability and toxic tort verdicts were unjustly made on the basis of junk science. According to Huber, junk science in the courts threatened not only justice but the workings of the American economy. This threat rested on two premises:

1. Juries are not competent to recognise flaws in scientific testimony, especially toxic tort or product liability suits where decisions on causation rested on complex scientific issues.

2. The result of junk science is the issuing of awards that deter manufacturers from introducing worthwhile products into the marketplace, out of fear of unwarranted tort liability for injuries that their products have not caused.

By requiring experts to provide relevant opinions grounded in reliable methodology, proponents of Daubert were satisfied that these standards would result in a fair and rational resolution of the scientific and technological issues that lie at the heart of product liability adjudication.

To summarise, five cardinal points Daubert asks from every new technique to be admissible in court are:

1. Has the technique been tested in actual field conditions, not just in a laboratory? (e.g. fingerprinting has been extensively tested and verified not only in laboratory conditions, but even in actual criminal cases. So it is admissible. Polygraphy, on the other hand has been well tested in laboratories but not so well tested in field conditions.)

2. Has the technique been subject to peer review and publication?

3. What is the known or potential rate of error? Is it zero, or low enough to be close to zero?

4. Do standards exist for the control of the technique's operation?

5. Has the technique been generally accepted within the relevant scientific community?

The Supreme Court explicitly cautioned that the Daubert list should not be regarded by judges as 'a definitive checklist or test . . . ' Yet, in practice, many judges regularly exclude scientific evidence when they, assuming the role of 'amateur scientist', determine it to be lacking on even a single Daubert point, instead of assessing the totality of such evidence.

Further reading

1 Berger, M.A. (2005). What Has a Decade of Daubert Wrought? (PDF). *American Journal of Public Health* 95 (S1) S59.

2 Huber, P.W. (1991). *Galileo's Revenge: Junk Science in the Courtroom*. New York: Basic Books. ISBN 0-465-02623-0.

3 Gottesman, M. (1998). For Barefoot to Daubert to Joiner: Triple Play or Double Error? *Arizona Law Review* 40, 753.

4 Owen, D.G. (2002). A Decade of Daubert. *Denver University Law Review* 80, 345.

5 Dixon, L. & Gill, B. (2002). *Changes in the Standards for Admitting Expert Evidence in Federal Civil Cases Since the Daubert Decision*. RAND Institute for Civil Justice.

6 Risinger, D.M. (2000). Navigating Expert Reliability: Are Criminal Standards of Certainty Being Left on the Dock? *Albany Law Review* 64, 99–152.

7 Neufeld, P. (2005) The (Near) Irrelevance of Daubert to Criminal Justice and Some Suggestions for Reform. *American Journal of Public Health* 95 (S1) S107.

8 Gatowski, S.I., Dobbin, S.A., Richardson, J.T., Ginsburg, G.P., Merlino, M.L. & Dahir, V. (2001). Asking the gatekeepers: A National Survey of Judges on

Judging Expert Evidence in a Post-Daubert World. *Law and Human Behavior* 25 (5), 433–458.

9 Rothman, K.J. & Greenland, S. (2005). Causation and Causal Inference in Epidemiology. *American Journal of Public Health* 95 (S1) S144.

10 Melnick, R. (2005). A Daubert Motion: A Legal Strategy to Exclude Essential Scientific Evidence in Toxic Tort Litigation. *American Journal of Public Health* 95 (S1) S30.

11 Jasanoff, S. (2005). Law's Knowledge: Science for Justice in Legal Settings. *American Journal of Public Health* 95 (S1) S49.

Appendix 2

Commercial and General Abbreviations for Bullet Configurations

ACC   Accelerator – sub-calibre bullet fitted into conventional cartridge with a plastic sabot.

ACP   Automatic Colt Pistol – used as a designation for cartridges designed specifically for self loading pistol cartridges, e.g. .380″ ACP, .45″ ACP. Can also be in lower case, e.g. .380″ acp or .45″ acp.

AP   Armour Piercing bullet, usually with a tungsten core.

API   Armour Piercing Incendiary – as above, but with the addition of an incendiary pellet in the nose.

BBWC   Bevel Base Wadcutter.

BRPT   Bronze Point – bronze insert in tip improves trajectory, velocity and energy transfer at extreme ranges. Tip expands rapidly when driven back through bullet.

BT   Boat-Tail.

CL   Core-Lokt – a Remington bullet with the core bonded to the jacket. Also has a progressively tapered jacket which initiates and controls expansion.

CORBON   Brand name for Glazer ammunition.

CP   Copper Plated – lead bullet dipped in copper; reduces lead fouling and is cheaper than copper coating.

DPX   A solid copper hollow point bullet made by Glazer.

EFMJ   Expanding Full Metal Jacket – Federal's answer to areas with restrictions on hollow points. A regular full metal jacket bullet, but with a rubber tip to the lead core. The tip of the jacket is grooved and collapses on striking the target, producing petal-like expansion and delivering energy without over-penetration.

ENCAP   Encapsulated – a bullet completely encapsulated with a metal jacket, usually by electroplating. Intended to reduce environmental lead contamination in training ranges.

EP   Expanding Point – Winchester developed bullet to assist expansion in small calibre hollow point bullets, e.g. .25″ ACP. Has a round lead ball inserted into the hollow point cavity to assist in feeding and expansion on striking target.

ERBT   Extended Range Boat-Tail – long-range bullet by Remington.

Forensic Ballistics in Court: Interpretation and Presentation of Firearms Evidence, First Edition. Brian J. Heard.
© 2013 John Wiley & Sons, Ltd. Published 2013 by John Wiley & Sons, Ltd.

Exp	Express cartridge – used on high-powered sporting rifle cartridges to designate a higher velocity and kinetic energy than the standard calibre. Initially used with the additional prefix 'Nitro' to distinguish between black powder and nitrocellulose-based propellants.	GD	Speer Gold Dot bullet.
		GDHP	Speer Gold Dot Hollow Point.
		GM	Gilding Metal – copper/zinc alloy for bullet jackets.
		GMCS	Gilding Metal-Clad Steel – steel bullet jacket coated with gilding metal.
FMJ	Full Metal Jacket – jacketed bullet with lead core exposed at base.	GS	Remington Golden Saber bullet.
		GSC	Custom turned copper bullets
FMJE	Full Metal Jacket Encapsulated – like FMJ, but also has the base covered and does not expose any of the lead core.	HBWC	Hollow Base Wadcutter – for better expansion on firing and to move the centre of weight of the bullet forwards.
FNSP	Flat Nose Soft Point – similar to the FPJ, but has lead-exposed point that expands on impact.	HC	Hard Cast – hard lead alloy.
		HE-IT	High Explosive Incendiary Tracer bullet.
FP	Flat-Pointed bullet.	GCK	Gas Check – metallic cup or disc is attached to bottom of lead alloy bullet. Decreases gas blow-by, increases velocity and reduces lead fouling.
FPJ	Flat-Point Jacketed – full metal jacketed bullet with a flat point. Most .40″ S&W and .30-30″ Winchester rounds have this design. The .30-30″ Winchester has a tubular magazine and uses a flat-point bullet to prevent accidental detonation of one round by the tip of another during recoil.		
		GDHP	Gold Dot Hollow-Point. Speer's hollow-point bullet with jacket bonded to lead core to prevent separation and control expansion and penetration.
FRAN	Frangible – prevents ricochet by breaking apart on contact. Usually made from lead, iron or tungsten dust, bonded with hard wax or an epoxy resin. Originally used in fairground mini range ammunition to prevent ricochet or penetration of the target. Has recently been developed for air marshals to avoid over-penetration and ricochet aboard airplanes. Metal dust other than lead is used in non-toxic ammunition for use in indoor ranges (see Chapter 4.4 on non-toxic ammunition).	GS	Golden Saber – Remington-designed controlled expansion bullet.
		GS	Grand Slam – Speer's design for hunting big game. Jacket is 45 per cent bigger at base to prevent roll-back and retain bullet's weight. Internal jacket flutes ensure proper expansion. Bullet's core is a ternary (three-part) alloy, which is poured into the jacket at 900°F to prevent jacket slippage.
		H&H	Holland and Holland cartridge designed for the company for their high powered sporting rifles.
FST	Winchester Failsafe Talon round.	HSHK	Hydra-Shok – Federal's handgun defence bullet. Unique centre-post design delivers controlled expansion. Notched jacket transfers energy efficiently and penetrates barriers while retaining stopping power.
GC	Metallic cup or disc is attached to bottom of lead-alloy bullet. Decreases gas blow-by, increases velocity and lead fouling in the barrel.		

JHC	Jacketed Hollow Cavity – jacketed bullet with hole in tip to promote expansion on impact. More often designated JHP, i.e. Jacketed Hollow Point.
KTW	A metal-penetrating round – originally made of sintered tungsten and later hardened brass-coated with green-coloured PTFE. Only sold to law enforcement agencies.
LHP	Lead Hollow-Point.
LRN	Lead Round Nose.
LSWC	Lead Semi-Wadcutter.
LSWC-GC	Lead Semi-Wadcutter Gas Checked.
LWC	Lead Wadcutter – bullet with completely flat nose to cut clean hole through paper targets.
LTC	Lead Truncated Cone – conical-shaped bullet with flat point.
MC	Metal Cased – jacketed bullet.
Mag	Magnum, to specify cartridges of a higher power than standard e.g. .41″ Rem Mag., .44″ Mag.
MK	MatchKing – bullets made to exact tolerances by Sierra for target shooting.
MOLY	Moly-Coated – bullet is coated with molybdenum disulphide to reduce friction and increase velocity.
NBT	Nosler Ballistic Tip – Nosler developed this bullet with a polycarbonate tip that protects the bullet from damage in the magazine resulting from recoil. The tip also stabilises the bullet for long-range shooting and ensures reliable expansion when the bullet hits its target.
NP	Nosler Partition – has two lead cores separated by bullet jacket. Top part of jacket is thin and promotes expansion of bullet. Bottom part of bullet has thicker jacket that retains bullet's weight, stops fragmentation and increases penetration.

NTLR	Non-Toxic Large Rifle (ammunition primer).
Nyclad	Federal's bullet totally coated with black nylon to reduce friction and reduce lead pollution in ranges.
PB	9×19 mm and 7.65×19 mm cartridges with Latin designation Parabellum (i.e. for war).
PEP	Positive Expanding Point – Winchester bullet for maximum impact on medium-size game.
PG	Partition Gold – Winchester's proprietary design delivers expansion and penetration on medium- and large-size game at a wide range of impact velocities. Rear core is hard lead alloy, locked in place with a heel crimp to prevent core slippage and maximise penetration. Patented steel cup reinforces and prevents core distortion at high-impact velocities.
PL	Power-Lokt – Remington's small-game bullet produces benchrest-level accuracy. Copper jacket is electrolytically bonded to lead core.
PnPT	Pneumatic Point.
PPL	Paper Patched Lead.
PSP	Plated Soft Point.
PSP, PTDSP	Pointed Soft Point.
+P	'Plus P' (10–15 per cent overpressure) – high-pressure cartridge for use in standard weapon where greater power is required.
+P+	'Plus P Plus' (20–25 per cent overpressure) – as above, but even more powerful. Only recommended for weapons with a strong steel frame and usually only sold to law enforcement agencies.
PP	Power-Point jacketed soft nose from Winchester delivers maximum energy on impact. Notches around jacket's mouth improve upset and ensure uniform, rapid expansion.

PSP   Pointed Soft Point – pointed bullet that retains velocity over long ranges. Soft nose initiates rapid bullet expansion. Jacket and core toughness vary according to calibre and weight of bullet.

PTHP   Platinum-Tipped Hollow Point – a Winchester design for handgun hunters.

PWC   Pointed Wadcutter – lubricated solid lead with pointed nose. Formed by swaging process with sharp shoulder for clean hole-punching in paper targets.

RN   Round Nose – ogival nose shape to bullet.

RNFP   Round Nose Flat Point – as above, but with flat point to ogive.

RNL   Round Nosed Lead – plain lead bullet with ogive-shaped bullet.

S&W   Designation for cartridges designed specifically for Smith and Wesson designed weapons, e.g. .38″ S&W revolver.

SBK   Sierra BlitzKing – used for 'varmint hunting'; has plastic tip inserted into bullet cavity, which expands on impact.

SFS   Supreme Fail Safe – hollow-point bullet with lead core and steel insert. Delivers controlled expansion, deeper penetration and bullet weight retention.

SLD   Solid – rifle bullet usually made from copper, bronze or brass alloy, but not lead. For thick skinned game, e.g. buffalo, elephant.

SMG   Sub-Machine Gun.

SMP   Semi-Pointed.

SP   Soft Point – jacketed bullet with exposed lead tip.

SP   Spire Point – long sharp-pointed bullet.

SPTZ   Spitzer – pointed bullet

ST   Silver Tip – Winchester trade name for bullet with an alloy aerodynamic tip.

SWC   Semi-Wadcutter – intermediate between a wadcutter and a round-nosed bullet.

SPCL   Soft Point Core-Lokt – locks progressively heavier jacketed midsection to lead core, preventing separation. Stays together on impact, expands in a controlled manner and mushrooms uniformly.

SPT   Spitzer – pointed bullet normally used in modern military rifles.

SST   Super Shock Tipped – Hornady's design incorporates a pointed polymer tip that improves ballistic coefficient and increases velocity, accuracy and downrange power. Specially designed jacket grips and controls expanding core, allowing maximum expansion while retaining mass and momentum.

SXT   Supreme Expansion Technology – Winchester's personal protection bullet. Designed with reverse-tapered jacket, has uniform expansion, greater accuracy and reliable firearm functioning.

TAP   Tactical Application Police – designed by Hornady specifically for law enforcement. Heavier bullet weight and polymer tip provide rapid expansion and excellent barrier penetration (without over-penetration).

TC   Truncated Cone – similar to an inverted cone, but with the top chopped off.

TCHP   Truncated Cone Hollow-Point – same as truncated cone, but with a hole in top to promote expansion in target.

THV   Tres Haute Vitesse – French for 'Very High Velocity'. Very lightweight and thin-spire pointed bullet, usually made from a bronze alloy. High speed and design result not only in huge wound

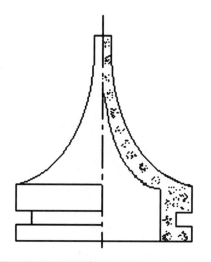

Figure A.2.1   THV bullet.

but also has good metal and BRV penetrative capabilities (Figure A.2.1).

TMJ   Total Metal Jacket – same as full metal jacket, except base is also jacketed.

TMWC   Target-Master Wadcutter – wadcutter bullets made to highest tolerances to achieve best accuracy possible.

UNI-Classic   RWS deformation bullet,
UMC LeadLess   Remington's range of non-toxic ammunition

V-Max   Varmint Express Ballistic Tip – Hornady's ballistic-tip 'varmint' bullet has a polymer insert that aids in rapid expansion once the bullet hits the target.

WinClean   Winchester's range of non-toxic ammunition.

WC   Wadcutter – Essentially a round-nosed bullet without the round nose. Gives a sharp edge for cutting clean holes in the target when target shooting.

XTP   Extreme Terminal Performance – Hornady bullet designed for controlled expansion at wide range of handgun velocities. Bullet's jacket and core expansion rates are the same, reducing separation and increasing trauma in target.

Z BULLET   Zinc alloy bullet made in various configurations by National Bullet Co.

Appendix 3

Some of the More Common Trade Names

A.A — Trade name of Azanza y Arrizabalaga, Spain Manufactured copies of cheap Belgian pistols.

Acme — Trade name of spur trigger revolvers made by Hopkins & Allen ca. 1885.

Acme Arms — Used by J. Stevens Arms Co. ca. 1882.

Acme Hammerless — Used by Hulbert Bros on Hopkins & Allen revolvers ca. 1893.

Adams Patent Small Arms Co, London. — Manufacturer of Adams designed firearms 1864–92.

Aetna — Spur trigger revolvers made by Harrington and Richardson ca. 1876.

Ajax Army — On revolvers sold by Meacham & Co. 1880.

Alamo — On revolvers sold by Stoeger from West Germany.

Allen — Trade name on revolvers made by Hopkins & Allen.

Alpine Industries — Makers of M1 carbines 1962–65.

Robert Adams — London gun maker 1809–1890, patented the first successful double-action revolver in 1851. His revolvers were used during the Crimean War, the Indian Mutiny, the U.S. Civil War and the Anglo-Zulu War.

AM — Abbreviation on Italian military arms meaning Air Force.

American International — Importers in Salt Lake City, Utah of .22 RF calibre machine guns, notably the AR180.

Amadeo — Trade name of Barthelet D. Amadeo of Eibar, Spain Manufactured copy of Galand, calibre 11 mm, marked 'Privilegiado A.P.E.G. Eibar'. Bayard pistols from 1907–39.

Anciens Establissments Pieper

Anschutz, Bruno — German manufacturer of sporting arms 1919–26.

Arizmendi — Trade name of F Arizmendi y Goenaga of Eibar, Spain. Manufactured copies of Belgian pistols as well as their own design.

Arminius — Trade name of Friederich Pickert pre-WWII, probably manufactured in East Germany. Now made by Weihrauch

Astra — Astra-Unceta y Cia. Formed 1908 in Eibar. Moved to Guernica, 1913. In 1926 name changed to Unceta y Cia and in 1953 to Astra Unceta y Cia

Auto Ordinance Corp — Developers of the Thompson SMG. New York City ca. 1920.

Baby Russian — Model name used by H. Kolb and Sedgeley on small revolvers.

Martin Bascaran — Made Spanish copies of cheap Belgian pistols 1919–27.

Baltimore Arms Co. — Maker of hammerless shotguns 1895–1902.

Bauer Firearms — Manufacturer of pocket pistols, 1972–84 Fraser, Michigan, USA.

Forensic Ballistics in Court: Interpretation and Presentation of Firearms Evidence, First Edition. Brian J. Heard.
© 2013 John Wiley & Sons, Ltd. Published 2013 by John Wiley & Sons, Ltd.

Beeman Airguns	Founded in 1972 and sold to S/R Industries of Maryland in 1993.
Beretta, Pietro	Italian manufacturer of shotguns, rifles and pistols back to 1680.
Bernadelli, Vincenzo	Italian manufacturer of sporting arms since 1865.
Bicycle	Trade name on revolvers made by Harrison & Richardson.
Isaac Blisset	Leadenhall Street, London, England, 1822–45. Double-barrelled side-lock hammer shotguns.
Bolumburu Gregorio	Belgian manufacturer of cheap quality self-loading pistols 1917–23.
Boy's Choice	Trade name used on revolvers from Hood Firearms ca. 1873.
John Brown	John Brown, a silversmith and gunsmith worked at Lincolns Inn Fields, 1805–1808. Very high quality flintlock pistols
Bulldog & British Bulldog	Trade name on revolvers made by Forehand & Wadsworth ca. 1871–90.
Cadet	Trade name on revolvers sold by Maltby & Curtis 1876–1910.
CETME	Centro de Estudios Tecnicos de Materiales Especiales of Madrid Spain. Name of military rifle made between 1958–1982.
Cogswell & Harrison	Gun makers in London 1770 to date and 1924–38 in Paris.
Cow Boy	Trade name of Fabrication Francaise.
Colt, London	Factory opened in January 1853 and was located at Pimlico on the bank of the river Thames, London. Over the next three years, it produced a total of 11,000 Model 1849 Pocket revolvers and 42,000 Model 1851 Revolvers. There were also some 700 3rd Model Dragoons with parts made in Hartford and assembled in London.
Colt, USA	Founded in 1847. Among the most famous products from Colt are the Walker Colt used by the Texas Rangers and the Single Action Army. Later well-known Colt revolvers include the Colt Python and Colt Anaconda. John

	Browning also worked for Colt for a time, and came up with the Colt M1900 pistol, leading to numerous pistol design, including the famous Colt M1911.
Crown Jewel	Trade name used on pistols by Norwich Falls Pistol Co. 1881–87.
Cumberland Arms	Trade name used by Grey & Dudley Hardware, Nashville, USA.
CZ	Trade name of Ceska Zbrojovka 1919 to date.
Daisy	Trade name on revolvers from Bacon Arms Co 1864–91.
Daly Arms Co.	Revolver maker in New York 1890.
Dan Wesson	Revolver manufacturer bought by CZ in late 1980s.
Georges Henry Daw	British percussion gun maker in the 1850s.
Destroyer Carbines	Spanish police carbines made by Gaztanaga y Cia, Eibar 1926 and more recently by Ayra Duria S.A. of Eibar.
Detonics	Manufacturer of pistols in Seattle, USA 1964 to present.
Dreadnaught	Trademark used by Hopkins and Allen, 1984.
Dreyse	Trade name of Rheinische Metallwaren und Maschinenfabrik. Needle gun in 1836.
DWM	Abbreviation for Deutsche Waffen und munitionsfabriken.
Eastern	Trade name used by Stevens Arms Co.
Egg, Henry W, Joseph and Durs.	1 Piccadilly, London. 1851–1880, makers of fine flintlock pistols, shotguns and rifles.
EIG	Importer of cheap firearms into the US from Italy between 1950 and 1970.
Electrique	Trade name used on electrically fired guns made by SMFM 1963.
El Gamo	Originated in 1880s, when known as Antonio Casas, S.A. making various lead products. 1945 specialised in air gun pellets, then high-quality air rifles and pistols.
EM-GE	Trade name on blank/tear gas/flare guns made by Moritz &

Gerstenberger (before 1939) or Gerstenberger & Eberwein (after 1939).

Empire State   Trade name on revolvers, double and single barrelled shotguns made by Meriden Firearms Co. 1895–1918.

Enfield   Royal Small Arms Factory (RSAF), Enfield, has produced British military rifles and muskets since 1804. It was built on the instructions of the Board of Ordnance on marshland at Enfield Lock, on the banks of the River Lea, around about the end of the Napoleonic War. It was privatised in 1984, along with a number of Royal Ordnance Factories to become part of Royal Ordnance Plc, which was later bought by British Aerospace (BAe), who closed the site in 1988.

Estrella   Trade name of Bonifacio Echeverria. Started business in 1905. In 1919, Bonifacio formally registered the Star trade name, and all subsequent weapons were marked as such.

Excel   Trade name used by Iver Johnson.

FAB   Trade name used by Rohn on revolvers.

Fabrica Nacional De Armas Mexico   Began production of weapons before WW1. Manufacturing H&K G3 rifles since 1980 for the Mexican army.

Federal Arms   Used by Sears Roebuck on revolvers made by Meriden Arms.

F.I.E.   Firearms Import and Export Co., Miami, Florida. Manufacturers and importers of cartridge and black powder weapons.

Finladia Firearms   Tikka Arms, Finland.

Finnish Lion   Target rifles made by Valmet of Finland.

FMG   Fab de Material de Guerra Ejercito of Santiago, Chile.

FN   Fabrique National d'Arms de Guerre, Herstal, Belgium from 1889 to date. Manufacturers of sporting and military arms. Noted for Browning designed weapons.

Forjas Taurus   Manufacturer of Taurus branded revolvers. Taurus produced its first revolver, the Model 38101SO, in 1941.

Fortuna Werke   Current manufacturer of sporting arms in Suhl, Germany.

Frommer   Fegyveres Gepygar Resvenytarsasag, Budapest. Later Femaru Fegyver-es Gepyar. Manufacturer of the Fromer STOP a long recoil .32 pistol.

Frontier Bulldog   Trade name on Fab d'Armes de Guerre.

FS   On grip of Fromer Stop pistols.

Galesi   Trade name of Industria Armi Galesi pistols. Founded in 1910, they began to produce pistols in 1914, following Italy's entry into World War I. The first design was a 6.35 mm blowback design based on the Browning 1906.

Game Getter   Trade name of Marble Arms.

Geco   August Genshaw, only manufactures ammunition now.

Golden Eagle   Trade name on guns made by Nikko Arms Co, Japan.

Grant, Stevens and Sons   Makers of sporting arms in London, England, 1841 until they merged with C. Lancaster and Lang and Hussey to form Joseph Lang and Co.

W.W. Greener   In 1829, William Greener, who had been working in London for Manton, a prominent gun maker, returned to his hometown of Newcastle and founded the W. Greener company. In November, 1844, he moved his business to Birmingham. During the period of 1845–58, Greener was appointed to make guns for the Prince Consort. Money obtained from supplying South Africa with two-groove rifles enabled the company to erect a factory on 'Rifle Hill', Aston, in 1859. This was around the time when the firm really began to prosper. Greener was a firm believer in the concept of muzzle-loaders and refused to make any breech-loaders. Hence, his son,

William Wellington Greener, struck out a line of his own (the W. W. Greener company) and produced his first breech-loader in 1864. When William Greener died in 1869, the two companies were amalgamated together as the W.W. Greener Company, and carried on by William Wellington Greener.

Guardian   Trade name on revolvers made by Bacon Arms Co.

Haenel, C.G. Waffen Und Fahrradfabrik   Manufacturers of sporting and military firearms from 1840 to 1945, when it became Ernst Thalman Werk, VEB.

Haerens To Jhus   Marking on Bayard/Bergman pistols made by Anciens Etablissments Pieper under Danish contract.

Halcon   Trade name on .22 rifles of Metalurgica Centro in Argentina.

James Hall   Birmingham, UK, 1820–33. Manufacturer of fine flintlock pistols.

Hammerli   Lenzburg, Switzerland from 1921 to date. Makers of high-quality target pistols and rifles.

Harrington and Richardson   Worcester, Mass, USA since 1874, now in Gardener, Mass. Manufacturers of sporting and military arms.

Hartford Arms   Manufacturers of handguns in Hartfort, Connecticut from 1929. Purchased by High Standard in 1932.

Herculese   Trade name used by J. Steven Arms Co. on shotguns.

Holland and & Holland   98 New Bond St, London, 1835 to present. Manufacturers of the finest quality shoguns and rifles.

Hopkins and Allen   Established in Norwich, Connecticut in 1868; taken over by Marlin-Rockwell in 1917; now owned by Numrich Arms Co. Made all types of sporting arms but best known for their early revolvers.

H&R   Abbreviation for Harrington and Richardson.

Husqvarna   Trade name for Husqvarna Vapenfabrik Akiebolak, makers of

a wide range of firearms since 1867 in Jonkoping, Sweden.

HW   Abbreviation and trade name on Herman Weirauch Sportenwaffenfabrik, on revolvers made in West Germany.

Hi Standard   Connecticut, USA. In 1932, Hi Standard, a drilling company, purchased the Hartford Arms and Equipment Company and began making .22″ calibre target pistols. Company closed in 1984. Reopened in 1993 in Houston, Texas.

Hy Score Arms Co.   One of the largest American air gun makers. Began production in 1948 copying a British air pistol design where the piston encircles the barrel.

IAB SpA.   Manufacturer of reproduction black powder and cartridge replica weapons in Italy.

IAG   Abbreviation for Industria Armi Galesi on self-loading pistols.

IBM   Abbreviation for International Business Machines. Made M1 Carbines during WWII at Poughkeepsie, NY.

ICI   After WWI, many of the UK ammunition and explosives manufacturers were brought together under Nobel Explosives to become Nobel Industries, which was a founding element of Imperial Chemical Industries Ltd (ICI) in 1926. Kynoch, along with names such as Eley, became brands of subsidiaries. With general downturn in ammunition requirements, the sidelines in sporting cartridges were discontinued by Imperial Metal Industries (IMI), of which ICI was part, in 1970. IMI became independent of ICI in 1977, still producing rimfireand shotgun cartridges for the sporting markets. The more economically viable production of shotgun and rimfire ammunition continued. The ammunition division was

	incorporated separately as Eley Limited in 1983.
I.M.I.	Abbreviation for Israeli Military Industries, Tel Aviv, Israel.
Indian Arms Co.	Current manufacturer of pistols in Detroit, Michigan.
Industria Armi Galesi	Manufacturer of pistols in Collebeato, Italy since 1914.
Inglis, John Co	WWII manufacturer of Browning HP 9 mm PB pistols and Bren M/Gs in Toronto, Canada.
Ingram	Trade name on SMG made by Police Ordinance of LA and Military Armament Co of Georgia, USA.
Ingram Gordon	In 1964 Gordon Ingram designed the M10 SMG in .45″ acp. Also produced M11 in 9 mm PB.
Inland	Division of General Motors made M-1 Carbines during WW II.
Interarms	Manufacturers of sporting arms since 1954.
Irwin-Pedersen	Manufacturer of M-I Carbines, Grand Rapids. None accepted for service use, although some were re-tooled by Saginaw and put into service.
Ithaca Gun Co	Manufacturer of sporting arms in Ithaca, NY.
Iver Johnson Arms & Cycle Works	Started as Johnson, Bye & Co in 1871 at Worcester, Mass. In 1883 became Iver Johnson and changed to current name in 1884. In 1891 moved to Finchburg, Mass. USA.
Jackson Hole Rifles	Manufacturer of take down rifles ca. 1972.
Jaga	Used by Frantisek Dusek on Czechoslovakian pistols.
Jager, Franz & Co	Gun makers in Suhl, Germany from 1923–29.
Jeffrey W & Son	Manufacturer of high quality sporting and military arms in Plymouth, England, 1866–1929
J.G.A.	Trade name of J.G. Anschutz.
J-9	Trade name used by Zavodi Crevena Zastava of Belgrade, Yugoslavia.
Johnson-Tucker Firearms	Made MI type carbines in St Louis, US, ca. 1965.
Just, Joseph	Manufacturer of sporting arms in Ferlach, Austria 1919–39.

K.G.F.	Abbreviation for Koenigliche Gewehrfabrik of Potsdam, Germany.
Killdeer	Trade name on single-shot rifles made by Western Arms Co. 1910.
Kimball	In 1958, the J. Kimball Arms Co. went into business (and out of business quite shortly) producing a .30 carbine calibre pistol that closely resembled a slightly scaled-up High Standard Field King.
Knockabout	Trade name on Mod. 311 shotguns made by Stevens Arms Co.
Kodiak Manufacturing Co.	North Haven, Connecticut. US manufacturer of rifles and shotguns ca. 1965.
Koishigawa	See Kokura Arsel, Japan.
Kokura Arsenal	Tokyo, Japan from about 1900 until end of WWII. Originally named Koishigawa.
Kolibri	Trade name used by Georg Grabner, Austria. The 2 mm Kolibri (also known as the 2.7 mm Kolibri Car Pistol or 2.7 × 9 mm Kolibri) is the smallest commercially available centre fire cartridge, patented in 1910 and introduced in 1914 by Franz Pfannl, an Austrian watchmaker, with financial support from Georg Grabner. It was designed to accompany the Kolibri semi-auto pistol or single shot pistol, both marketed as self-defence weapons.
Kongsberg	Government arms manufacturer in Kongsberg, Norway.
Krico	Trade name used by Kreigeskorte of Stuttgart-Hedelfingen, West Germany, on current sporting arms.
Krieghoff, Heinrich	Manufacturer of military and sporting arms from 1929 to 1945 in Suhl, Germany and from 1945 until present in Ulm, Germany.
Kruschitz	Trade name on custom arms made in Vienna ca. 1956.
K.T.G.	Shotgun manufacturer in Hitachi, Japan.
La Industria Orbea	Trade name of Orbea Hermanos, Eibar, Spain.

Lancaster, Charles & Co.	London, England, 1867 to 1900; successor to Charles William Lancaster. Best known for the manufacture of very high-quality sporting rifles and big game hunting pistols. Merged with Stephen Grant & Sons and Lang and Hussey in 1900 to become Joseph Lang & Co. Ltd.
Lang, Joseph & Co.	See above.
Lefever Sons & Co	Started in Syracuse in 1976 and in 1926 purchased by Ithaca Gun Co.
Le Francais	Trade name of Mre. Francais d'Armes et Cycles. Manufacturer of a tip-up barrel .32 acp pistol.
L&H Gun Co.	Manufactured military-style firearms with surplus parts 1972–74 in San Antonio Texas. Purchased by Springfield Armoury.
Liliput pistol	The 4.25 mm Liliput pistol is one of the smallest semiautomatic handguns made (the Kolibri is generally considered the smallest). The Liliput was manufactured by Waffenfabrik August Menz in Suhl, Germany from approximately 1920 to 1927.
Lithgow	Royal Australian Small Arms Factory, NSW, Australia, making military arms. From 1959 until the early 1990s, the Australians used the British L-1A1 (licensed to the Australian company of the Lithgow Small Arms Factory) as their standard personal weapon, when it was replaced by the F-88 (the Australian designation for the Steyr AUG).
Llama	Llama firearms are produced by the firm of Gabilondo y Cia located in Elgoibar, Spain. In 1931, Gabilonda Y Cia decided to do its part in revitalizing the reputation of the lagging Spanish firearms industry. To this end, they began making almost exact copies of the Colt/Browning M1911 design. The name Llama (pronounced Yama) was chosen for this line of pistols to separate it from earlier production of 'Ruby style' pistols of WWI
	vintage. The Ruby pistols did not have the quality control they needed and, as a result, earned a very bad reputation for Spanish firearms and Gabilondo y Cia. The new line of Llama pistols was produced in 9 mm Long, .38″ ACP and .45″ ACP.
Long Branch	Canadian Arsenals Ltd of Long Branch, Ontario. Manufacturer of military arms.
Lovell Arms Co.	1840-91, Boston, Mass., USA. Became J.P. Lovell & Sons about 1870. Possibly absorbed by Iver Johnson in 1868 but allowed to operate under its own name.
Luger	Trade name of Stoeger Industries. Used on P08 pistols and copies which are sold by Stoeger.
Lynx	Trade name on revolvers made in South Africa
M.A.B.	Abbreviation for Mre. D'Armes Automatiques Bayone. Manufacturer since 1921 of automatic pistols based on the Browning mechanism. Used during WWII by German forces (some models exist with German marks) and also by the French army. Now used as surplus pistols for the French police.
M.A.C.	Abbreviation for Military Armaments Corp. Manufacturer of M10 and M11 SMG.
Mamba	Trade name on pistols made by Relay Products of Johannesburg, S. Africa.
Mannlicher-Schoenauer	Trade name on rifles made by Daimler Puch of Steyr, Austria used on rotary magazine bolt action rifle adopted by both the Greek and Austrian Armies in 1903.
Joseph Manton	From 1760–1835 was a much celebrated British gunsmith who was to revolutionise sport shooting, vastly improve the quality of weapons and father the modern artillery shell.
Manufrance	Trade name for Mre. Francais d'Armes et Cycles.

Manurhin | Trade name for Manufacture de Machines du Haut-Rhin, France, who, at the end of the WWII, started producing Walther handguns (PP, PPk and P38) They produced the M73 pistol for the French police, but it was too expensive to manufacture in numbers. In order to produce a more affordable handgun, Manurhin signed an agreement with Sturm Ruger using Ruger's investment casting technology and knowhow. They did also start the production of a new Revolver, called the M-88. This revolver kept the cylinder and barrel of the MR-73, but the frame was the one from the Ruger Security Six. The French police was then issued this gun.

Marble Arms Manufacturing | From 1898 to 1908 manufacturing the 'Game Getter' rifles and shotguns.

Marksman | Trade name on rifles made by H. Pieper of Liege ca. 1900.

Marlin Firearms | 1870 established as J.M. Marlin. In 1881 became Marlin Firearms Co, in 1915 Marlin Rockwell and in 1926, Marlin Firearms Co again. Made sporting and military rifles and shotguns.

Mars | Long-recoil very high-powered pistol designed by Gabbett-Fairfax and made by Webley and Scott of Birmingham, England, ca. 1895. 19015 available in 8.5 mm, 9 mm and .45″ (both long & short chambering),

Marson, Samuel & Co | Manufacturer of sporting and military arms in Birmingham, England, 1840 on.

Martini Henry | The Martini-Henry (also known as the Peabody-Martini-Henry) was a breech-loading lever-actuated rifle adopted by the British, combining an action worked on by Friedrich von Martini (based on the Peabody rifle developed by Henry Peabody), with the rifled barrel designed by Scotsman Alexander Henry. It first entered service in 1871 replacing the Snider-Enfield, and variants were used throughout the British Empire for 30 years. It was the first British service rifle that was a true breech-loading rifle using metallic cartridges.

Mathiew Arms Co | Manufacturer of rifles in Oakland, California, 1950 to 1963.

Mauser Werke AG. | Established 1864, manufacturer of sporting and military rifles. Their designs were built for the German armed forces, and have been exported and licensed to a number of countries in the later 19th and early 20th century, as well as being a popular civilian firearm. In the late 20th century, Mauser continued making sporting and hunting rifles. In the 1990s, it became a subsidiary of Rheinmetall. Mauser Jagdwaffen GmbH was split off and continues making rifles.

Melior | Trade name on pistols made by Robar et Cie.

Mikros | Trade name of Mre. D'Armes des Pyrenees on pistols from 1934–39 and 1958 to date.

Minneapolis Firearms Co. | Made palm pistols ca. 1891.

MKE | Trade name of Kirikkale Tufek Fb. Turkey. Used on Walther PP copies.

Charles Moore | London, England from 1820–1843, produced fine quality pistols.

Mossberg O.F. & Sons | Manufacturer of sporting arms from 1892 (Oscar F. Mossberg) and 1919 (OF Mossberg).

Nagoya | Japanese military weapon plant to 1948.

National Postal Meter | Manufactured M-1 carbines.

New Nambu | On copies of Colt M1911A1 made in Japan by Shin Chau Kogyo of Tokyo.

Newton Arms Co. | Made rifles in Buffalo, NY from 1914. Closed in 1918 and reorganised in 1918 as Newton Rifle Co. Finished trading in 1931.

Nitro Proof/Special   Used on shotguns made by J. Stevens Co.

Niva   Trade name of Kohout & Spol on Czechoslovakian pistols.

Norinco, China   The China North Industries Corporation, official English name Norinco, manufactures vehicles (trucks, cars and motorcycles), machinery, optical-electronic products, oil field equipment, chemicals, light industrial products, explosives and blast materials, civil and military firearms and ammunition, etc. Norinco is also known outside of China for its high-tech defence products, many of which are adaptations of Soviet equipment. Norinco produces precision strike systems, amphibious assault weapons and equipment, long-range suppression weapon systems, anti-aircraft & anti-missile systems, information & night vision products, high-effect destruction systems, fuel air bombs, anti-terrorism & anti-riot equipment and small arms.

North American Arms Co.   Quebec, Canada, manufacturer of 1911A1 pistols.

Numrich Arms Co.   West Hurley, NY. Current manufacturers of sporting and black powder arms, machine guns and parts. Present owners of Auto Ordinance and Hopkins and Allen.

NWM   Abbreviation of Nederlandische Wapenen Munitiefabrik in Holland. Sporting and military arms to present.

Oak Leak   Trade name of J. Stevens Arms Co. on shotguns.

Ojanguran Y Vidosa   Handgun manufacturer in Eibar, Spain, 1922–38.

Orbea   Orbea Hermanos, manufacturer of handguns in Eibar, Spain, 1916–22.

Omnipol   Czechoslovakian arms export organisation in Prague.

Owen   The Owen Machine Carbine was an Australian sub-machine gun designed by Evelyn (Evo) Owen in 1939. The Owen was the only Australian-designed service firearm of World War II and was the main sub-machine gun used by the Australian Army during the war.

Oy Tikkakoski   Rifle manufacturer in Tikkakoski, Finland from 1963. Used trade names Tikka and Ithaca LSA.

Pancor Corporation   Produced the Pancor Jackhammer, a gas-operated automatic weapon. It is one of very few fully automatic shotguns and, although patented in 1987, it never entered full-scale production.

Paragon   Trade name used by Hokins and Allen on revolvers ca. 1886.

Parker Bros   Meriden, Mass, USA, 1868, produced shotguns until taken over by Remington Arms in 1934.

Parker-Hale   Parker Hale Ltd. was a United Kingdom firearms, air rifle and firearms accessory manufacturer, located in Petersfield, Hampshire. It was purchased by John Rothery Wholesale Ltd in late 2000 and ceased firearm production, although cleaning kits and accessories continue to be produced. The company had over 115 years of history and produced pistols, rifles, air guns and accessories of varying sorts.

Parkhurst, William   Arms maker in Bristol, England, ca. 1923

Pedersen Custom Guns   Division of O.F. Mossberg & Sons.

Perfection Automatic Revolver   Trade name used by Forehand Arms Co, ca. 1890.

Perla   Trade name used on Czechoslovakian pistols.

Phoenix Arms Co   Makers of pocket pistols, Lowell, Mass, USA, ca. 1920.

Pieper, Henri   Liege, Belgium from 1884–1907, when company became Ancions Etablisments Pieper.

Pinkerton   Used by Gaspar Arizaga, Spain on pistols.

Poly Tech   PolyTech Arms Corp, in association with Norinco, China produce commercial weapons.

The PolyTech has been imported in both pre- and post-ban variations until the 1998 importation bans. Many people like the gun and say that is the best Chinese AK imported in to the United States.

PZK   Abbreviation for Posumavska Zbrojovka.

Quackenbush   Henry Quackenbush, manufacturer of rifles and air guns in Herkimer, NY ca. 1880. Dennis Quackenbush started making large bore air guns suitable for big game hunting, 1992.

Quality Hardware and Machine   Made M-1 carbines in Chicago, USA.

R.A.   Abbreviation of Trade name Republic Arms, gun makers in Johannesburg, SA.

RA   Abbreviation on Italian military arms meaning Regia Aeronautica (Air Force).

Radom   Polish VIS M35 9 mm PB pistol.

Ralock   Used by BSA, Birmingham, England on rotating block self loading .22″ calibre rifles

Ranger Arms   Rifle maker in Texas, 1972 on.

Retzola   The Retzola brothers of Belgium made their appearance in about 1890, with the inevitable imitation of 'Velo-Dog' type revolvers. Had strong links with gunsmiths in Eibar, Spain. Continued to build automatics at low prices until the US Civil War.

RE   Abbreviation on Italian military arms, meaning Regia Esercito (Royal Army).

Remington Arms   Established in 1816 by Eliphalet Remington. In 1831 became E. Remington & Sons. In 1888 became Remington Arms Co., in 1910 Remington Arms UMC Co, and finally in 1925, again Remington Arms Co.

RG   Abbreviation for Rohm Gesellschaft on West German guns.

Rheinmetall   Trademark of Rheinische Metallwaren Fabrik.

Riverside Arms Co   Trade name used by Stevens Arms & Tool Co.

Robar et de Kirhove   Arms maker in Liege until 1958.

Robin Hood   Trade name used by Hood Firearms Co about 1882.

Rochester Defence Co   Made M-1 carbines during WWII.

Romanski   Current manufacturer of target arms in Obendorf, Germany.

Rossi, Maedeo S.A.   Began manufacture in 1889 and continues to date, making high quality shotguns, rifles and revolvers.

Rubi   Cheap quality revolvers and self-loading pistols.

Ruby   The semi-automatic .32 acp Ruby pistol is best known as a French World War I sidearm, the Pistolet Automatique de 7.65 millim. genre 'Ruby'. It was closely modelled after the Browning M1903 by Belgian Fabrique Nationale de Herstal, and was produced primarily by the Spanish Gabilondo y Urresti-Eibar firm (the official 'Gabilondo Ruby').

RWS   Abbreviation of Rheinische Westfalische Sprengstoff, ammunition makers since 1931.

Sarasqueta, Victor   Sporting arms manufacturer in Eibar, Spain from 1934.

Sarsilmaz   Turkish arms manufacturer established by Abdüllatif in 1880. Produces weapons and equipment for the Turkish military.

Sauer, J. P. & Sohn   J.P. Sauer & Sohn GmbH, established in 1751, is the oldest gun manufacturer in Germany, manufacturing high-quality shotguns, rifles and pistols.

Sears   Trade name on weapons made for Sears, Roebuck & Co.

SFM   Abbreviation for Societie Francaise des Muntions de Chasse of St Etienne, France. Notable for its THV high-velocity ammunition.

Sharps Arms Co.   Manufacturer of replica Sharps rifles in 1969 until purchased by Colt in 1970.

Simplex   The Bergmann Simplex Pistol was a German semi-automatic pistol

	produced from 1901 to 1914 and was chambered for the 9 mm Bergmann cartridge.
SMFM	French manufacturer of electrically fired weapons, 1965.
Spencer Arms	Windsor, Connecticut, USA, makers of repeating shotguns.
Spencer rifle	Designed by Christopher Spencer in 1860. It was a magazine-fed, lever-operated rifle chambered for the .56–56″ rimfire cartridge.
Springfield	US Government armoury in Springfield, Mass, USA from 1782.
Springfield Arms	Sporting arms manufacturers in Springfield, Mass. since 1850. Now part of Savage Arms Co.
Squibman	Trade name on arms made by Squires Bingham of the Philippines, 1930 on.
S&S	Trade name of J.P. Sauer & Sohn.
Standard Arms Co.	Manufacturer of rifles in Wilmington, Del. US 1909–12.
Star	Trade name of Bonafacio Echeverria, Spain. Pistols and revolvers.
J. Stevens Arms and Tool Co.	Established in 1864, absorbed by Page-Lewis Arms in 1926, then by Savage Arms Co in 1936.
Sterling Arms	Manufacturers of pistols and rifles. Established 1968.
Stoeger Industries	Manufacturer since 1924 of good quality shotguns of all types.
Swift Rifle	Manufacturer of military arms in London ca. 1943, most notably the military Swift Training Rifle.
Tanque	Trade name of guns made by Ojanguren y Vidosa, Spain.
Taurus	Trade name of Forjas Taurus of Brazil. Manufactures high quality revolvers and pistols.
TDA	Trade name of Thermodynamic Systems revolvers.
Techni-Mec	Trade name of shotguns made by Fabbrica d'Armi di Isidoro Rizzini of Bresica, Italy. Founded in 1971 by Guido Rizzini and his brothers. Makers of high-quality shotguns.
Terrible	Trade name on pistols made by Hijos de Calixto Arrizabalaga.
TGE	Abbreviation of Tokyo Gas and Electric, used on Baby nambu pistols.

Tikka	Trade name on high quality rifles made by Oy Tikkakoski, Finland.
Titan	Trade name on pistols imported into the USA from Bresica, Italy. Now made in US by FIE
Tokagypt	Trade name on 9 mm copy of TT3 for Egyptian Arms by femaru Fegyver es Gepgyar of Hungary.
Tokarev	Russian TT33 7.62 × 25 mm pistol.
Tulsky Oruzheiny Zavod	Russian manufacturers of high-quality shotguns.
Uberto	Current manufacturer of sporting arms in Ponte Zanano, Italy. Best known for their reproduction Colt single action revolvers.
UD42	The United Defence M42 was an American sub-machine gun in World War II. It was produced from 1942 to 1943 by United Defence Supply Corp. for possible issue as a replacement for the Thompson sub-machine gun and was used by agents of the Office of Strategic Services (OSS). Made in both 9 mm Luger Parabellum and .45″ ACP prototypes, the 9 mm version was the only one to ever see widespread production.
UMC	Abbreviation for Union Metallic Cartridge Co., ammunition makers.
Union Firearms	Toledo Ohio, USA, from 1903 until purchased by Ithaca. Manufacturer of shotguns and revolvers.
Unique	Trade name used by C.S. Shattuck on revolvers ca. 1882.
Unique	Trade name used by Mre. D'Armes des Pyrenees, France.
UnitedStatesArms Corp.	Manufactures of revolvers in Riverhead NY since 1976.
Universal Sporting Goods	Manufacturer in WWII of M-I carbines.
US Arms and Cutlery	Rochester, NY. Manufacturer of knife pistols ca. 1875.
US & S	Abbreviation for Union Switch & Signal of Swissvale, USA, on 1911A1 pistols made in 1943.
US Small Arms Co	Chicago, ca. 1917, manufactured knife pistols.

Valtion Kivaari Tehdas	Finnish state rifle factory. Made Lahti pistol in 1935.
Valmet	Manufactures rifles for Finnish Defence Forces.
Våpensmia	Manufacturer of NM149 sniper rifle for the Norwegian Army. Based on the M98 bolt action.
VB	Abbreviation for Vincenzo Bernadelli on pistols.
Vestpocket	Trade name found on revolvers marked Rosco Arms Co.
Vincenzo Bernadelli	Manufacturer of fine shotguns, rifles and pistols since 1721.
Voere	Current sporting arms manufacturer in Kufstein, Austria.
Volcanic Rifle	In 1854 Horace Smith and Daniel Wesson began manufacturing a lever action magazine-fed pistol called the Volcanic. In 1856 it was joined by the Volcanic Repeating Rifle. They were built in their plant at Norwich, USA.
Vyatskie Polyany Machine-Building Plant "Molot	Russian manufacturers of target rifles and shotguns.
Walam	Trade name on copies of Walther PP made by Femaru Fegyver es Gepgyar in Budapest, Hungary.
Walther, Carl	Manufacturer of sporting and military arms since 1886 in Zella-Mehlis, Germany until 1945, now in Ulm, Germany.
Weatherby	Weatherby, Inc. is an American gun manufacturer founded in 1945 by Roy Weatherby. The company is best known for its high-powered Magnum cartridges, such as the .257″ Weatherby Magnum and the .460″ Weatherby Magnum. Company headquarters is in the northern San Luis Obispo County town of Paso Robles, California.
Webley	The Webley Revolver (also known/referred to as the Webley Break-Top Revolver or Webley Self-Extracting Revolver) was, in various marks, the standard issue service pistol for the armed forces of the United Kingdom, the British Empire and the Commonwealth from 1887 until 1963.
Webley & Scott	Webley and Scott is an arms manufacturer based in Birmingham, England. Webley produced handguns and long guns from 1834. The company ceased to manufacture firearms in 1979 and now produces air pistols and air rifles.
Weihrauch	Weihrauch & Weihrauch GmbH & Co. KG is a German manufacturer of target and sporting air rifles and air pistols. The company also manufactures a small range of cartridge rifles and pistols. In North America they are often distributed under the 'Beeman' brand name. Weihrauch air rifles have a reputation for being rugged and solidly-built, but heavy; an accessorised HW 77 can weigh as much as 10 lbs.
Wesson Firearms	Manufacturers of shotguns in Springfield, Mass. 1864–68.
Wesson, Dan	Daniel B. Wesson, who founded Wesson Firearms Co., Inc. in 1968 was the great-grandson of D. B. Wesson, co-founder of Smith & Wesson. Dan Wesson produces innovative revolver and pistols of very high quality. In the 1980s Dan Wesson Arms began to produce revolvers chambered for the .357, .375, and .445 SuperMag cartridges. In 2000 they added .414 Supermag, and .460 Rowland.
Westley Richards	Westley Richards is one of the oldest surviving traditional English gun makers. It was founded in 1812 by William Westley Richards. Over the years invented some of the most widely used inventions, like the Anson & Deeley boxlock action and the Droplock. which equals in status James Purdey's self-opening and Holland & Holland's removable locks.
William Powell & Son, Ltd	Since 1812, William Powell & Son, Ltd have made exclusive shotguns in Birmingham, England.
Winchester Repeating Arms Co.	New Haven, Connecticut, USA, 1857 to date. In 1857, Oliver Winchester reorganised the Volcanic Repeating Arms Co. into

the New Haven Arms Co. and, in 1866 it became the Winchester Repeating Arms Co. In 1869, absorbed Fogerty Repeating Rifle Co and American Rifle Co., the Spencer Repeating Arms Co. in 1870 and Adrionack Arms in 1874.

WRA   Abbreviation for Winchester Repeating Arms

XL   Trade name used by Hopkins & Allen, 1883.

XXX Standard   Trade name used on revolvers by J.M. Marlin, 1877.

Yamamoto Firearms   Current manufacturer of shotguns in Kochi, Japan.

Teodoro Ybarzábal   Belgian manufacturer of 9 mm Galand-type revolvers.

Young America   Trade name on revolvers made by Harrington & Richardson, ca. 1900.

Zabala   Spanish manufacturer of shotguns.

Zastava Arms   Serbian arms manufacturer Zastava Arms makes clones of the Russian AK-47 Kalashnikov.

Zigana   Turkish manufactured 9 mm PB pistol.

Zoli, Antonio   Manufacturer of shotguns in Bresica, Italy.

Z-M Weapons   A firearm design and manufacturing firm based in Bernardston, Massachusetts. The company specialises in the AR-15, M16, and its own LR-300 rifle.

Appendix 4

Important dates in the History of Firearms from 1247

Event	Date
The first record of the actual use of gunpowder in Europe is a statement by Bishop Albertus Magnus in 1280 that it was used at the Siege of Seville in:	1247
Roger Bacon gives an account of gunpowder in his *Opus Majus* (actually, his account was written in cryptic form (See, T. *Explosives*, Pelican Books, 1942).	1267
Hand Cannon had appeared in the field of battle during the reign of Edward III in:	1364
Handguns were known in Italy in 1397, and in England they appear to have been used as early as:	1375
The first mechanical device for firing the handgun made its appearance in:	1424
We hear of armour being penetrated by bullets and the handgun showing signs of becoming a weapon capable of rudimentary precision by:	1425
Henry VII organised the corps of Yeomen of the Guard, half of whom were to carry bows and arrows, while the other half were equipped with harquebuses. This represents the first introduction of firearms as an official weapon of the Royal Guard.	1485
Rifling was invented in:	1498
The first wheel lock or 'rose lock' was invented somewhere about:	1509
Firearms were recognised as hunting arms as early as 1515, and a book (*Balleates Mosetuetas y Areabuces Pablo del Fucar*, Naples, 1535) on sporting firearms appeared in 1535.	1535
Rifled arms have been made since:	1540
The hair trigger was a German invention of about:	1540
The invention of the typical Spanish lock is attributed by some writers to Simon Macuarte II, about:	1560
The snap-haunce lock, the forerunner of the true flintlock, was invented about, or considerably earlier than:	1580
The standard flintlock gun came in about:	1630
The London Gun makers' Company initiated proofs when it was first incorporated, but it is not clear whether private proofs or a trade proof house common to the Company was used (a crowned 'A' was given as the mark).	1637
The screw or cannon barrel pistol came in probably prior to:	1640
The bayonet was introduced by the French; it was a long narrow blade with a wooden plug handle and was simply dropped into the muzzle of the musket.	1640

Forensic Ballistics in Court: Interpretation and Presentation of Firearms Evidence, First Edition. Brian J. Heard.
© 2013 John Wiley & Sons, Ltd. Published 2013 by John Wiley & Sons, Ltd.

The London Gun makers' Company enjoyed powers which enabled them to enforce proof when the second charter was granted in: 1672

A ring attachment was added to the bayonet so that it no longer served as a muzzle plug. 1680

The earliest known English breech-loading rifle was made by Willmore, who was apprenticed to Foad in: 1689

The 'Brown Bess' was known in Ireland as a 'King's Arm' from its use by William III at the Battle of the Boyne. 1690

The whole English army was equipped with flintlocks in: 1690

Snap-haunces continued to be made on the Continent until about: 1700

In the reign of Queen Anne, the 'Brown Bess' was known as the 'Queen's Arm' in Ireland. 1702–1714

The socket bayonet had appeared and was adopted in the British service about: 1710

The letters G.R. were adopted as a mark in the reign of George I (1714–27), but successive Georges did not add any variant. 1714–1830

The broad arrow, as a sign of government property, was adopted during the reign of George I, and the word TOWER is marked on the lock plate of many of these arms. 1714–1727

The French established their 'Manufacturers Royales' at Charleville, St. Etienne and Maubeuge in: 1718

The large box lock type of pistol made its appearance about: 1730

A few hammerless flintlock sporting guns were made by Stanislaus Paczelt, of Prague in Bohemia, about: 1730

The use of pistols for duelling purposes became general as the practice of carrying the rapier or small sword died out between: 1750–1765

The duelling pistol was entirely unknown until about: 1760

Note: meetings were fought with horse pistols prior to this date. The horse pistol shows a marked development into the true duelling pistol from: 1760–1775

Double shotguns were rather peculiar arms, usually of the under-and-over revolving barrel type until about: 1760

Duelling pistols became officially standardised weapons –then it was laid down that they should be 9- or 10-inch barrelled, smooth bore flintlocks of one-inch bore, carrying a ball of 48 to the pound. 1777

The top rib in double-barrelled guns appeared about: 1780

Spring bayonets are common on blunderbusses and pistols of the period subsequent to the date of the patent (John Waters, Pat. No. 1284) in: 1781

The first patent for single trigger locks for double arms (James Templeman, Pat. No. 1707) was in: 1789

Single trigger pistols, with side-by-side, and also under-and-over barrels, were made by Egg about: 1789

The acorn pattern trigger guard extension toward the barrel used up to about: 1790

Joseph Manton's first patent (No. 1865) introduces the 'break-off' breech, into which the barrel fits with a lump instead of being secured by a tang and screw, as previously used. 1792

The swivel ramrod attached to the piece by a stirrup appeared about 1800

The 'First Baker Rifle' was issued in: 1800

The half-stocked pistol, with the lower rib beneath the barrel fitted to carry the ramrod came in during: 1800

The 'Second Baker Rifle' was introduced in: 1807

Alexander Forsyth patented the detonating or percussion principle in: 1807

The first serious military breech-loader was an American invention, Colonel John H. Hall's patent. This was made first as a flintlock, then as percussion, and is the first breech-loader officially adopted by any army. The flintlocks were made till 1832, the percussion model from 1831. 1811

The copper percussion cap is not definitely alluded to in the patent records until 1823, but appears to have been invented about: 1814–1816

The saw handle was very popular, both in flint and percussion pistols, about: 1815–1825

The true flintlock revolver is the very rare weapon made by Collier about: 1820

Flints were converted to percussion cap, and the flint principle lost favour from: 1820

The percussion cap came into general use on private arms about: 1826

The Delvigne (French) service rifle was invented in: 1826

The 'Third Baker Rifle' was issued about: 1830

The back action lock made its appearance about: 1830

The Robert rifle was invented by Robert, a gunsmith of Paris, in: 1831

The percussion cap system of ignition was in common use before it was adopted for the service weapon. It was tested at Woolwich in: 1843

Coach pistols supplied to the guard of public stage coaches are extremely rare, but were made with flintlocks and brass lock plates until: 1835

Percussion cap locks fitted with a pierced platinum disc below the nipple gradually fell into disuse and are seldom found in arms subsequent to: 1835

Colt claims the ratchet motion, locking the cylinder, and centre fire position of the nipples as particular points of his specification. 1835

Colt did not know that the revolving principle was an old European idea until he visited England in: 1835

The Enfield percussion carbine – .65 inch calibre with hinged spring triangular bayonet folding below the barrel – was made for the constabulary service in: 1835

Dreys released the first needle fire rifle in: 1836

The true pinfire cartridge emerged about: 1840

It was not until 1840 that we definitely find a breech-loading needle gun cartridge, patented (Wm. Bush, Pat. No. 8513) in: 1840

The Brunswick rifle superseded the Baker model about: 1840

Duelling declined in England after: 1840

The period of decadence of duelling was noticeable for the production of rather short-barrelled pistols. 1840–1850

A few service arms were converted to the percussion cap system in 1839, and it was officially adopted in: 1842

The service percussion musket was mainly experimental until: 1844

A double-barrelled, 26-inch barrel, .67″ calibre arm was issued for constabulary use in: 1845

The Prussians concentrated on experiments with the needle gun in 1844, and it was used in the war of: 1848

The shotgun, or fowling piece, began its separation from the musket in the latter half of the 18th century, and divorce was completed by: 1850

The Minie (English) service rifle was introduced in: 1850

Minie's patent for the self-expanding bullet was purchased and adopted by the British Government for the Enfield rifle in: 1851

Muzzle-loading was so unassailably established we do not find a single breech-loading cartridge weapon shown by a British firm at the Great Exhibition of: 1851

Colt delivered a lecture on Colt revolvers before the Institute of Civil Engineers during his visit to London in: 1851

Charles Lancaster brought out his central fire under lever gun with extractor and the first true centre fire cartridge in: 1852

Colt procured a factory at Thames, Bank, Pimlico, London, and produced replicas of his standard pistols, marked on the barrel 'Address Col. Colt, London' during the period: 1853–1857

The Pritchett bullet, a plain lead cylindroconoidal plug with a shallow base depression, was selected as the best type of bullet for the new Enfield rifle in: 1853

Note: Later this was superseded by the Enfield bullet

During the Crimean War, 25,000 Enfield rifles were made in America. This war was the last war in which all combatants used muzzle-loaders. 1854–1856

There never was an official British state-maintained arms factory until the government established Enfield as a government factory, when the Birmingham gun makers struck for 1855

higher wages in the middle of the Crimean War.

Whitworth rifles were produced in:	1857
Duelling continued in India to the date of the Mutiny.	1857–1858
The first recorded European revolver for central fire cartridges appears to be that patented by Perrin and Delmas in:	1859
The first effective and widely used magazine repeater was undoubtedly the Spencer carbine, patented in the USA in:	1860
Tyler F. Henry brought out the Henry rifle in:	1860
In the American Civil War, both breech and muzzle loader were used.	1860–1865
Breech-loaders were coming into general use by:	1861
The first central fire repeater appears to have been Ball's carbine made by the Lamson Arms Co., Windsor, Vermont, USA, in:	1863
For all practical purposes, metallic cartridges were not widely introduced until:	1863–1864
The first cartridge repeater shotgun appears to have been the Roper of:	1866
The Snider service rifle was issued in:	1866
The Henry was merged into Winchester in:	1866
Claims have been made for an American origin for choke boring, but these have never been proved, and there is no doubt that it was the invention of Pape of Newcastle in:	1866
Duels were fought in Ireland till as late as:	1868
The Martini-Henry rifle was issued in:	1869
The first European magazine military arm was the Swiss Vetterli rifle of:	1869–1871
In 1866, the Chassepot was authorised and all branches of the French army were equipped with the weapon by:	1870
The Franco-German War was almost entirely a breech-loading affair.	1870–1871
The first true hammerless gun appears to have been that of Murcott in:	1871–1871
The first bolt-action military repeater seems to be the Edge rifle (Pat. No. 3643) of:	1874–1875
Anson and Deeley Box Lock shotgun action.	1875
First double action revolver.	1877

Lee patented his box magazine in:	1879
The French adopted the Lebel rifle in:	1886
The Gras-Kropatschek rifle was issued for the French Marine in:	1886–1887
Winchester repeating shotguns were first introduced in:	1887
The Maxim was officially adopted in the army as a machine gun in:	1887
The Lee-Metford rifle was adopted by Great Britain in:	1888
The first automatic weapon to appear on the market was the Borchardt pistol in:	1893
The Bergmann pistol appeared in:	1894
The first Mannlicher automatic pistol introduced	1894
The Mauser combination automatic pistol or carbine, the wooden holster serving as a stock attachment was introduced in:	1898
The Browning automatic pistol of .32″ calibre, made its appearance about:	1898
Webley Fosberry .455″ self loading revolver introduced.	1901
The Winchester Firearms Company brought out the first widely sold automatic rifle in:	1903
The Webley self-loading .455″ pistol was adopted for the British Navy in:	1905
German 9 mm PB Luger introduced.	1908
Broom Handled 7.63 mm Military Mauser introduced.	1912
Browning 9 mm PB HP introduced.	1935
British .303 Bren machine gun.	1936
German MG42 7.92 × 57 mm introduced.	1938
British Lanchester 9 mm PB sub-machine gun introduced.	1940
British Sten Mk I 9 mm PB SMG introduced.	1941
Thompson M1 .45ACP SMG introduced.	1942
Kalashnikov AK47 7.62 × 39 mm assault rifle introduced.	1947
Israeli 9 mm PB Uzi SMG introduced.	1953
British Sterling 9 mm PB SMG introduced.	1953
Chinese 7.62 × 25 mm Type 54 introduced. This is a direct copy of the Russian TT.	1954
.44″ Remington Magnum introduced.	1955
Chinese Type 58 7.62 × 39 mm assault rifle introduced. This is an exact copy of the Russian AK47.	1956
.454″ Casull Cartridge introduced.	1959

Czechoslovakian 7.65 mm ACP Skorpion introduced.	1960
H&K MP5 9 mm PB introduced.	1965
Beretta 92 introduced.	1976
Steyr-Manlicher AUG 5.56 × 45 or 7.62 × 51 mm NATO.	1978
Israeli .257″ Magnum Desert Eagle introduced.	1982
Glock 17 9 mm PB introduced.	1983
Barrett M82A1 .50″ Browning long range sniping rifle introduced in:	1983
Enfield L85A1 5.56 × 45 mm NATO introduced in:	1985
Israeli .50″ Action Express Desert Eagle introduced in:	1991

Appendix 5

Dates for the Introduction of Various Cartridges by Calibre

Calibre	Date
.17″ Remington	1971
.17″ Rem Fireball	2007
.204″ Ruger	2004
.218″ Bee	1938
.204″ Ruger	2004
.22″ Short	1857[1]
.22″ Long	1871
.22″ Daisy Caseless	1962
.22″ LR	1887
.22″ WRF	1890
.22″ Win Auto	1959
.22″ Rem Jet	1960
.22″ Hornet	1930
.22″ PPC	1974
.22-250 Rem	1965
.220 Swift	1935
.221″ Fireball	1963
.222″ Rem	1950
.222″ Rem Mag	1958
.223″ Rem (5.56 mm)	1955
.223″ Win SSM	2003
.224″ BOZ (British)	2006
.225″ Win	1964
.299″ Cruz	2006
.243″ Win	1955
.243″ Win SSM	2003
.25 Win SSM	2005
.25″ ACP (6.25 mm)	1906

Calibre	Date
.25-3000	1915
.25-06 Rem	1969
.25-20 Win	1894
.25-35 Win	1895
.250″ Savage	1915
.256″ Win Mag	1961
.257″ Roberts	1934
.264″ Win Mag	1958
.270″ WSM	2001
.270″ Win	1925
.280″ Rem	1957
.280″ British (EN1)	1948
.284″ Win	1963
.30″ Carbine	1940
.30″ Luger	1900
.30″ Rem	1906
.30″ Herrett	1973
.300″ H&H Mag	1925
.300″ Savage	1920
.300″ Win Mag	1963
.300″ WSM	2001
.30-06 Springfield	1906
.30-30 Win	1895
.303″ British	1888
.303″ Savage	1899
.30-40 Kraig	1892
.307″ Win R	1982
.308″ Win	1954
.308″ Norma Mag	1960
.32″ ACP (7.65 mm)	1900
.32″ Short Colt	1875
.32″ Long Colt	1875
.32″ Win	1905

[1] Oldest commercial cartridge being loaded today.

Forensic Ballistics in Court: Interpretation and Presentation of Firearms Evidence, First Edition. Brian J. Heard.
© 2013 John Wiley & Sons, Ltd. Published 2013 by John Wiley & Sons, Ltd.

.32″ S&W Rev	1870	.45″ Win Mag	1978
.32″ S&W Long	1896	.455 Webley	1889
.32″ Win Spl	1895	.45-70 US Govt.	1873
.32″ H&R	1984	.454″ Casull	1954
.32-20 Win	1882	.458″ Win Mag	1956
.325″ WSM	2005	.460″ Weatherby Mag.	1958
.343″ WSSM	2003	.470″ Nitro Express	1907
.338″ Win Mag	1958	.476 Enfield	1880
.338″ Lapua (8.6 × 70 mm)	1983	.480″ Ruger	2001
.348 Win	1936	.50″ Action Express	1988
.35″ Rem	1906	.500″ S&W Magnum	2003
.350″ Rem Mag	1965	.50″ Remington Army	1867
.351″ Win SL	1907	.50″ Browning M/G	1921
.357″ Mag	1935	.50-90 Sharps	1872
.357″ Sig Auto	1994	.600″ Nitro Express	1903

Metric

.358″ Win	1955	4.6 × 30 mm German	2000
.358″ Norma Mag	1959	4.7 × 33 mm H&K D11	
.357″ H&H Mag	1912	Caseless	1989
.357″ Sig	1994	5 mm Rem RF Mag	1968
.375″ Win	1978	5.45 × 39 mm Russian M74	1974
.38″ Dardick	1958	5.56 × 45 mm NATO	1960
.38″ ACP	1900	5.56 × 45 mm Rem	1963
.38″ Short Colt	1875	5.56 × 45 S-109	1979
.38″ Long Colt	1875	5.6 × 45 mm GP90 Swiss	1987
.38″ S&W	1876	5.7 × 28 mm Belgium	1990
.38″ Spl	1902	6 mm Rem	1963
.38″ Super	1922	6 mm PPC	1975
.38″ Super Auto	1929	6.5 mm JDG	1978
.380″ ACP (9 mm Short)	1908	6.5 × 39 Grendel	2003
.38-40 Win	1878	6.5 mm Rem Mag	1966
.38-55 Win.	1884	6.5 × 50 mm Arisaka	1897
.40″ S&W	1990	6.5 × 55 mm Swedish	1895
.400″ Corbon	1997	6.5 × 68 mm	1939
.408″ Chey Tac	2001	6.8 × 43 mm Rem SPC	2003
.41″ Action Express	1986	7 × 57 mm Mauser	1892
.416″ Rem Mag	1988	7 mm Exp Rem	1979
.416″ Barrett	2006	7 mm-08 Rem	1980
.44″ S&W	1869	7 mm Rem Mag	1962
.41″ Rem Mag	1964	7 mm WSM	2002
.41″ Action Express	1986	7.5 × 55 mm Schmidt Rubin	1889
.44″ Spl	1907	7.62 × 39 mm Russian	1943
.44″ Rem Mag	1955	7.62 × 51 mm USA	1950
.44″ AMP	1971	7.62 × 51 mm NATO	1953
.444″ Marlin	1964	7.62 × 54 mm R	1891[2]
.44-40 Win	1873	7.65 mm Browning (.32 ACP)	1899
.450″ Marlin	2000	7.65 mm PB (7.65 mm Luger)	1900
.450″ Adams Revolver	1868	7.7 × 58 mm Arisaka	1939
.450″ Mars	1902	7.92 × 33 mm Kurtz (German)	1938
.450″ Nitro Express	1895		
.45″ GAP Austrian	2003		
.45″ ACP	1905		
.45″ Colt (.45 Long Colt)	1873		

[2] Oldest cartridge still in official military use.

7.92 × 57 mm Mauser	1888
7.92 × 107 mm DS	1934
8 × 57 mm	1905
8 × 68S	1939
8 mm Rem Mag	1978
9 mm PB (9 mm Luger)	1902
9 mm Browning Short	1812
9 mm Win Mag	1978
9 mm Federal Rev	1989
9 × 57 mm Mauser	1894
10 mm Auto	1983

In the above table, the following abbreviations apply[3]:

ACP	Automatic Colt Pistol
Auto	Automatic, i.e. for self-loading pistol
Win	Winchester – cartridge designed by the company
Rem	Remington – cartridge designed by the company
S&W	Smith & Wesson – cartridge designed by the company
H&H	Holland and Holland – cartridge designed by the company
Sig	Sig Sauer – cartridge designed by the company
Mag	Magnum
Rev	Revolver
Exp	Express cartridge
Spl	Special
Win SSM	Winchester Super Short Magnum

---

[3] See Appendix 2 for list of ammunition abbreviations.

Appendix 6
Some Trademarks Found on Guns

Gun marks can include proof marks, but for this appendix they are restricted to manufacturer's marks, inspector's marks and arsenal marks.

There are many thousand of these and it would take several books even to begin to list them. However, they do present a very valuable aid to the forensic firearms examiner as they can provide information as to a weapon's age, its history and its country of origin and manufacturing factory.

In addition to gun marks, there are thousands of **trade names** which can reveal similar details to that of gun marks. As with gun marks, to list all the trade names is beyond the scope of this book.

Some examples of both gun marks and trade names are listed for general reference purposes.

Probably the most authoritative book available on these subjects is *Gunmarks* (1979) by Byron, David. Crown Publishers (abebooks.co.uk). ISBN 10: 0517538482.

Other useful books would include:

- Carey, A. M. (1967). *English, Irish and Scottish Firearms Makers: Middle Sixteenth Century to the End of the Nineteenth Century.* Arms and Armour P.

- Carey, A. M. (1967). *American Firearms Makers: When, Where, and What They Made, from the Colonial period to the End of the Nineteenth Century.* Arms and Armour P.

- Whisker, J.B. (1992). *Arms Makers of Colonial America.* Susquehanna University Press.

- Mathews, J.H. (1962–1973). *Firearms identification*, Vols I, II & III. Springfield, IL, USA, Thomas.

A.6.1 Examples of gun marks

Lions

Trademark on Danish Madsen machine guns.

Relay Products of Johannesburg, SA; trademark on Mamba pistols.

Aguirre y Aranzabal of Eibar, Spain; trademark on shotguns and rifles.

Trademark on pistols by Harrison & Richardson revolvers.

Forensic Ballistics in Court: Interpretation and Presentation of Firearms Evidence, First Edition. Brian J. Heard.
© 2013 John Wiley & Sons, Ltd. Published 2013 by John Wiley & Sons, Ltd.

Birds

 Mre. Liegeoise d'Armes a Feu of Liege, Belgium; trademark.

 US Springfield Armoury: Inspector's mark on 1911 pistols.

 Gebruder Merkel of Sujhl, Germany; trademark on rifles and shotguns.

 On WWII German Nazi pistols.

Crests

 Ethiopian crest.

 Bulgarian crest.

 Argentinean crest.

 BSA of Birmingham, England; trademark

 Armi Famars, Brescia, Italy; trademark on shotguns

 Herter's Inc. of Waseca, USA; trademark

 Iver Johnson, Fitchburg, USA; trademark on shotguns

 Stevens Arms and Tool Co., USA; on butt plates

Geometric designs

 Tula Weapons Factory, Russia; commercial trademark

 Russian gripmark on pistols

 Gerstenberger u Eberwein, W. Germany; gripmark on revolvers

 Harrington and Richardson, Mass., USA; gripmark on revolvers

 Japanese, Kokura Arsenal mark, 1928–35.

 Meridian Firearms Company of Conn., USA; gripmark on revolvers.

In borders

 Marlin Firearms Co. Conn., USA; gripmark on revolvers.

 Israeli mark on arms for export.

 Israeli mark on arms for export.

 Vilimec of Kdyne, Czechoslovakia; gripmark.

In circles

 US inspection mark of W. Penfold on M1911 pistols.

 Trocaola, Aranabal y Cia of Eibar, Spain; revolver gripmark.

 Ceska Zbrojovka of Czechoslovakia; gripmark.

 Sears Roebuck & Co.; gripmark on revolvers.

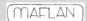 Smith & Wesson of Springfield, Mass., USA; trademark on revolvers & self-loading pistols.

J.P. Sauer & Sohn; trademark on pistols.

Appendix 7

General Firearms Values Conversion Table

To Convert From:	To:	Multiply By:
Feet/sec	metres/sec	0.3048
Feet/sec	miles/hour	0.6818
Metres/sec	ft/min	196.85039
Metres/sec	ft/sec	3.2808399
Foot pounds	ergs	1.35582×10^7
Foot pounds	Joules	1.35582
Foot pounds	kg metres	0.138255
Joules (Int)	foot pounds	0.737684
Joules (Int)	foot poundals	23.73428
Gravitational constant	cm (sec $\times$ sec)	980.621
Gravitational constant	ft (sec $\times$ sec)	32.1725

Metres	Inches	39.3701
Metres	Kilometres	0.001
Metres	Miles, statute	0.000621
Metres	Millimetres	1000
Metres	Millimicrons	1×10^9
Micron	Centimetres	0.0001
Micron	Inches	3.9370079×10^{-5}
Metres	Yards	1.0936
Miles	Kilometres	1.6093
Miles	Metres	1609.3
Millimetres	Inches	0.03937
Yards	Centimetres	91.44
Yards	Metres	0.9144

A.7.1 Length

To Convert From:	To:	Multiply By:
Centimetres	Feet	0.0328
Centimetres	Inches	0.3937
Decimetres	Inches	3.937
Feet	Centimetres	30.48
Feet	Decimetres	3.048
Feet	Metres	0.3048
Inches	Centimetres	2.54
Inches	Millimetres	25.4
Kilometres	Feet	3280.8
Kilometres	Metres	1000
Kilometres	Miles	0.62137
Kilometres	Yards	1093.6

A.7.2 Weight

To Convert From:	To:	Multiply By:
Grams	Drams (avoirdupois)	0.5644
Grams	Grains	15.432
Grams	Kilograms	0.001
Grams	Micrograms	1×10^6
Grams	Milligrams	1000
Grams	Ounces (avoirdupois)	0.03527
Grams	Pounds (avoirdupois)	0.002205
Kilograms	Drams (avoirdupois)	564.38
Kilograms	Grains	15432.36
Kilograms	Grams	1000
Kilograms	Ounces (avoirdupois)	35.27396

Forensic Ballistics in Court: Interpretation and Presentation of Firearms Evidence, First Edition. Brian J. Heard.
© 2013 John Wiley & Sons, Ltd. Published 2013 by John Wiley & Sons, Ltd.

Kilograms	Pounds (avoirdupois)	2.20462	Pounds (avoirdupois)	Grains	7000
Ounces (avoirdupois)	Drams (avoirdupois)	16	Pounds (avoirdupois)	Grams	453.59
Ounces (avoirdupois)	Grains	437.5	Pounds (avoirdupois)	Kilograms	0.4536
Ounces (avoirdupois)	Grams	28.3495	Pounds (avoirdupois)	Ounces (avoirdupois)	16
Ounces (avoirdupois)	Pounds (avoirdupois)	0.0625			
Pounds (avoirdupois)	Drams (avoirdupois)	256			

Appendix 8
Hearing Loss

A.8.1 Introduction

Hearing loss among firearms examiners is a major problem. Those regularly firing sawn-off 12-bore shotguns and high powered military or hunting rifles are particularly at risk for no matter what hearing protection is utilised each shot will produce some permanent damage. The likelihood of a compensation claim for such hearing loss is, even with modern hearing protection aids, a very real possibility. This chapter is, therefore, included as a primer on the subject.

Before delving further into this subject, some background information on how the inner ear works is appropriate.

A.8.2 How we hear

Sound waves enter the outer ear and travel through a narrow passageway called the ear canal, which leads to the eardrum. The eardrum vibrates from the incoming sound waves and sends these vibrations to three tiny bones in the middle ear. These bones are called the malleus, the incus and the stapes.

The bones in the middle ear amplify, or increase, the sound and send the vibrations to the snail-shaped cochlea, or inner ear. The cochlea is a fluid-filled organ with an elastic membrane that runs down its length and divides the cochlea into upper and lower parts. This membrane is called the 'basilar'

membrane because it serves as the base, or ground floor, on which key hearing structures sit.

The vibrations cause the fluid inside the cochlea to ripple, and a travelling wave forms along the basilar membrane. This motion causes bristly structures on top of the hair cells to bump up against an overlying membrane and deflect to one side.

As the bristles, or stereocilia, move, pore-like channels on their surface open up. This allows certain chemicals to rush in that generate an electrical signal. The auditory nerve carries the signal to the brain, which translates it into a 'sound' that we recognise and understand.

Hair cells near the base of the cochlea detect higher-pitched sounds, such as a cell phone ringing. Those nearer the apex, or centremost point, detect lower-pitched sounds, such as a large dog barking. It is these hair cells at the base of the cochlea that receive most damage by high-frequency and high-volume sounds, such as the discharge of a firearm. Damage to these hair cells is irreversible and results in a permanent loss of hearing.

After exposure to excessive levels of high-frequency sound, a ringing in the ears, called tinnitus, can also be experienced. This can also be permanent.

A.8.3 Frequency

Pitch is measured in frequency of sound vibrations (cycles) per second, called Hertz (Hz). A low pitch

Forensic Ballistics in Court: Interpretation and Presentation of Firearms Evidence, First Edition. Brian J. Heard.
© 2013 John Wiley & Sons, Ltd. Published 2013 by John Wiley & Sons, Ltd.

such as a deep voice or a tuba makes fewer vibrations per second than a high voice or violin. The higher the pitch of the sound, the higher the frequency. Generally, noise-induced hearing loss occurs at a pitch of about 2,000–4,000 Hz.

Young children, who generally have the best hearing, can often distinguish sounds from about 20 Hz, such as the lowest note on a large pipe organ, to 20,000 Hz, such as the high shrill of a dog whistle that many people are unable to hear.

Human speech, which ranges from 300–4,000 Hz, sounds louder to most people than noises at very high or very low frequencies. When hearing impairment begins, the high frequencies are often lost first, which is why people with hearing loss often have difficulty hearing the high-pitched voices of women and children.

Loss of high frequency hearing can also distort sound, so that speech becomes difficult to understand, even though it can be heard. Hearing impaired people often have difficulty detecting differences between certain words that sound alike, especially words that contain S, F, SH, CH, H, or soft C sounds, because the sound of these consonants is in a much higher frequency range than vowels and other consonants.

A.8.4   Hearing loss

It is generally accepted that a continuous noise level of 85 db (decibels) is the maximum safe level for long term exposure to steady noise level within the frequency range of about 600–1,200 Hz. The very brief gunfire noises are another matter.

Leading hearing specialists stipulate that about 150 db is the maximum peak limit for gunfire noises without impairment of speech perception, and 140 db maximum without impairment of good hearing of music and the like.

It should be noted that decibels are a logarithmic scale and that the sound energy doubles with each 3 db increase.

Tables A.8.1 to A.8.4 list data describing the peak sound pressure levels produced by firearms of various calibres. With the introduction of muzzle breaks and porting, the risks of hearing loss dramatically increase.

Table A.8.1   Shotgun Noise Data

Calibre	Barrel length	Sound level
.410″	28″ (71 cm) barrel	150 dB
.410″	26″ (66 cm) barrel	150 dB
.410″	18″ (41 cm) barrel	156 dB
20-bore	28″ (71 cm) barrel	152 dB
20-bore	22″ (55 cm) barrel	154 dB
12-bore	28″ (71 cm) barrel	151 dB
12-bore	26″ (66 cm) barrel	156 dB
12-bore	18″ (41 cm) barrel	161 dB
12-bore	12″ (30 cm) barrel	168 dB
12-bore	8″ (20 cm) barrel	172 dB

Table A.8.2   Centre Fire Rifle Data

Calibre	Barrel length	Sound level
.223″	18″ (41 cm) barrel	155 dB
.243″	22″ (55 cm) barrel	155 dB
.30-20	20″ (51 cm) barrel	156 dB
7 mm Magnum	20″ (51 cm) barrel	157 dB
.308″ Win	24″ (61 cm) barrel	156 dB
.30-06	24″ (61 cm) barrel	158 dB
.30-06	18″ (41 cm) barrel	163 dB
.375″ Magnum	18″ (41 cm) barrel	162 dB
.375″ Magnum	18″ (41 cm) barrel with muzzle brake	170 dB

Table A.8.3   Centre Fire Pistol Data

Calibre	Sound level
.25″ ACP	155 dB
.32″ Long	152 dB
.32″ ACP	153 dB
.380″	157 dB
9 mm	159 dB
.38″ S & W	153 dB
.38″ Special	156 dB
.357″ Magnum	165 dB
.41″ Magnum	163 dB
.44″ Special	155 dB
.45″ ACP	157 dB

Table A.8.4   Some Reference Sound Levels

Approx. Decibel Level	Example
0	Faintest sound heard by human ear.
30	Whisper, quiet library.
60	Normal conversation, sewing machine, typewriter.
90	Lawnmower, shop tools, truck traffic.
100	Chainsaw, pneumatic drill, snowmobile.
115	Sandblasting, loud rock concert, car horn.
140	Jet engine; noise causes pain and even brief exposure injures unprotected ears. Considered to be the threshold of pain.

Dr. Krammer[1] states that the damage caused by one shot from a .357 Magnum pistol, which can expose a shooter to 165 dB for 2 msec, is equivalent to over 40 hours in a noisy workplace.

A.8.5   Hearing protectors

These come in two basic forms – **earplugs** and **earmuffs** – and are designed to decrease the intensity of sound that reaches the eardrum.

Hearing protectors should be in standard use on any range, although their use is not always compulsory. However, shooters tend not to use hearing protection on outdoor ranges, due to the misconception that the sound levels will be lower.

Properly fitted earplugs or muffs reduce noise by 15–30 dB. The better earplugs and muffs are approximately equal in sound reduction, although earplugs are better for low-frequency noise and earmuffs for high-frequency noise.

Simultaneous use of earplugs and muffs usually adds 10–15 dB more protection than either used alone. Combined use should be considered when noise exceeds 105 dB. Note that for such situations, it may be that there is no type of hearing protection that will stop a very loud noise from causing permanent damage.

---

[1] Dr Krammer, Ball State University, Muncie, Indiana, USA.

Types available

Expandable foam plugs are made of a formable material designed to expand and conform to the shape of each person's ear canal. Basically, they are rolled flat, inserted into the ear and then allowed to expand to form a tight fit. Simple and highly effective, but only intended for single use due to contamination by ear wax.

Pre-moulded, reusable plugs: pre-moulded plugs are made from silicone, plastic or rubber and are manufactured as either 'one-size-fits-most' or are available in several sizes. Many pre-moulded plugs are available in sizes for small, medium or large ear canals.

It should be noted that a person may need a different size plug for each ear. The plugs should seal the ear canal without being uncomfortable. This takes trial and error with the various sizes. They can be custom-made for an individual.

Canal caps often resemble earplugs on a flexible plastic or metal band. The earplug tips of a canal cap may be a formable or pre-moulded material. Some have headbands that can be worn over the head, behind the neck or under the chin. Newer models have jointed bands, increasing the ability to properly seal the earplug.

The main advantage that canal caps offer is convenience. Some people find the pressure from the bands uncomfortable. Not all canal caps have tips that adequately block all types of noise. Generally, the canal caps that resemble stand-alone earplugs appear to block the most noise.

Earmuffs come in many models, designed to fit most people. They work to block out noise by completely covering the outer ear. Muffs can be 'low profile', with small ear cups, or large to hold extra materials for use in extreme noise. Some muffs also include electronic components to help users to communicate, while blocking impulsive noises when they reach a certain threshold.

Workers who have heavy beards or sideburns, or who wear glasses, may find it difficult to get good protection from earmuffs. Hair, and the arms of the glasses, break the seal that the earmuff cushions make around the ear.

Fine fibreglass wool: originally marketed by Bilsom, this is an extremely fine grade of fibreglass wool which is rolled up and pushed into the ear canal. While it is extremely effective, concerns have been aired over the practice of placing fibreglass, no matter how fine, into such a sensitive area. This may no longer be available.

Miscellaneous devices

Manufacturers are receptive to comments from hearing protection users, and this has led to the development of new devices that are hybrids of the traditional types of hearing protectors.

Because many people like the comfort of foam plugs but do not want to roll them in dirty environments, a plug is now available that is essentially a foam tip on a stem. This plug is inserted in the same way as a pre-moulded plug, but without rolling the foam.

Cotton wool/rolled-up paper is often used, but it is of very little use, as an attenuation of only around 7 dB can be achieved. Likewise for bullets or cartridge cases pushed into the ear canal.

A.8.6   Extreme conditions

For those situations where extreme noise pollution is anticipated, such as when firing multiple shots from sawn-off 12-bore shotguns, additional precautions have to be taken.

The problem with extremely high impulse sound is that it is also transmitted to the inner ear via the facial bones and the teeth. While some attenuation may occur due to tissue and muscle, damage to the hearing can still be caused. The use of a Makralon face shield to deflect the sound, lining the ear muff with additional layers of foam and wearing ear plugs will, if all used together, significantly reduce the risk.

Further reading

1 Henselman, L.W., Henderson, D., Shadoan, J., Subramaniam, M., Saunders, S. & Ohlen, D. (1995). Effects of Noise Exposure, Race, and Years of Service on Hearing in U.S. Army Soldiers. *Ear & Hearing* 16 (4), 382–91.
2 Ylikoski, M.E. & Ylikoski, J.S. (1994). Hearing loss and handicap of professional soldiers exposed to gunfire noise. *Scandinavian Journal of Work, Environment and Health* 20 (2), 93–100.
3 Christiansson, B.A.C. & Wintzell, K.A. (1993). An audiological survey of officers at an infantry regiment. *Scandinavian Audiology* 22, 147–152.
4 Pelausa, E., Abel, S. & Dempsey, I. (1995). Prevention of Hearing loss in the Canadian Military. *The Journal of Otolaryngology* 24 (5): 271–280.
5 Paul, D.R., Chai, S.L. & Thomas, M. (1979). Hearing in Military Personnel. *Annals of The Academy Of Medicine, Singapore* 8 (2), 164–171.
6 Noise Induced Hearing Loss and Its Prevention: http://www.medicinenet.com

Appendix 9
A List of Handgun Cartridges

2.7 mm Kolibri – The smallest commercially available centre fire cartridge ever made.

2.34 mm – Rimfire ammunition used in MTH's Swiss Mini Gun.

3 mm Kolibri

4 mm Practice Cartridge GECO

4 mm Practice Cartridge M. 20

4.25 mm Liliput

.17 Mach 2

.17 Hornady Magnum Rimfire

4.5 × 26 mm

4.6 × 30 mm

.22 BB

.22 CB

.22 Short

.22 Long

.22 Long Rifle

.22 WMR (.22 Magnum)

.22 Reed Express

.22 Remington Jet (.22 Jet, .22 Centre fire Magnum)

.221 Remington Fireball

5.45 × 18 mm

5.7 × 28 mm

.25 ACP (6.35 mm Browning)

.25 NAA

.256 Winchester Magnum

7 mm Nambu

7 mm Bench Rest Remington (7 mm BR)

7.65 mm Brev.

7.62 × 25 mm Tokarev

7.62 × 38 mmR (7.62 × 38 mm Nagant)

7.63 × 25 mm Mauser

7.65 × 25 mm mm Borchardt

7.65 × 22 mm Parabellum (7.65 × 22 mm Luger)

7.65 mm Longue (7.65 mm MAS, 7.65 mm Long)

7.65 mm Mannlicher (7.63 mm Mannlicher in Austria, 7.65 mm Mannlicher in Germany, and 7.65 × 21 mm in the United States)

.32 ACP (7.65 × 17 mm Browning SR)

.32 NAA

.32 S&W

.32 S&W Long (.32 Colt New Police)

.320 Revolver

.32 Short Colt

.32 Long Colt

.32 H&R Magnum

.32-20 Winchester (.32 WCF, .32-20 Marlin, .32 Colt Lightning)

8 mm French Ordnance (8 mm Lebel Revolver)

8 × 22 mm Nambu

.38 Short Colt

.38 Long Colt

.38 S&W (.38 Colt New Police, .38 Super Police)

.38 Calibre

.380 Revolver

.38 Special (9 × 29 mmR)

.357 Magnum (9 × 31 mmR)

.357 Super Magnum

.357 Remington Maximum

9 × 18 mm Makarov

9 × 18 mm Police (9 mm Ultra)

9 mm Browning Long (9 × 20 mm Browning SR)

9 mm Glisenti

9 × 19 mm Parabellum (9 mm Luger, 9 × 19 mm NATO)

9 × 21 mm IMI

9 × 23 mm Steyr

9 mm Largo (9 mm Bergmann-Bayard, 9 × 23 mm Largo)

9 mm Winchester Magnum

9 × 25 mm Dillon

.380 ACP (9 × 17 mm Browning Short)

Forensic Ballistics in Court: Interpretation and Presentation of Firearms Evidence, First Edition. Brian J. Heard.
© 2013 John Wiley & Sons, Ltd. Published 2013 by John Wiley & Sons, Ltd.

.38 Auto (.38 ACP)
.38 Super Auto
.357 SIG
9.8 mm Auto Colt
.38-40 Winchester (.38 WCF)
.375 Super Magnum
.400 Corbon
.40 Smith & Wesson (10.0 × 21 mm)
.40 Super
10 mm Auto
10.4 mm Italian Revolver
.41 Action Express
.41 Remington Magnum
.414 JDJ
.414 Super Magnum
.44-40 Winchester (.44 WCF)
.44 Special
.44 S&W Russian
.44 Remington Magnum
.44 Auto Mag
.44 Webley (.442 RIC)
.445_SuperMag (.4295 RIC)
11 mm French Ordnance
.45 Schofield (.45 S&W Schofield, .45 S&W)
.45 Colt
.45 Super
.450 Revolver (.450 Adams)

.45 Webley
.455 Webley (.455 Webley Mk I, .455 Revolver, .455 Colt, .455 Colt Mk I)
.455 Webley Mk II (.455 Revolver Mk II, .455 Colt Mk II, .455 Eley)
.455 Webley Automatic
.45 GAP
.45 ACP (.45 Auto)
.45 S&W
.45 Winchester Magnum
.454 Casull
.458 Devastator
.460 S&W Magnum
.460 Rowland
.475 Linebaugh
.475 Wildey Magnum
.480 Ruger
.476 Eley (.476 Enfield Mk3)
.499 Linebaugh
.50 Action Express
.500 S&W Special
.500 S&W Magnum
.50 Remington (M71 Army)
.50 GI
.500 Linebaugh
13 mm Gyrojet
.577 Boxer

Appendix 10
A List of Rifle Cartridges

Inches

.17 Remington
.17 Remington Fireball (based on the wildcat .17 Mach IV)
.204 Ruger
.218 Bee
.219 Zipper
.22-250 Remington (.22-250 Ackley Improved)
.22 Hornet
.22 PPC
.22 BR Remington
.220 Russian
.220 Swift
.221 Remington Fireball
.222 Remington
.222 Remington Magnum
.223 Remington (.223 AI)
.223 WSSM
.224 Weatherby Magnum
.225 Winchester
.244 Remington (6 mm Remington)
.240 Weatherby Magnum
.243 Winchester (.243 AI)
.243 WSSM
.244 H&H Magnum
.250-3000 Savage
.256 Winchester Magnum
.256 Newton
.25-06 Remington
.25-20 Winchester
.25-35 Winchester (6.5 × 52R)
.25 Remington

.25 WSSM
.257 Roberts (.257 Roberts +P) (.257 Roberts Ackley Improved)
.257 Weatherby Magnum
.260 Remington
.264 Winchester Magnum
.270 Weatherby Magnum
.270 Winchester
.270 WSM (Winchester Short Magnum)
.276 Pedersen
.280 British
.280 Remington (a.k.a.7 mm Express Remington)
.280 Ross (a.k.a.280 Rimless Nitro Express)
.284 Winchester
.30 Carbine
.30 Newton
.30 Remington
.30-30 Winchester
.30-06 Springfield
.30-40 Krag(.30 Army)
.30-378 Weatherby Magnum
.300 Savage
.300 Remington SA Ultra Mag
.300 WSM (Winchester Short Magnum)
.300 Winchester Magnum
.300 H&H Magnum
.300 Weatherby Magnum
.300 Remington Ultra Magnum
.303 British
.303 Savage
.307 Winchester

Forensic Ballistics in Court: Interpretation and Presentation of Firearms Evidence, First Edition. Brian J. Heard.
© 2013 John Wiley & Sons, Ltd. Published 2013 by John Wiley & Sons, Ltd.

.308 Marlin Express
.308 Norma Magnum
.308 Winchester (7.62 × 51 mm NATO)
.32-20 Winchester (.32 WCF, .32-20 Marlin, .32 Colt
    Lightning)
.32-40 Ballard
.32-40 Winchester
.32 Remington
.32 Winchester self loading
.32 Winchester Special
.325 WSM (Winchester Short Magnum)
.33 Winchester (.33 WCF)
.338-378 Weatherby Magnum
.338 Federal
.338 Lapua Magnum
.338 Remington Ultra Magnum
.338 Winchester Magnum
.340 Weatherby Magnum
.348 Winchester
.35 Newton
.35 Remington
.35 Whelen
.35 Winchester
.350 Remington Magnum
.351 Winchester Self-Loading
.356 Winchester
.358 Norma Magnum
.358 Winchester
.375 H&H Magnum
.375 Ruger
.375 Remington Ultra Magnum
.375 Weatherby Magnum
.375 Whelen (.375-06)
.375 Winchester
.376 Steyr
.378 Weatherby Magnum
.38-40 Winchester
.38-55 Winchester
.40-60 Remington
.400 H&H Magnum
.401 Winchester Self Loading
.404 Jeffery (10.75 × 73)
.405 Winchester
.408 CheyTac
.416 Remington Magnum
.416 Rigby
.416 Weatherby Magnum
.44-40 Winchester
.44 Remington Magnum
.444 Marlin
.45-70 Government
.450 Bushmaster

.450 Marlin
.450 Rigby
.458 Winchester Magnum
.460 Weatherby Magnum
.465 H&H Magnum
.470 Nitro Express

Metric

5.45 × 39 mm
5.6 × 50 mm Magnum
5.6 × 52R (.22 Savage Hi-Power)
5.6 × 57 mm
5.6 × 57R mm
5.6 × 61 SE (5.6 × 61 Vom Hofe Super Express)
5.56 × 45 mm NATO
5.7 × 28 mm
5.8 × 42 mm DBP87
6 × 45 mm
6 mm BR Remington
6 mm PPC
6 mm Remington (.244 Remington)
6.5-284
6.5 mm Remington Magnum
6.5 × 50 mm Arisaka
6.5 × 52 mm Mannlicher-Carcano
6.5 × 53 mmR Dutch
6.5 × 54 mm Mannlicher-Schoenauer
6.5 × 55 mm
6.5 × 68 mm (also known as the 6.5 × 68 RWS, 6.5 × 68
    Schüler or the 6.5 × 68 Von Hofe Express)
6.8 mm Remington SPC
7 mm calibre
7 mm-08 Remington
7-30 Waters
7 mm BR Remington
7 mm Express Remington (a.k.a. .280 Remington)
7 mm Remington Magnum
7 mm Remington SA Ultra Mag
7 mm Remington Ultra Magnum
7 mm STW
7 mm Weatherby Magnum
7 mm WSM (Winchester Short Magnum)
7 × 33 mm Sako
7 × 57 mm Mauser (.275 Rigby)
7 × 61 mm Sharpe & Hart
7 × 64 mm Brenneke
7.5 × 55 mm Schmidt Rubin

7.5 × 57 mm MAS mod. 1924 7.5 × 54 mm MAS mod.
  1929
7.62 mm calibre
7.62 × 25 mm Tokarev
7.62 × 38 mmR
7.62 × 39 mm
7.62 × 45 mm vz. 52
7.62 × 51 mm NATO (.308 Winchester)
7.62 × 54R (rimmed) (7.62 Russian)
7.63 × 25 mm Mauser
7.65 mm Parabellum
7.65 × 53 mm Mauser (7.65 Argentine)
7.65 × 53 mmR
7.7 × 58 mm Arisaka
7.92 × 33 mm Kurz
7.92 × 57 mm Mauser (8 mm Mauser or 8 × 57 IS)
8 mm Lebel
8 mm Remington Magnum
8 × 50 mmR
8 × 56 mm Mannlicher-Schoenauer
8 × 56 mmR
8 × 60 mm Spitz
8 × 68 mm S
9 × 45 mm
9 × 56 mm Mannlicher-Schoenauer
9 × 57 mm Mauser
9.3 × 57 mm
9.3 × 62 mm
9.3 × 64 mm Brenneke
9.3 × 66 mm Sako
9.3 × 72 mmD
9.3 × 74 mmR
9.5 × 57 mm Mannlicher-Schoenauer (.375 Rimless
  Nitro Express × 2-1/4″)
11 × 60 mm Mannlicher
4.5 mm mkr
5 mm Craig
5 mm/35 SMc
6-06
6-284
6 mm BRX
6 mm Dasher
6 mm XC
6 × 45 (6 mm/223)
6 × 47 Swiss Match (6 mm/222 Mag)
6.5 Grendel
6.5 × 47 Lapua
7 mm Dakota
7.82 Lazzeroni Patriot
7.82 Lazzeroni Warbird
10 × 35 Vetterli

Very large calibre (.50 and larger)

Inches

.50-70 Government
.50-90 Sharps
.50-140 Sharps
.50 Alaskan
.50 Beowulf
.50 BMG
.50 Peacekeeper
.500 Black Powder Express
.500 Jeffrey Nitro Express
.500 Nitro Express 3″
.500/450 Nitro Express
.500/465 Nitro Express
.505 Gibbs
.510 DTC Europ
.510 Fat Mac
.510 Whisper
.550 Magnum
.550 Nitro Express
.577 Nitro Express
.577 Tyrannosaur(.577 T-Rex)
.577 Snider
.577/450 Martini-Henry
.585 Nyati
.600 Nitro Express
.600/577 REWA
.600 Overkill
.700 Nitro Express
.729 Jongmans
.950 JDJ

Metric

12.7 × 99 mm Multi-Purpose
12.7 × 108 mm
14.5 × 114 mm
14.5 mm JDJ
15.2 mm Steyr Armor Piercing Fin Stabilised Discarding
  Sabot (APFSDS)
20 × 110 mm Hispano
30 × 165 mm
30 × 173 mm

Appendix 11

Air Weapon Legislation

This appendix is included so that the air weapon legislation for various countries can be compared. A similar appendix for firearms legislation has not been included, due to the complexities of such and the fact that it would probably exceed the total length of this book.

A.11.1 Australia

Australian laws are controlled and administered by each State and Territory, with each classifying 'air', 'CO_2' and 'mechanical propulsion' used in air rifles and BB rifles as 'Category A' firearms. This places them in the same class as break-action shotguns and rimfire rifles, requiring a licence for ownership. Air pistols and BB pistols are classified as 'Category H' for all handguns (see reference 1 below). Anyone found in Australia possessing an unlicensed air rifle or pistol faces the same charge as a person who unlawfully possesses a firearm. However, it is allowed in most areas of Australia for an unlicensed person (from age 12) to use a firearm under direct supervision of a licensed person. It is important to check with the State or Territory Police Firearms section, as the laws vary across Australia. Air rifle and air pistol pellets are considered to be 'ammunition components' and can only be purchased, possessed and used by a licensed person. The same storage requirements for firearms also applies to air guns.

The 'Category A' and 'Category H' firearm licence can be issued to a 13 year old person (or a minor from age 12) after proof of being a member of a licensed shooting club. However, they must complete and pass an air gun safety awareness/safe handling and target shooter obligations course as required by the firearms laws, and have had background checks conducted by the police.

A.11.2 Brazil

The Brazilian legislation that regulates the manufacture, import, export, trade, traffic and use of air guns divide them into two groups:

- air guns by spring action of up to 6 mm calibre;

- air guns by spring action of calibre exceeding 6 mm, or pre-compressed gas in any calibre.

Air guns in the first group may be purchased by anyone over 18. Air guns in the second group can only be purchased by people registered in the army. Transportation depends on authorisation and usage is allowed only in places approved by the army. Air guns of any kind may not be carried openly (1, 2).

A.11.3 Canada

Air guns with both a muzzle velocity greater than 152.4 metres per second (500 feet per second) and a

Forensic Ballistics in Court: Interpretation and Presentation of Firearms Evidence, First Edition. Brian J. Heard.
© 2013 John Wiley & Sons, Ltd. Published 2013 by John Wiley & Sons, Ltd.

muzzle energy greater than 5.7 Joules (4.2 foot-pounds) are firearms for purposes of both the Firearms Act and the Criminal Code. Usually, the manufacturer's specifications are used to determine the design muzzle velocity and energy. Air rifles that meet these velocity and energy criteria are classified as non-restricted firearms, while air pistols are classified as restricted if their barrel is longer than 105 mm, or prohibited if their barrel length is 105 mm or less. The lawful possession of these air guns requires that the owner have a valid firearms licence and that the air gun be registered as a firearm.

Air guns that meet the Criminal Code definition of a firearm, but are deemed not to be firearms for certain purposes of the Firearms Act and Criminal Code, are those that have a muzzle velocity of less than 152.4 metres per second (500 feet per second) and a maximum muzzle energy of 5.7 Joules (4.2 foot pounds). Such air guns are exempt from licensing, registration and other requirements under the Firearms Act, and from penalties set out in the Criminal Code for possessing a firearm without a valid licence or registration certificate. However, they are considered to be firearms under the Criminal Code if they are used to commit a crime.

The simple possession, acquisition and use of these air guns for lawful purposes is regulated by provincial and municipal laws and by-laws. For example, some provinces may have set a minimum age for acquiring such an air gun. Air guns are exempt from the specific safe storage, transportation and handling requirements set out in the regulations supporting the Firearms Act. However, the Criminal Code requires that reasonable precautions be taken to use, carry, handle, store, transport, and ship them in a safe and secure manner (3).

Silencers for all firearms, including air guns, are prohibited in Canada.

A.11.4   Cyprus

Air rifles are covered by Cypriot law 113-1-2004, which is the same law that covers all firearms possession, and they are classified in the same category as break-action shotguns.

All air rifles must be registered to the owner at the local police station. Only persons without criminal record over the age of 18 are allowed to register and possess firearms, including air rifles. When an air rifle is sold on, a transfer application must be made at the local police station.

Only rifles of calibre .177″/4.5 mm are allowed – any other calibre is strictly forbidden. Only air guns that are legally classified as rifles are allowed. Pistols are forbidden unless they are for Olympic sport and conform to Olympic specifications. In order to acquire a pistol for Olympic sports, the owner must be a member of the Cyprus Shooting Sport Federation and have a written statement from them in order to be allowed to import the pistol.

Air rifles may have either folding or adjustable stock, and there is no minimum or maximum barrel or rifle length, but they must be legally classified as rifles. There is no power limit or muzzle velocity restrictions on air rifles. Air rifles can be PCP or spring-powered and can be either single shot or magazine fed. Semi-automatics are allowed, provided that only one pellet leaves the barrel on each pull of the trigger. Fully automatic air rifles are not allowed.

In order to combat rampant poaching, lasers, torches and silencers are also forbidden. Air rifle owners are allowed to use a barrel weight on the end of the barrel, provided that this does not dampen the sound emitted. People found in possession of silencers and/or unregistered air rifles are criminally prosecuted under the same laws that cover the illegal possession and transportation of firearms and explosives.

With regards to hunting with an air rifle, the current law the law states that air rifles can only be used for target shooting, so shooting any live animal with an air shooter is not using the rifle to hunt.

A.11.5   Czech Republic

In the Czech Republic, anyone over age of 18 can acquire an air gun with a muzzle energy not exceeding 16 Joules (12 foot pounds). Children over age of 10 have to be supervised by an adult when shooting. The only restriction on shooting place is the requirement of public safety. Since firearms can be used only at the officially licensed shooting ranges, air guns became popular to practise target shooting at or near the home.

Air guns with a muzzle energy over 16 Joules (12 foot pounds) require the same licence as firearms and police registration. Such air guns can be used only at the shooting ranges (**4**).

A.11.6   Denmark

In Denmark, air guns can be owned by anyone over the age of 18. There are no restrictions regarding muzzle energy.

A.11.7   Finland

Finland is contemplating mandatory licensing of high powered air guns (**5**).

A.11.8   Germany

In Germany, air guns producing a muzzle energy up to 7.5 Joules (5.53 foot pounds) can be owned by persons from the age of 18 years and freely acquired, provided they bear the 'F-in-pentagon mark' (Figure A.11.1) that indicates a muzzle energy not exceeding 7.5 Joules (5.5 foot pounds) kinetic energy. Carrying air guns in public necessitates a carry permit. Only the transportation of unloaded and non-accessible air guns (or carrying unloaded during a biathlon) is considered a 'permissible carry' (§ 12 Abs. 3 Nr. 2, Nr. 3 WaffG).

Shooting is permitted on licensed ranges (§ 27 Abs. 1, § 12 Abs. 4 2 Nr. 1 WaffG) and on enclosed private property, if it is assured that the projectiles cannot possibly leave the shooting area (§ 12 Abs. 4 Nr. 1a WaffG). The minimum age for air gun

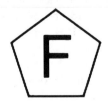

shooting in Germany is 12 years under supervision (§ 27 Abs. 3 S. 1 Nr. 1 WaffG), but exceptions may be granted to younger children upon request, supported by suitable references from a doctor and by a licensed shooting federation (§ 27 Abs. 4 WaffG).

Air weapons exceeding 7.5 Joules muzzle energy (e.g. field target guns) are treated like firearms and therefore require a relevant permit for acquisition and possession. Proof of need, a clean criminal record and the passing of a knowledge and handling test are required (§ 4 Abs. 1 WaffG) to gain the permit.

A purchase authorisation is not required for air guns that were manufactured and introduced onto the market before 1 January 1970 in Germany or before 2 April 1991 in the territory of the former East Germany (WaffG, Appendix 2, Section 1, Subsection 2, 1.2). They can, regardless of their muzzle energy or the absence of an 'F-in-pentagon' mark, be freely acquired and possessed.

The storage requirements for firearms do not apply to air guns (cf. § 36 Abs. 1 S. 1 WaffG). However, they must be stored in a place that is inaccessible to minors.

A.11.9   Hong Kong

In Hong Kong, under the Firearms and Ammunition Ordinance HK Laws Chap. 238, 'any air rifle, air gun or air pistol from which any shot, bullet or missile can be discharged with a muzzle energy greater than 2 Joules (1.48 foot pounds)' are considered 'arms'. As such, a permit is required for possession (which would otherwise be illegal), otherwise there are penalties up to a fine of $100,000 and 14 years in jail. Ammunition of the lead 'Diablo' type is treated as ammunition, requiring a firearms licence.

A.11.10   Italy

In Italy, any mechanism that produces a muzzle energy higher than 1 Joule (0.74 foot pounds) and lower than 7.5 Joules (5.53 foot pounds) is considered a 'low-power air gun'. The sale of such instruments is open to anyone over 18 years of age without licence or registration, but it can take place only in authorised gun shops, where the owner must require the purchaser to provide an ID card as a proof of age.

Any device developing a muzzle energy equal to, or higher than, 7.5 Joules is considered a 'high-power air gun', requiring police licensing and registration for purchase and detention just like any firearm. Bows, crossbows and similar weapons are exempt from this rule. The muzzle energy of such devices is certified by a governance office called 'Banco di Prova' (6). Air guns developing less than 1 Joule of muzzle energy are categorised as 'airsoft', which are considered by law to be toys, with no restriction whatsoever to their trade, except that they can never be modified to achieve a higher muzzle energy and must be only able to shoot 6 mm plastic pellets.

A.11.11   Israel

In Israel, all barrelled arms shooting metallic ammunition are considered firearms and therefore require a special government licence to own. Airsoft arms are defined as 'dangerous weapons'. While they are not licensed as firearms, they may only be sold to recognised airsoft clubs. Since civilians do not automatically have the right to carry firearms in Israel (citizens have to comply with certain conditions and prove 'necessity'), only people who fulfil the restrictive criteria for owning and carrying pistols may purchase an air rifle or pistol. Members of recognised shooting clubs are excepted and may own air rifles or pistols, and other sporting firearms, after proving two years of competitive activity. The Ministry of the Interior sometimes changes the qualifications for purchasing and owning air guns.

A.11.12   Japan

In Japan, any air gun that fires a metallic projectile is restricted as a firearm, so only airsoft-type guns are readily available.

A.11.13   Malta

In Malta, all air-driven guns for target sport (this includes air guns, airsoft and paintball guns) are subject to a Target Shooter B licence. This licence can be issued to an 18 year old person after proof of being a member of a licensed shooting club, completed and passed an air gun safe handling and Target shooter obligations course as required by the Maltese Arms Act law, and had background checks by the police.

The licensed target shooter is obliged by Maltese law to have a shooting sports insurance policy to cover the shooting practice. A licensed target shooter then can purchase, keep and carry and use an air gun, airsoft gun or paintball gun, but only at an authorised/licensed range. There is no restriction in muzzle velocity of air guns.

Minors from 14 years of age can be issued with a special permit from the police commissioner to practise air rifle or air pistol target shooting only. This permit is issued to the junior with full responsibility of the minor's parent or guardian, both of which must follow the same procedures until the licence can be issued.

Air guns issued under a target shooter's licence are intended for sport target shooting only. The air gun licence for hunting is a different licence, which is controlled by hunting laws and regulations. This is issued only for wild rabbit hunting.

A.11.14   Netherlands

In the Netherlands, air guns can be owned by persons from the age of 18 years and can freely be acquired. Until 1997, there were limitations on muzzle velocity and kinetic energy, similar to the German law, but these restrictions were lifted for practical reasons. Carrying air guns in public and the possession of air guns (and toy guns) that resemble firearms is prohibited. The expression 'to resemble' is nowadays given a very broad interpretation, so that just about any air gun can be considered as resembling a firearm. Whether an air gun is considered to resemble a firearm too closely is decided by the police or, when it comes to that, by the court. It is impossible to predict the outcome of such court cases. Air guns may be kept in private homes but must be inaccessible for persons under 18. Commercial sales of air guns may only take place in licensed gun shops. It is illegal to own an air gun that was 'produced or modified so that it can more easily be carried concealed'. Generally, this is considered the case if the barrel has been shortened or the weapon has a folding or telescoping stock (**7**).

A.11.15   New Zealand

In New Zealand any member of the public over the age of 18 may own and fire most air rifles without a firearms licence (**8**), provided they use the air rifle in a safe environment with a responsible attitude (**9**).

Minors 16 and over, but under the age of 18, require a firearms licence to possess an air rifle. However, they may use an air rifle under adult supervision without this licence.

Air guns cannot be fully automatic, and there is provision under the NZ Arms Laws to specify 'especially dangerous air guns' (**10**). Only pre-charged pneumatic rifles (over 762 mm long) have now been specified in this category (**10**), so a firearms licence is now a requirement for possession and use (**11, 12**). The change was made as a consequence of two fatal shootings by .22″ calibre semi-automatic air rifles (**13**).

A.11.16   Philippines

In the Philippines, air guns can be legally owned by citizens of ten years old and above. Registration of air guns is required by the payment of a one-time but non-transferable registration fee.

A.11.17   Poland

In Poland, it is possible to freely acquire air guns with a muzzle energy not exceeding 17 Joules (13 foot pounds). Air guns with muzzle energy over 17 Joules must be registered at a local police station no later than five days after purchase (gun licence is not needed) (**14**).

A.11.18   Spain

In Spain, it is possible for any person over the age of 14 to freely acquire an air rifle with a muzzle energy not exceeding 18 foot pounds (24 Joules) (roughly 1,000 ft/s or 300 m/s muzzle velocity in 0.177 calibre).

A.11.19   Sweden

In Sweden, it is possible to freely acquire air guns with a muzzle energy not exceeding 10 joules (7.4 foot pounds). Air guns with muzzle energy over 10 Joules must be registered (a gun licence is needed).

A.11.20   United Kingdom

Air pistols generating more than 6 foot pounds (8.1 Joules) and air rifles generating more than 12 foot pounds (16.2 Joules) of energy are considered firearms (**15**) and, as such, require possession of a Firearms Certificate (FAC). Pistols and rifles below these energy levels do not require licensing and may be purchased by anyone over the age of 18.

The UK Violent Crime Reduction Act, 2006, prohibits online or mail-order sale of new air guns; transactions must be finalised face-to-face, either at the shop where purchased, or through a registered firearms dealer (to which an item may be posted and the transfer completed). The sale and transfer of second-hand air guns is not affected by these restrictions.

From 10 February 2011, The Crime & Security Act, 2010 (S.46), made it an offence '...for a person in possession of an air weapon to fail to take reasonable precautions to prevent any person under the age of eighteen from having the weapon with him . . . ' (**16**). This legislation essentially relates to the storage of air guns and the requirement of owners to prevent unauthorised access by children. Failure to do so renders owners liable for a fine of up to £1,000 (**17**).

Any person on private property without permission is trespassing; possession when doing so of even a low-power air weapon with no ammunition makes this the serious crime of armed trespass, subject to heavy penalties (**18**).

A.11.21   United States

The sale or possession of an air gun is usually unregulated in most US states. A few states and municipalities restrict or prohibit air gun sales or possession in some manner, including: San Francisco; New York City; Camden, New Jersey and Newark, New Jersey; Johnson City, Tennessee; Chicago; Philadelphia, Pennsylvania; and the States of Illinois and Michigan (**19**). Additionally, ordinances in many cities prohibit the discharge of air guns outdoors, outside of an approved range.

Firearms legislation references

1 'Decreto no. 3.665, de 20 de novembro de 2000.'
2 'Portaria COLOG no. 2, de 26 de fevereiro de 2010.'
3 http://www.rcmp-grc.gc.ca/cfp-pcaf/fs-fd/air_gun-arme_air-eng.htm
4 Gun law 119/2002 Sb. of the Czech Republic.
5 'Air gun permits planned, but not for airsoft or paintball'. blog.anta.net. 11 June 2008. ISSN 1797-1993.
6 Official website of the Banco Nazionale di Prova per le Armi da Fuoco portatili e le Munizioni commerciali (National Testing Board for Firearms and Commercial ammunition) – in Italian.
7 Arms and ammunition law – Dutch.
8 'Do I need a licence for an air gun?' NZ Police website.
9 'Careless use of firearm, air gun, pistol, or restricted weapon', Arms Act 1983 No 44.
10 'Arms (Restricted Weapons and Specially Dangerous Air guns) Order 1984'.
11 'High-powered air rifles now require license', The Beehive.
12 'Important information...', NZ Police.
13 'Crackdown on killer air rifles'. NZPA. 14 July 2010.
14 Polish Weapons and Ammunition Act.
15 UK air gun law.
16 UK legislation concerning the prevention of air guns falling into the hands of those under 18 years of age.
17 UK Air gun legislation as reported in Press Release issued by BASC.
18 Marple Rifle & Pistol Club, Gun Law in the UK.
19 'Michigan Compiled Laws, Chapter 8, Revised Statutes of 1846, Chapter 1, section 8.3t: 'Firearm' defined'. Michigan Legislature.

Index

Forensic Ballistics in Court: Interpretation and Presentation of Firearms Evidence, First Edition. Brian J. Heard.
© 2013 John Wiley & Sons, Ltd. Published 2013 by John Wiley & Sons, Ltd.